Opportunities and Challenges in Digital Healthcare Innovation

Kamaljeet Sandhu
University of New England, Australia

IGI Global
PUBLISHER of TIMELY KNOWLEDGE

A volume in the Advances in Medical Technologies and Clinical Practice (AMTCP) Book Series

Published in the United States of America by
IGI Global
Medical Information Science Reference (an imprint of IGI Global)
701 E. Chocolate Avenue
Hershey PA, USA 17033
Tel: 717-533-8845
Fax: 717-533-8661
E-mail: cust@igi-global.com
Web site: http://www.igi-global.com

Library of Congress Cataloging-in-Publication Data

Library of Congress Cataloging-in-Publication Data

Names: Sandhu, Kamaljeet, 1970- editor.
Title: Opportunities and challenges in digital healthcare innovation / Kamaljeet Sandhu, editor.
Description: Hershey, PA : Medical Information Science Reference, [2020] | Includes bibliographical references and index. | Summary: "This book addresses opportunities and obstacles in digital healthcare innovation"-- Provided by publisher.
Identifiers: LCCN 2019051439 (print) | LCCN 2019051440 (ebook) | ISBN 9781799832744 (hardcover) | ISBN 9781799832751 (ebook)
Subjects: MESH: Medical Informatics | Biomedical Technology | Delivery of Health Care
Classification: LCC R855.3 (print) | LCC R855.3 (ebook) | NLM W 26.5 | DDC 610.285--dc23
LC record available at https://lccn.loc.gov/2019051439
LC ebook record available at https://lccn.loc.gov/2019051440

This book is published in the IGI Global book series Advances in Medical Technologies and Clinical Practice (AMTCP) (ISSN: 2327-9354; eISSN: 2327-9370)

British Cataloguing in Publication Data
A Cataloguing in Publication record for this book is available from the British Library.

For electronic access to this publication, please contact: eresources@igi-global.com.

Advances in Medical Technologies and Clinical Practice (AMTCP) Book Series

Srikanta Patnaik
SOA University, India
Priti Das
S.C.B. Medical College, India

ISSN:2327-9354
EISSN:2327-9370

Mission

Medical technological innovation continues to provide avenues of research for faster and safer diagnosis and treatments for patients. Practitioners must stay up to date with these latest advancements to provide the best care for nursing and clinical practices.

The **Advances in Medical Technologies and Clinical Practice (AMTCP) Book Series** brings together the most recent research on the latest technology used in areas of nursing informatics, clinical technology, biomedicine, diagnostic technologies, and more. Researchers, students, and practitioners in this field will benefit from this fundamental coverage on the use of technology in clinical practices.

Coverage

- Clinical Nutrition
- Clinical Studies
- Patient-Centered Care
- Diagnostic Technologies
- Telemedicine
- Biomechanics
- Clinical High-Performance Computing
- E-Health
- Biometrics
- Nutrition

IGI Global is currently accepting manuscripts for publication within this series. To submit a proposal for a volume in this series, please contact our Acquisition Editors at Acquisitions@igi-global.com or visit: http://www.igi-global.com/publish/.

The Advances in Medical Technologies and Clinical Practice (AMTCP) Book Series (ISSN 2327-9354) is published by IGI Global, 701 E. Chocolate Avenue, Hershey, PA 17033-1240, USA, www.igi-global.com. This series is composed of titles available for purchase individually; each title is edited to be contextually exclusive from any other title within the series. For pricing and ordering information please visit http://www.igi-global.com/book-series/advances-medical-technologies-clinical-practice/73682. Postmaster: Send all address changes to above address.

Titles in this Series

For a list of additional titles in this series, please visit:
http://www.igi-global.com/book-series/advances-medical-technologies-clinical-practice/73682

Mobile Devices and Smart Gadgets in Medical Sciences
Sajid Umair (The University of Agriculture, Peshawar, Pakistan)
Medical Information Science Reference • © 2020 • 363pp • H/C (ISBN: 9781799825210) • US $245.00

Applications of Deep Learning and Big IoT on Personalized Healthcare Services
Ritika Wason (Bharati Vidyapeeth's Institute of Computer Applications and Management (BVICAM), India) Dinesh Goyal (Poornima Institute of Engineering and Technology, India) Vishal Jain (Bharati Vidyapeeth's Institute of Computer Applications and Management (BVICAM), India) S. Balamurugan (QUANTS IS and Consultancy Services, India) and Anupam Baliyan (Bharati Vidyapeeth's Institute of Computer Applications and Management (BVICAM), India)
Medical Information Science Reference • © 2020 • 248pp • H/C (ISBN: 9781799821014) • US $275.00

Communicating Rare Diseases and Disorders in the Digital Age
Liliana Vale Costa (University of Aveiro, Portugal) and Sónia Oliveira (University of Aveiro, Portugal)
Medical Information Science Reference • © 2020 • 412pp • H/C (ISBN: 9781799820888) • US $295.00

Artificial Intelligence Paradigms in Smart Health Informatics Systems
Abdel-Badeeh M. Salem (Ain Shams University, Egypt) and Senthil Kumar A V (Hindusthan College of Arts and Science, India)
Medical Information Science Reference • © 2020 • 300pp • H/C (ISBN: 9781799811015) • US $265.00

Incorporating the Internet of Things in Healthcare Applications and Wearable Devices
P. B. Pankajavalli (Bharathiar University, India) and G. S. Karthick (Bharathiar University, India)
Medical Information Science Reference • © 2020 • 288pp • H/C (ISBN: 9781799810902) • US $285.00

Impacts of Information Technology on Patient Care and Empowerment
Roger W. McHaney (Kansas State University, USA) Iris Reychev (Ariel University, Israel) Joseph Azuri (Maccabi Healthcare Services, Israel) Mark E. McHaney (U.S. Air Force, USA) and Rami Moshonov (Assuta Medical Centers, Israel)
Medical Information Science Reference • © 2020 • 452pp • H/C (ISBN: 9781799800477) • US $295.00

Handbook of Research on Clinical Applications of Computerized Occlusal Analysis in Dental Medicine
Robert B. Kerstein, DMD (Tufts University School of Dental Medicine, USA & Private Dental Practice Limited to Prosthodontics and Computerized Occlusal Analysis, USA)
Medical Information Science Reference • © 2020 • 1356pp • H/C (ISBN: 9781522592549) • US $765.00

IGI Global
PUBLISHER of TIMELY KNOWLEDGE

701 East Chocolate Avenue, Hershey, PA 17033, USA
Tel: 717-533-8845 x100 • Fax: 717-533-8661
E-Mail: cust@igi-global.com • www.igi-global.com

I dedicate this book to the memory of my mother and father.

Editorial Advisory Board

Table of Contents

Preface xiv

Acknowledgment xix

Chapter 1
Advances for Artificial Intelligence in Health Data Analytics to Drive Digital Systems Innovation..... 1
Kamaljeet Sandhu, University of New England, Australia

Chapter 2
Digital Health Innovation Enhancing Patient Experience in Medical Travel 13
Anita Medhekar, Central Queensland University, Australia

Chapter 3
An Affordance Perspective on the Enabling and Disruptive Effects of Social Media Tools on Self-Management of Chronic Illness 36
Nwakego Isika, The University of Melbourne, Australia
Antonette Mendoza, The University of Melbourne, Australia
Rachelle Bosua, Open University of the Netherlands, The Netherlands

Chapter 4
Supporting a Value-Based Healthcare Paradigm With Digital Health and Wellness Personalised Monitoring Solutions 57
Nilmini Wickramasinghe, Swinburne University, Australia & Epworth HealthCare, Australia
Steve Goldberg, Inet International Inc., Canada

Chapter 5
Digital Transformation Leadership for Smart Healthcare Organizations: House of Success Model ... 72
Dina Ziadlou, Colorado Technical University, USA

Chapter 6
Professional Practices for Digital Healthcare 97
Sisira Edirippulige, Centre for Online Health, The University of Queensland, Australia
Buddhika Senanayake, Centre for Online Health, The University of Queensland, Australia

Chapter 7
Digital Employability Skills and Training Needs for the Indian Healthcare Industry 113
Esha Jain, The NorthCap University, Gurugram, India

Chapter 8
My Digital Healthcare Record: Innovation, Challenge, and Patient Empowerment 131
Anita Medhekar, Central Queensland University, Australia
Julie Nguyen, Central Queensland University, Australia

Chapter 9
Digital Recognition of Breast Cancer Using TakhisisNet: An Innovative Multi-Head Convolutional Neural Network for Classifying Breast Ultrasonic Images 151
Loris Nanni, Università di Padova, Italy
Alessandra Lumini, University of Bologna, Italy
Gianluca Maguolo, University of Padova, Italy

Chapter 10
Workforce Readiness and Digital Health Integration 170
Buddhika Senanayake, Centre for Health Services Research, The University of Queensland, Australia
Nirupama Tyagi, Centre for Health Services Research, The University of Queensland, Australia
Xiaoyun Zhou, Centre for Health Services Research, The University of Queensland, Australia
Sisira Edirippulige, Centre for Health Services Research, The University of Queensland, Australia

Chapter 11
Process Analytics Model Approach in Healthcare: The Technological Perspective 186
S. Santhosh Kumar, Department of Computer Science, Alagappa University, India
A. Sumathi, Department of CSE, SRC, SASTRA University (Deemed), India

Chapter 12
Investigating Diabetic Subjects on Their Correlation With TTH and CAD: A Statistical Approach on Experimental Results 197
Rohit Rastogi, Dayalbagh Educational Institute, Agra, India & ABES Engineering College, Ghaziabad, India
Devendra K. Chaturvedi, Dayalbagh Educational Institute, Agra, India
Parul Singhal, ABES Engineering College, Ghaziabad, India
Mayank Gupta, Tata Consultancy Services, Noida, India

Compilation of References 221

About the Contributors 256

Index 260

Detailed Table of Contents

Preface xiv

Acknowledgment xix

Chapter 1
Advances for Artificial Intelligence in Health Data Analytics to Drive Digital Systems Innovation..... 1
Kamaljeet Sandhu, University of New England, Australia

Artificial intelligence in health (AIH) and health data has become a focus of attention for customers of health services, organizations providing health services, and the government organization monitoring the performance and outcome for health services. These three groups have vested interests in how, where, and when the health data can be used and delivered to facilitate and streamline the delivery and process for health services from adopting AIH. The driving force in AIH for health data analytics stems from the discovery of new information, analysis that seeks to provide a clear understanding of a problem, interpretation in making clear sense of the problem, and communication of meaningful data patterns that can be effectively used in finding solutions to drive digital systems innovation. Modern technology provides an important platform for the health data transformation at different stages of the process to deliver different kinds of health services adopting artificial intelligence.

Chapter 2
Digital Health Innovation Enhancing Patient Experience in Medical Travel 13
Anita Medhekar, Central Queensland University, Australia

Digital health technological innovations are disrupting every sector of the economy, including medical travel/tourism. Global patients as medical tourists are using patient-centric digital health technologies, enhancing patient/medical tourists experience and making it more transparent and engaging with healthcare providers and medical tourists. Digital communication tools such as e-mail, online appointments, smartphones, instant messaging applications, social media tools, user-generated content by online patient communities, tele-medicine, tele-radiology, my-Health records, Skype consultation, WhatsApp, health video, electronic health records, health data analytics tools, and artificial intelligence-enabled health technologies enhance the medical travel decision-making process, reduce cost, improve patient care and transparency of communication, and engage the relationship between the patient and the healthcare provider with positive outcomes, medical tourist experience, and empowerment.

Chapter 3
An Affordance Perspective on the Enabling and Disruptive Effects of Social Media Tools on Self-Management of Chronic Illness 36
Nwakego Isika, The University of Melbourne, Australia
Antonette Mendoza, The University of Melbourne, Australia
Rachelle Bosua, Open University of the Netherlands, The Netherlands

This chapter examines the appropriation of social media tools by chronically ill adults to better understand and manage their illness using an affordance perspective. Despite the continued attention that information systems scholars have directed to studies on affordances and social media, there seems to be limited discussion on the negative, disruptive effects that social media could have on accomplishment of illness management goals. Accordingly, the authors argue that social media affordances could have both positive, enabling effects on illness management outcomes or negative, disruptive effects.

Chapter 4
Supporting a Value-Based Healthcare Paradigm With Digital Health and Wellness Personalised Monitoring Solutions 57
Nilmini Wickramasinghe, Swinburne University, Australia & Epworth HealthCare, Australia
Steve Goldberg, Inet International Inc., Canada

Especially in the US, many are advocating for the incorporation of a value-based system for healthcare delivery including bundled payments for services in an attempt to address escalating healthcare costs. The following proffers the role for digital health solutions to support health and wellness management and the need to develop suitable sustainable business models. However, this approach brings a focus onto comorbidities and chronic conditions, which often need to be addressed or at least better managed before surgery can take place. This opens up the opportunity to examine the potential for digital health solutions such as mobile apps and serious games to provide an enabling or support role for individuals to better manage their chronic conditions. It also brings up the need for better, flexible models to assist health and wellness solution development.

Chapter 5
Digital Transformation Leadership for Smart Healthcare Organizations: House of Success Model ... 72
Dina Ziadlou, Colorado Technical University, USA

The digital transformation has revolutionized the contexts of healthcare organizations in all aspects, and those hospitals that tend to create a smart digital environment are require to perceive vital factors of digital transformation. The author has created a framework called "House of Success" Model to elaborate on the significant organizational factors contributing to developing a smart healthcare organization in the digital era. This model consists of digital transformation, as the foundation of the house; quadruple aims, as the roof of the house and the ultimate goal of the transformation; and leadership and management, as the pillars of the house. Moreover, the house of success model has four rooms including change management and change leadership, people leadership, digital technology leadership, and the global partnership that resulted in building up a prosperous digital transformation outlook toward sustainable effectiveness development.

Chapter 6
Professional Practices for Digital Healthcare 97
Sisira Edirippulige, Centre for Online Health, The University of Queensland, Australia
Buddhika Senanayake, Centre for Online Health, The University of Queensland, Australia

Digital health is quickly becoming an integral part of healthcare services. Research evidence suggests that digital health can benefit stakeholders involved in healthcare including patients and care providers. As digital health continues to integrate into routine healthcare, practitioners may require new knowledge, skills, and competencies to make the best use of it and to be able to communicate with an increasingly digitally enabled consumer. While much effort has been made to systematic education and training relating to digital health, which is an important aspect in developing the digital health workforce, it is important that governments and health systems consider digital health education and training as an important element in the process of implementing digital health within health services. Digital health education must be given its due recognition and support so that the future heath workforce has an opportunity to develop required knowledge and skills relating to digital health.

Chapter 7
Digital Employability Skills and Training Needs for the Indian Healthcare Industry 113
Esha Jain, The NorthCap University, Gurugram, India

The utilization of computerized innovation in wellbeing applications is encountering a huge blast in huge part because of growing human services costs and the impediments of one-on-one treatment to meet the psychological well-being needs of the populace. Specifically, cell phone applications for wellbeing have become popular, which gives chances to grow current consideration past the customary facility setting. The objectives of this study were to identify the employability skills and training needs in the digital healthcare industry. Results showed that all the eight skills are important for the training of line service staff (e.g., communication, ICT, work engagement, teamwork, cognitive). As per the response, handling situations is one of the most critical skills required to perform the job followed by self-management, planning and organizing, and analytical skills. However, the type and requirement of skills vary from person to person.

Chapter 8
My Digital Healthcare Record: Innovation, Challenge, and Patient Empowerment 131
Anita Medhekar, Central Queensland University, Australia
Julie Nguyen, Central Queensland University, Australia

In the 21st century, the digital revolution is disrupting every sector of the economy. Australia has adopted the digital healthcare technological revolution such as My Health Record (MyHRC) to improve healthcare practice for clinicians/medical professionals and empower consumers to provide positive health management experience with a patient-centred approach to digital health revolution and digital literacy. My Health Record has its benefits, but it has been a challenge for the healthcare practitioners, hospital staff, as well as patients as consumers to accept, embrace, and uptake digital technologies and manage their healthcare records amidst concerns of slow adoption by the patient, data privacy, and implications of the secondary use of their personal data by non-government entities.

Chapter 9
Digital Recognition of Breast Cancer Using TakhisisNet: An Innovative Multi-Head Convolutional Neural Network for Classifying Breast Ultrasonic Images 151
Loris Nanni, Università di Padova, Italy
Alessandra Lumini, University of Bologna, Italy
Gianluca Maguolo, University of Padova, Italy

In this chapter, the authors evaluate several basic image processing and advanced image pattern recognition techniques for automatically analyzing bioimages, with the aim of designing different ensembles of canonical and deep classifiers for breast lesion classification in ultrasound images. The analysis starts from convolutional neural networks (CNNs) in a square matrix that is used to feed other CNNs. The novel ensemble, named TakhisisNet, is the combination by sum rule of the whole set of the modified CNNs and the original one. Moreover, the performance of the system is further improved by combining it with some handcrafted features. Experimental results obtained on the well-known OASBUD breast cancer dataset (i.e., the open access series of breast ultrasonic data) and on a large set of bioimage classification problems show that TakhisisNet obtains very valuable results and outperforms other approaches previously tested in the same datasets.

Chapter 10
Workforce Readiness and Digital Health Integration 170
Buddhika Senanayake, Centre for Health Services Research, The University of Queensland, Australia
Nirupama Tyagi, Centre for Health Services Research, The University of Queensland, Australia
Xiaoyun Zhou, Centre for Health Services Research, The University of Queensland, Australia
Sisira Edirippulige, Centre for Health Services Research, The University of Queensland, Australia

The benefits that digital health may offer include clinical, administrative, research, and educational. Research shows that if used in the right circumstances, digital health may increase access to healthcare services, improve clinical outcomes, safety, and quality of care. Digital health also has the potential to improve organisational efficiencies by reducing duplication and unnecessary diagnostic testing. From a healthcare consumer perspective, there is an expectation that healthcare services need to be provided in a more flexible and cost-effective way as in other spheres such as banking, commerce, and media. This is another important driver for consideration to integrate digital health in healthcare services. As digital health continues to be used in routine healthcare services, practitioners may require new knowledge, skills, and competencies to make the best use of this innovative method. Education and training relating to digital health have been recognised as a priority for developing the future healthcare workforce.

Chapter 11
Process Analytics Model Approach in Healthcare: The Technological Perspective 186
S. Santhosh Kumar, Department of Computer Science, Alagappa University, India
A. Sumathi, Department of CSE, SRC, SASTRA University (Deemed), India

Process analytics involves the relationship between the doctor, diagnostic centers and patient. The primary advantages of using process analytics in healthcare are expert guidance, global medical assistance, and possible alternate treatment mechanisms. The secondary advantages are the analysis of the same type of disease complications and the creation of a disease-based healthcare data repository. This chapter focuses on the process model-based approach for healthcare analytics. The two emerging techniques Big data and IoT are needed to be incorporated with the process model for storing and analyzing the healthcare data. The first category assists administrators with identifying areas to streamline operations and concretely increase savings. Research and development are crucial aspects of healthcare, providing new innovative solutions and treatments that can be properly tracked, measured, and analyzed.

Chapter 12
Investigating Diabetic Subjects on Their Correlation With TTH and CAD: A Statistical Approach on Experimental Results 197
Rohit Rastogi, Dayalbagh Educational Institute, Agra, India & ABES Engineering College, Ghaziabad, India
Devendra K. Chaturvedi, Dayalbagh Educational Institute, Agra, India
Parul Singhal, ABES Engineering College, Ghaziabad, India
Mayank Gupta, Tata Consultancy Services, Noida, India

Digital technology is modernizing healthcare. Large volumes of data refer to big data by digitising health information that can quickly be processed by machines. Digital healthcare analysis is the ability to diagnose and suggest ways to reduce costs; provide quality patient care and outcomes, available 24/7; reach to patients located in vast distant geographical areas; and avert preventable diseases. Artificial intelligence (AI) is an autonomous real-time machine system in comparison to natural information analyzed by humans. Diabetes is a serious, under-reported, life-threatening disease affecting millions of people of all ages, and researchers have identified it to be a major public health problem that is approaching epidemic proportions globally. The purpose of this study is to investigate diabetes analysis from CAD and other diseases using the latest advanced digital technologies to analyze information extracted from IoT and big data and stress correlation (TTH) on human health.

Compilation of References 221

About the Contributors 256

Index 260

Preface

Digital healthcare innovation has been a recent topic of high attention, as there is very little understanding on the opportunities and challenges it has posed for government, private and public institutions and their customers, and other stakeholders. There is no doubt that digital healthcare if successfully implemented offers many benefits such as effective cost savings, delivery and monitoring of health services on wearable and mobile devices such as smartphones and websites 24/7, boosting efficiency for delivery of health services, and to people at distant places, eliminates paper-based record systems, real time delivery and access to vast volumes of important health data and portability over the internet, and easy customer access to personal data and health records.

Digital healthcare is one of the most important transformation in healthcare as it has been demonstrated that the health services can be offered digitally at different places and as well at patients home thus reducing the pressure on health institutions such as hospitals which have been overloaded with patients. Digital healthcare systems not only relieve the pressures of public hospital infrastructure but are also providing advanced care and interactive models of patients care that support personalised, accurate, and well-informed high-quality medical treatment. This means higher safety, better quality of care and faster treatment for patients at offsite locations such as home, which also have led to patient empowerment in adopting digital healthcare.

Digital healthcare innovation and transformation emphasises that the healthcare data will enable the use of critical information to drive healthcare improvements that can revolutionise the functioning of healthcare institutions. Modern scientific technologies such as Artificial Intelligence in healthcare, Autonomous machine learning, Healthcare data analytics, and many others, are amalgamating in driving the innovation for advanced digital healthcare. Today medical scientist and practitioners are adopting advanced digital technologies to discover new cure for chronic diseases such as diabetes, cancer, and many others, which in the past was not possible due to lack of high-quality healthcare data. Patients are exchanging digital health information with loved ones and carers on social media from different global locations which has led to newer ways to providing the best treatment.

Digital healthcare connectivity has offered people new opportunities and choices, to have quick access to reach medical practitioners overseas for affordable healthcare which is fast expanding internationally as a global healthcare business model/medical tourism to access the best quality healthcare from the convenience of their homes and via live video conferencing with practitioners. Healthcare is no longer constrained with in the walls of a health institution such as a hospital, rather it has shown that digital healthcare can reach far off locations where there are no hospitals, and patients can interact with medical practitioner via tools such as telehealth and video conferencing. Patients benefiting the most who are living in remote rural and regional communities where there are no healthcare services and hospitals.

In Queensland state of Australia, the first of its kind to offer custom-built mobile clinic fitted with advanced digital medical devices in a truck to perform critical healthcare services such as stress testing, cardiac ultrasound, Holter monitoring, and a whole suite of other non-invasive cardiac and respiratory tests, and other essential services which are delivered to rural and remote patients to save lives where there are no hospital infrastructure.

In the past delivering health services to rural and remote communities was challenging with small population spread across diverse areas. Digital transformation has closed that gap and modern health systems are today well connected to reach patients for providing quality care across health service providers and eliminate the issues of physical distance and isolation and delivering better healthcare in rural and remote communities. Through digital healthcare transformation, medical practitioners have learnt newer ways to adapt to digital platforms, provide best healthcare professional practices, learning innovative skills for analysing patient's data in real time, learning newer techniques for accessing patient's healthcare records via software systems and analyse data across different systems. This has made the medical workforce ready to embrace new digital technologies by integrating into their healthcare work practices. The leadership to drive digital healthcare have also shown to have adopted a proactive approach, as many healthcare projects are being designed based on digital healthcare delivery, such projects are also leading to eliminating processes that were time consuming and wasteful, physically constrained & resource draining, and expensive, and turning around into cost effective and instant real time delivery to a wider geographic region.

The chapters in this book unravel important information, piece by piece, so that the readers can clearly understand, that is driving the requirements for digital healthcare transformation. Prominent researchers have deeply engaged and examined areas of digital healthcare models, leadership, management, & strategy and have provided the readers with a clear understanding of important issues and challenges being studied, such as problems, literature and theory, research methodology, new research data findings, solutions and recommendations, and future research direction for Digital Healthcare Innovation that adds to the discovery of new knowledge and direction for further research.

The journey for developing and completing this book is a long one in which all authors have made a valuable contribution to the body of new research knowledge, and adopted new research techniques to study the problems, and found innovative solutions to address those complicated problems. This study will be very useful for many researchers to build on new findings that have been reported in this book. This book will also serve as a valuable tool for many students, health practitioners, government, managerial staff and other professionals to learn about new developments in digital healthcare innovation from a global perspective. International scholars have presented studies showing important new findings, which demonstrates the far-reaching impact for digital healthcare innovation, and which suggests that digital healthcare is continuously evolving into new ecosystems in different parts of the world via internet.

ORGANIZATION OF THE BOOK

A brief description of each of the chapters follows:

Chapter 1 demonstrates the role of Artificial Intelligence in Health (AIH) and health data has become a focus of attention for customers of health services, organizations providing health services, and the government organization monitoring the performance and outcome for health services. These three groups have vested interest in how, where, and when the health data can be used and delivered to facilitate and streamline the delivery and process for health services from adopting AIH. The driving force in AIH for health data analytics stems from the discovery of new information, analysis that seeks to provide a clear understanding of a problem, interpretation in making clear sense of the problem, and communication of meaningful data patterns that can be effectively used in finding solutions to drive digital systems innovation. Modern technology provides an important platform for the health data transformation at different stages of the process to deliver different kinds of health services adopting artificial intelligence.

Chapter 2 articulates that Digital health technological innovations are disrupting every sector of the economy, including medical travel/tourism. Global patients as medical tourists are using patient centric digital health technologies, enhancing patient/medical tourists experience and making it more transparent and engaging with healthcare providers and other medical tourists. Digital communication tools such as e-mail, on-line appointments, smart-phones, instant messaging application, social media tools, user-generated content by online patient communities, tele-medicine, tele-radiology, my-Health records, Skype-consultation, WhatsApp, health video, electronic health-records, health-data analytics tools and Artificial Intelligence enabled health technologies enhances medical travel decision making process, reduce cost, improves patient-care, transparency of communication, and engaged relationship between the patient and the healthcare provider with positive outcomes, medical tourist experience and empowerment.

Chapter 3 examines the appropriation of social media tools by chronically ill adults to better understand and manage their illness using an affordance perspective. Despite the continued attention that information systems scholars have directed to studies on affordances and social media, there seems to be limited discussion on the negative, disruptive effects that social media could have on accomplishment of illness management goals. Accordingly, the authors argue that social media affordances could have both positive, enabling effects on illness management outcomes or negative disruptive effects.

Chapter 4 illustrates the role of a value-based healthcare system, especially in the US, many are advocating for the incorporation of a value-based system for healthcare delivery including bundled payments for services in an attempt to address escalating healthcare costs. The following proffers the role for digital health solutions to support health and wellness management and the need to develop suitable sustainable business models. However, this approach brings a focus onto co-morbidities and chronic conditions which often need to be addressed or at least better managed before surgery can take place. This opens up the opportunity to examine the potential for digital health solution such as mobile Apps and serious games to provide an enabling or support role for individuals to better manage their chronic conditions. It also brings up the need for better, flexible models to assist health and wellness solution development.

Chapter 5 reports that digital transformation has revolutionized the contexts of healthcare organizations in all aspects and those hospitals that tend to create a smart digital environment require to perceive vital factors of digital transformation. The author has created a framework called "House of Success" Model to elaborate on the significant organizational factors contributing to developing a smart healthcare organization in the digital era. This model consists of digital transformation, as the foundation of the house, Quadruple Aims, as the roof of the house and the ultimate goal of the transformation, and leadership and management, as the pillars of the house. Moreover, the house of success model has four rooms including change management and change leadership, people leadership, digital technology leadership, and the global partnership resulted in building up a prosperous digital transformation outlook toward sustainable effectiveness development.

Chapter 6 demonstrates the role of digital health which is fast becoming an integral part of healthcare services. Research evidence suggests that digital health can benefit stakeholders involved in healthcare including patients, and care providers. As digital health continues to integrate into routine healthcare, practitioners may require new knowledge, skills, and competencies to make the best use of it and to be able to communicate with an increasingly digitally-enabled consumer. While much effort has been made to systematic education and training relating to digital health which is an important aspect in developing the digital health workforce. It is important that Governments and health systems consider digital health education and training as an important element in the process of implementing digital health within health services. Digital health education must be given its due recognition and support so that future heath workforce has opportunity to develop required knowledge and skills relating to digital health.

Chapter 7 explores the utilization of computerized innovation in wellbeing applications is encountering a huge blast in huge part because of growing human services costs and the impediments of one on one treatment to meet the psychological well-being needs of the populace. Specifically, cell phone applications for wellbeing have become quickly popular, which gives chances to grow current consideration past the customary facility setting. The objectives of this study were to identify the employability skills and training needs in the digital healthcare industry. Results showed that all the eight skills are important for the training of line service staff viz. communication, ICT, work engagement, teamwork, cognitive. As per the response, handling situations is one of the most critical skills required to perform the job followed by self-management, planning and organizing, and analytical skills. However, the type and requirement of skill vary from person to person.

Chapter 8 examines digital revolution which is disrupting every sector of the economy. Australia has adopted digital healthcare technological revolution such as My Health Record (MyHRC) to improve healthcare practice for clinicians/medical professionals and empower consumers to provide positive health management experience, with a patient-centred approach to digital health revolution and digital literacy. My Health Record has its benefits, but it has been a challenge for the healthcare practitioners, hospital staff as well as patients as consumers to accept, embrace and uptake digital technologies and manage their healthcare records amidst concerns of slow adoption by the patient, data privacy and implications of the secondary use of their personal data by non-government entities.

Chapter 9 evaluates several basic image processing and advanced image pattern recognition techniques for automatically analyzing bioimages, with the aim of design different ensembles of canonical and deep classifiers for Breast lesion classification in ultrasound image. The analysis starts from convolutional neural networks (CNNs), tries in a square matrix that is used to feed other CNNs. The novel ensemble, named TakhisisNet, is the combination by sum rule of the whole set of the modified CNNs and the original one. Moreover, the performance of the system is further improved by combining it with some handcrafted features. Experimental results obtained on the well-known OASBUD Breast cancer dataset (i.e. the Open Access Series of Breast Ultrasonic Data) and on a large set of bioimage classification problems show that TakhisisNet obtains very valuable results and outperforms other approaches previously tested in the same datasets.

Chapter 10 presents the benefits that digital health may offer include clinical, administrative, research and educational. Research shows that if used in right circumstances, digital health may increase access to healthcare services, improve clinical outcomes, safety and quality of care. Digital health also has potential to improve organisational efficiencies by reducing duplication and unnecessary diagnostic testing. From healthcare consumers' perspective, there is an expectation that healthcare services to be provided in a more flexible and cost-effective ways as in other spheres such as banking, commerce and media. This is another important driver for consideration to integrate digital health in healthcare services. As digital health continues to be used in routine healthcare services, practitioners may require new knowledge, skills, and competencies to make the best use of this innovative method. Education and training relating to digital health has been recognised as a priority for developing future healthcare workforce. By reviewing current literature, this chapter tries to shed light on the opportunities that digital health may offer and the workforce readiness as a priority for maximising those opportunities.

Chapter 11 reveals that increased old age population and the occurrence of acute and chronic illness to the early age population in the world lead to an increase in healthcare assistance. The healthcare industry is relying on technological support for advance treatment and improved medical care. The chronic diseases require periodical treatment during the lifetime of a patient which indulges to store patient records electronically. The digitization of patient data enables a reduction in the steps within the overall healthcare system. The process analytics involves the relationship between the doctor, diagnostic centers and patient. The primary advantages of using process analytics in healthcare are expert guidance, global medical assistance, and possible alternate treatment mechanisms. The secondary advantages are the analysis of the same type of disease complications and the creation of a disease-based healthcare data repository. This chapter focuses on the process model-based approach for healthcare analytics.

Chapter 12 proposes that digital technology is modernizing healthcare. Large volumes of data refer to Big Data by digitising health information that can quickly be processed by machines. Digital Healthcare analysis is the ability to diagnose and suggest ways to reduce costs, provide quality patient care & outcomes, available 24/7, reach to patients located in vast distant geographical areas, and avert preventable diseases. Artificial intelligence also referred as AI, is an autonomous real time machine system in comparison to natural information analyzed by humans. Diabetes is a serious, under-reported, life-threatening disease, affecting millions of people of all ages, and researchers have identified it to be a major public health problem that is approaching epidemic proportions globally. The purpose of this study is to investigate diabetes analysis from CAD and other diseases using the latest advanced digital technologies to analyze information extracted from IoT and Big Data and Stress Correlation (TTH) on human health.

Acknowledgment

I would like to acknowledge the help and contribution of all people, more specifically, to the authors and reviewers that took part in the review process. Without their support, this book would not have become a reality. All the authors have made valuable contribution by making many revisions to their chapters, presenting their interesting research to readers of this book.

Reviewers provided continuous and important feedbacks to the authors for improvements in their chapters, coherence, and content presentation of chapters.

I would like to personally thank all the authors and reviewers who have worked very hard to complete this book successfully. At every step we worked together as a highly coordinated and focused team.

In this journey we became very good and close colleagues, and this book has brought us all together from different parts of the world, and we have a valuable working relationship and I look forward to working with this great team again in another interesting book project to come soon.

I would like to personally thank staff at IGI-Global, development editors, who have provided the highest level of service. They continually and convincingly been very helpful & supportive in this research at every stage of the book development process, without their persistent help this publication would not have been possible.

I would like to thank my family, including my father and mother who passed away leaving beautiful memories and the importance for higher education and new learning that was ingrained in my very early life and which later was built into my ability to provide this advanced scholarly work to the advancement of new knowledge. This book is a tribute to my dear mum for all her love, support, belief, kindness, and trust, she had provided which transformed me into an author for scholarly research. I would not have achieved this book success without it.

Kamaljeet Sandhu
University of New England, Australia

Chapter 1
Advances for Artificial Intelligence in Health Data Analytics to Drive Digital Systems Innovation

Kamaljeet Sandhu
https://orcid.org/0000-0003-4624-6834
University of New England, Australia

ABSTRACT

Artificial intelligence in health (AIH) and health data has become a focus of attention for customers of health services, organizations providing health services, and the government organization monitoring the performance and outcome for health services. These three groups have vested interests in how, where, and when the health data can be used and delivered to facilitate and streamline the delivery and process for health services from adopting AIH. The driving force in AIH for health data analytics stems from the discovery of new information, analysis that seeks to provide a clear understanding of a problem, interpretation in making clear sense of the problem, and communication of meaningful data patterns that can be effectively used in finding solutions to drive digital systems innovation. Modern technology provides an important platform for the health data transformation at different stages of the process to deliver different kinds of health services adopting artificial intelligence.

INTRODUCTION

Digital technologies such as Artificial Intelligence (AI) can offer limitless possibilities to improve health services, from personal fitness to building stronger health systems for entire countries (Dzenowagis et al 2018, World Health Organisation). Despite the opportunities for Artificial Intelligence in Health (AIH) to solve many problems, the development and application of AIH has been very limited. The reasons for that are AIH is a time consuming, expensive, experts from health & IT having very limited or no understanding of where and how it can be applied to solve problems, and also the lack of medical and

DOI: 10.4018/978-1-7998-3274-4.ch001

healthcare data analytics that is needed for functioning AI systems. Consumers of healthcare services have raised important concerns: about their health information privacy, and access to the personal data, use of health data by institutions such as health insurance companies, unauthorized access to medical data and records, and cybersecurity. Jiang et al. (2017) argue that Artificial intelligence (AI) aims to mimic human cognitive functions. It is bringing a paradigm shift to healthcare, powered by increasing availability of healthcare data and rapid progress of analytics techniques.

In a case study by Anderson and Anderson (2019) it was discovered that Automation bias refers generally to a kind of complacency that sets in when a job once done by a healthcare professional is transferred to an AI program. The authors see nothing ethically or clinically wrong with automation, if the program achieves a virtually 100% success rate. If, however, the success rate is lower than that—92%, as in the case presented—it's important that there were assurances that the program has quality input; in this case, that probably means that the AI program "learned" from a cross section of patients of diverse ages, gender, and races.

Digital Systems Innovation for Health Data Analytics have faced obstacles in systems implementation & consumer acceptance of AI health services. Research suggests that digital health innovation has been a challenge and a slow process for acceptance when AI is not fined tuned to deliver specialized health services. At the same time AIH offers tremendous opportunities in Health Data Analytics for consumers of health services & service providers, such as health information portability, personalization of health information by consumers, easy access and usefulness of health information, better management of data records by institutions & government, and management of information by healthcare staff for patients' engagement and care. AI for Health Data Analytics is the key for driving a Digital Systems for Health Innovation. This research seeks to identify the digital health innovation opportunities and obstacles adopting AIH, develop a framework & a conceptual model for digital health innovation, that empowers consumer of digital health to use AIH to make informed decisions and choices.

DIGITAL SYSTEMS INNOVATION FOR HEALTH DATA ANALYTICS ADOPTING AIH

Researchers have long argued that the adoption rate of Electronic Health Record (EHR) systems is an important indicator of the degree of national e-health (Bonomi 2016). More recently adavnces have been made adopting AIH to d-health systems. This is also a measurement in the success of creating, sharing, distribution, of data analytics. Health Data is essential for digital innovation systems to function. Hambleton and Aloizos (2019) argue that the healthcare industry is one of the last industries to be disrupted by digital technologies especially focusing on AIH. It arguably has the most to gain, particularly from timely, accurate communication and clinical improvements, especially medication safety adopting AIH. At a time when governments of different countries willing to provide quality healthcare to their citizens on a digital platform, AIH can provide innovative solutions to severe healthcare problems. For example: Singapore government have made digital health a top priority for their citizens (RIE2020). Jha et al. (2008) state that health information technology in general and EHRs in particular, are tools for improving the quality, safety and efficiency of health systems in countries. They observed that in UK, Netherlands, Australia, and New Zealand generally used EHRs among general practitioners (each country>90%); Germany was far behind (40–80%); and there was a small minority of doctors in the U.S. and Canada who used EHRs (10–30%). They also explained that it is difficult for hospitals to obtain quality data

Table 1. Comparison of digital systems with paper-based systems

Digital AI Systems	Level of Customer Engagement & Managerial Implications: Digital AI Systems	Paper-based Systems	Level of Customer Engagement & Managerial Implications: Paper-based Systems
Digital AI Health Systems	High Engagement	Paper-based Health Systems	Low Engagement
Digital AI Health Records	Easy to use & useful, Fast access, Quick records, High Data Portability, Better Decisions, Highly Cost effective	Paper-based Health Records	Not easy to use, less useful, Slow access, Slow record, No Data portability, Slow Decisions, Least cost effective

and that only a small fraction of hospitals (<10%), of the countries analyzed had the key components required by an EHR. As shown in Table 1 digital systems have many benefits over paper-based systems.

Despite having many benefits, EHR is not uniformly used for national and international healthcare (Bonomi 2016). Data portability within country and across different states pose a real problem due to different jurisdiction applications on data transfer and ownership. Even though the data belongs to consumers of EHR, it's not clear about the use and transfer of such records with or without consumers knowledge. The next section seeks to review the literature and propose a conceptual model for digital health innovation. The next section builds on the literature review and the conceptual model.

LITERATURE REVIEW AND CONCEPTUAL MODEL FOR AIH

Research suggests that the use of electronic medical record has the potential to help improve safety, quality, and the cost efficiency of healthcare services (Mohammed & Younus 2017; Agarwal et al 2010). Not only EHR provide better management of consumer health data online, it also provides instant data portability across internet, for providing better access to physician for patient medical treatment, which can be streamlined adopting AIH. Digital AIH is about electronically connecting up the points of care so that health information can be shared securely. This is the first step to understanding how digital AIH can help deliver safer, better quality healthcare (ADHA 2019).

Bonomi (2016) discovered that successful implementation of Digital AIH Innovation leads to better access to medical records with detailed past and present clinical information regardless of space or time in order to support more informed decision-making; improvement of safety: digital records reduces the number of possible medical errors and prevents the loss of documents or misreading them of the entered data; improvement of healthcare quality and access to past and present information therefore reference to a larger number of data which facilitates decision-making and promotes the quality of services; improvement of healthcare: it optimizes treatments, consolidates and standardizes information, and links together the various areas of the health system and reduces administrative and management costs (Patrick et al 2016). The information is automatically updated and can be promptly obtained by authorized personnel. At the same time there are various reasons for the obstacles that hinder the implementation of AIH due to lack of universal standards or guidelines; Difficulty in economic returns; operational problems (i.e. data input); and reluctance to change to a digital platform due to many health institutions preferring to operate on a paper-based platform or a hybrid systems which is part paper and part digital which complicates the healthcare system and making ir uneconomical.

Mohammed & Younus (2017) report that Paper-based records are still by far the most common method of recording patient information for most hospitals and practices in the U.S. most of the doctors still find their ease of data entry and low cost hard to part with. However, as easy as they are for the physicians to record medical data at the point of care, they require large amount of storage space compare to record in electronic form. Data portability from paper records is a slow, time consuming, and a costly process and in circumstances of emergency time can be a critical factor for patients' medical diagnosis and care, compared to digital data that can be made available instantly when needed anywhere and anytime.

Fragidis & Chatzoglou (2018) found that the main reasons which are responsible for adopting a specific Digital Health Innovation implementation approach are usually political. Further, it is revealed that the most significant success factor of a nationwide Digital Health system implementation process is the commitment and involvement of all stakeholders (Yoo et al 2010). On the other hand, the lack of support and the negative reaction to any change from the medical, nursing and administrative community is considered as the most critical failure factor for AIH especially with issues around patients data privacy, lack of data security, data transparency, and data sharing.

An issue that should never be overlooked or underestimated is the alignment between the functionality of the new Digital Health system and users' requirements. Management and maintenance and funding for a national digital health system is also an important area that sometimes hinder the development, due to several issues such as political, cultural, technical, digital data interoperability, sharing analysing data from different systems, and lack of digital leadership expertise as shown in Figure 1.

Ginsburg et al (2018) argue that recent developments in data analytics also suggest barriers to change that might be more substantial in the healthcare field than in other parts of the economy. The authors further emphasise that compared to other industries, the slow pace of innovation reflects challenges that are unique to healthcare in implementing and applying "big data" tools (Krumholz 2014). These barriers include the nature of healthcare decisions, problematic data conventions, institutionalized practices in care delivery, and the misaligned incentives of various actors in the industry. To address these barriers, federal policy should emphasize interoperability of health data and prioritize payment reforms that will encourage providers to develop data analytics capabilities.

Ginsburg et al (2018) study shed deeper insight and found that despite the immense promise of health analytics, the industry lags behind other major sectors in taking advantage of cutting-edge tools. Most healthcare organizations, for example, have yet to devise a clear approach for integrating data analytics into their regular operations. One study even showed that 56 percent of hospitals have no strategies for data governance or analytics. Therefore, in such scenarios the effective role of AIH is diminished.

Summarising key points in AIH for Digital Health Innovation as shown in Figure 1, requires consolidation of several important concepts that will lead to development of Digital Health Innovation and its Acceptance by the consumers.

Figure 1. AIH for digital systems innovation in health data analytics

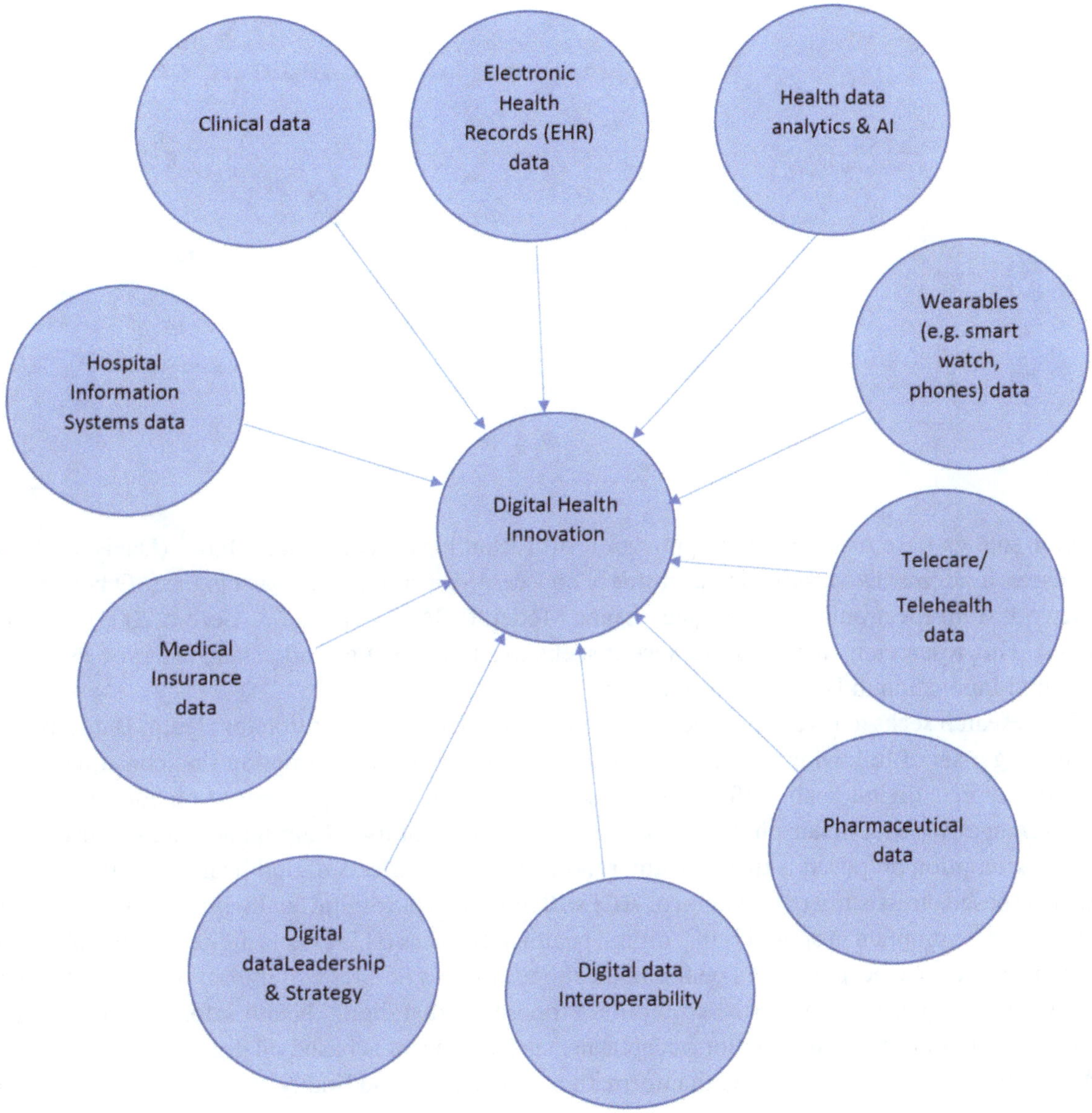

Cripps and Standing (2012) reported that while much of the recent attention on EHRs has been on the establishment and integration of computer systems, little attention has been paid to privacy and security in the health context. From a technical standpoint, consumers have voiced their concerns about their medical records being stored and used in electronic form citing issues including loss, theft, and misuse of what they consider private and personal information. It has been suggested that the emphasis on privacy and security in digital health information as a requirement for building consumer trust in these systems. Some digital health information systems lack bullet proof security that leads to online information being vulnerable for unauthorised access and use. Figure 2 shows high digital connectivity among Australians and that 84% went online for searching health information.

Figure 2. Key statistics about digital connectivity in Australia

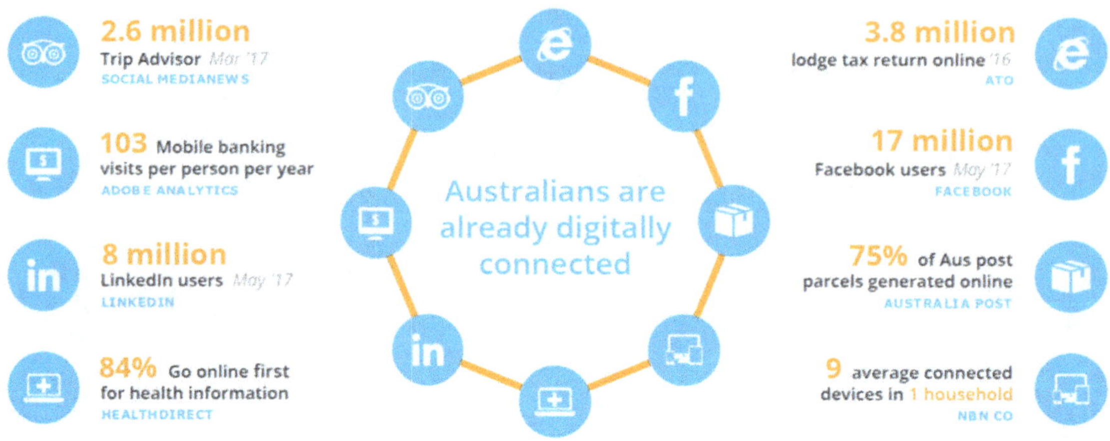

2.6 million
Trip Advisor Mar '17
SOCIAL MEDIANEWS
103 Mobile banking visits per person per year
ADOBE ANALYTICS
8 million
LinkedIn users May '17
LINKEDIN
84% Go online first for health information
HEALTHDIRECT
Australians are already digitally connected
3.8 million
lodge tax return online '16
ATO
17 million
Facebook users May '17
FACEBOOK
75% of Aus post parcels generated online
AUSTRALIA POST
9 average connected devices in 1 household
NBN CO

Prior studies have examined the application of Technology Acceptance Model (Davis 1989) and this research adopts TAM variables usefulness and ease of use and user acceptance. Other research framework from Electronic Servives Acceptance Model, E-SAM, (Sandhu & Corbitt 2008) have been adapted. This research is important because it seeks to adopt TAM to understand the process for AIH for Digital Innovation in Health Data Analytics.

This research seeks to investigate the drivers for AIH in Digital Innovation for Health Data Analytics by studying a set of following hypotheses. This study proposes the assumption that consumer experience (H1) affects digital health information ease of use. Such a concept is based on consumer having (positive/negative) experience oh AIH will impact on the ease of use of digital health information. The second assumption proposed is that consumer motivation (H2) affects digital health usefulness, such a concept is based on consumer motivation of AIH will impact on the digital health information usefulness.

The third assumption proposed is that digital health usefulness (H3) affects digital health information acceptance, such a concept is based on digital health usefulness of AIH will impact on the digital health information acceptance. The fourth assumption proposed is that digital health information ease of use (H4) affects digital health information acceptance, such a concept is based on digital health ease of use in AIH will impact on the digital health information acceptance. And finally, the fifth assumption is that digital health information acceptance (H5) affects digital health innovation, such a concept is based on digital health information acceptance of AIH will impact on the digital health innovation.

The proposed AIH conceptual model for Digital Health Innovation is shown in Figure 3.

RESEARCH METHODOLOGY

The main purpose of this research is to examine the variables that influence consumer acceptance of digital health information that leads to innovation for digital health from adopting AIH. The participants in this study having access & knowledge about digital health and are users of technology and have access to digital data, on their smart phones, tablets, and laptop. Mixed methodology using combination

Figure 3. AIH model for digital health innovation

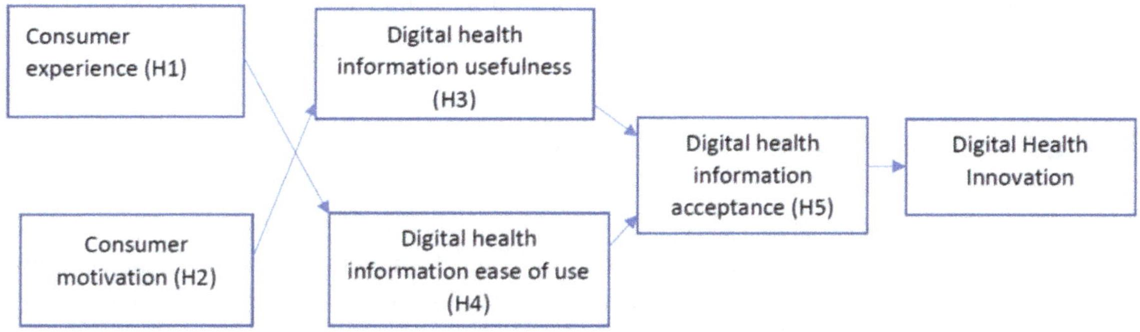

of qualitative research (e.g. interviews, focus group data for case studies, institutional data records) and empirical analysis (e.g. survey data for statistical analysis & PLS modelling, institutional data records) are adopted in this research. Adopting the two different methods provides deeper insights into the research for Digital Innovation for Health Data Analytics.

A set of key interview questionnaires (open and exploratory) in Digital Innovation for Health Data Analytics will be asked and recorded from the eighteen respondents. The interviews will be transcribed, and data analyzed for important findings and for further development of the survey's instruments. A number of following multiple Case Analysis were conducted to examine and improve on the survey instruments that would then lead to identifying important variables in this study.

A set of survey questionnaire will examine thirty-five respondents' attitude towards acceptance of digital health information and innovation. The questionnaire will be set on a Likert scale for responses to be measured on a scale from low (1) to high (5). The survey data will be analyzed using SPSS software to make meaningful sense of the data using descriptive statistics and confirmatory factor analysis. Partial Least Square modelling (Chin 2010) will be adopted for examining and testing the conceptual model for hypotheses path testing and validation and for measuring the variables developed in this study. The next section is into the three Case Analysis.

CASE ANALYSIS

Case Study 1: AIH Empowering Customers With Digital Health Information

Customers interact with vast amounts of information online, whether it is visiting websites, social media, travel arrangements, online learning, emails, and the activities are endless. Customer's interaction with digital health information has been slow. Digital health information access has been restricted due to number of reasons, such as people's health privacy, non-availability or limited and restricted access to one's health data from health organisations perspectives such as hospitals and government institutions, and as well as bureaucracy towards data access within health institutions.

Over the year's government and health institutions maintained digital health data records for people, but in the last few years' technology such as World Wide Web has made it easy for consumers to get access to digital data online from AIH. Health institutions and governments have been least prepared towards knowing how to make the health data available to consumers from an AIH platform. Some organisations are struggling to meet the demands of the consumers, whereas other have not yet started planning or implementing strategies in AIH for the delivering digital health data to their customers. Customers should have access to their digital health data.

Case Study 2: Digital Health Transformation

Health institutions such as hospitals, have for a long-time maintained records (paper and digital) of customers, with very limited or restricted access to customers. Though paper records demonstrate what information the customers "need to know", such as medical history, medications, doctors & hospital visits, and financial transaction, whereas access to other information which the intuition considers "sensitive" are not available to customers. Hospitals and institutions policies differ on information access to customers, which in today's time does not take into account the technology adoption by customers for digital information availability online.

Hospital institutions are also faced with legislations that they have to follow, and which have not been updated for recent times. Hospital and government institutions have been slow adopters of digital health technologies. Many institutions in regional areas lack AIH technological capabilities and infrastructure due to lack of funding, and availability of skilled personnel that can steer the digital health innovation project. And hence reliance on the old paper-based record system as the only option for driving and maintaining a paper-based health record system.

Case Study 3: Digital Health Innovation

Innovation has been studied in different disciplines, but its understanding in digital health has been limited especially from AIH perspective. For an idea or a concept to lead to innovation must meet the following requirements: (1) provide newer ways for a method, idea, or a product, to be usefully adopted; (2) needs to be cost effective; (3) can be applied widely; (4) have technological element; and (5) outcomes can be measured. To bind Digital Health Innovation together with AIH, means linking Digital Technology, AI, Health, and Innovation, as one. Research has shown that Digital Technology has a track record of widescale penetration and adoption across several industries such as social media, shared economy, travel, tourism, online learning, and many more.

Digital AI Technology has shown to have the potential to transform Health by injecting the element of Innovation, as customers are the biggest driver of technologies. Digital Health Innovation can not only provide newer ways for customers to interact with digital health information on an AIH platform, it can also transform health organisations business models for doing business. Customers are not only information users, they are also content creators as seen on social media, which is user driven, which is unique and distinctive, which have learning lessons for health institutions to develop digital systems that can cater to customers creating content in digital health and engaging with that content being facilitated and managed by autonomous AI. For a long time, "health" has had an "image" of being serious, sad, when people are sick, however with the integration of AI in health (AIH) that can quickly change to a more "positive" image.

This "image" is quickly changing around the world, when people engage with digital health information online, driven by AI such as wearing smart watches, smart phones, and monitoring health devices, that tracks their steps, calories, heart beats, blood pressure, and gym workouts, which also is linked to studies about better health and image for individuals to stay fit and active and taking control of their health. With the availability and engaging with newer data to customers digital health innovation can slow down several diseases such as obesity, diabetes, heart attacks, by people taking control of their health, which also means low medical insurance bills for the government, and the savings can be invested into other innovations that can further drive digital health innovations like a ripple effect. The next section is about conclusions, limitations, and future research directions.

SUMMARY OF THE RESULTS FROM STATISTICAL ANALYSIS

The statistical evidence revealed that consumer experience and empowerment from AIH were the key drivers for the adoption of digital health and need for information was considered significant to make a decision to use or not to use digital healthcare. Consumer motivation in AIH enhanced the use of digital healthcare, but it was not known the level of impact it had on their attitude towards newer technologies implementing digital healthcare (e.g. smartphones, smartwatches, etc.). Digital health information usefulness was highly valued as a core driver for AIH, further it also had emphasis and differentiates on different ways the usefulness could be spread across different areas of digital healthcare transformation in AIH, as consumer expected usefulness to be multifaceted that can be made available on a wide variety of AIH digital platforms to boost healthcare.

The data disclosed that Digital health ease of use though was a primary driver, nevertheless the use of technology such as AIH being simplified in terms of ease, had an important interplay with other distinct features by easily interfacing with digital healthcare. Consumers reported that AIH had made easier to transform their healthcare records and that Digital health information acceptance lead to making important decisions and participation in their healthcare management, which also demonstrates a level of autonomy consumers enjoyed in managing their healthcare digitally. The evidence revealed that Digital health innovation was highly dependent on modern technology for transformation oh AIH, which meant as newer technologies were integrated into healthcare, more pronounced versions of digital health innovation were discovered for advanced AIH, similarly lower integration of technology also had an impact, which lead to fewer innovations being discovered. Statistical data shows that there is a strong bond between modern IT such as AIH and Healthcare that leads to amalgamation of these two important elements to transform digital healthcare innovation.

SOLUTIONS AND RECOMMENDATIONS

This study has shown that the to drive Digital Systems Innovation it is important to have a an AIH to facilitate the different processed for health services. AIH provides many solutions to complex problems in healthcare, AIH is a long process and reliant on the expertise of specialized personnel's such as medical practitioners (e.g. doctors, nurses, & other healthcare staff), IT practitioners having an expert understanding on implementing and delivering on AIH projects, and leadership with in organisations that have an understanding and motivation to drive AIH, and consumer groups that have vested interest to use an AIH system. It should be noted that AIH projects are for long term and will deliver on the benefits after the system has been fined tuned to meet various requirements of different user groups. There will be problems that will require solutions which can make the AIH system better for improved functionality.

FUTURE RESEARCH DIRECTIONS

Future studies should focus on important issues that will drive AIH systems not only from a technical perspective but also from a user perspective, for example, make the AIH system user interaction seamless without flaw, embedding usefulness and ease of use elements within AIH interaction, consumer experience and motivation should be studied in more depth to understand how AIH can provide better health services and excellent experience for the health consumers and also increase their motivations to interact easily with AIH. The different elements of enjoyment to interact with the AIH systems needs closer attention to be implemented. Future studies should also focus on different user groups requirements that will interact with an AIH systems from different socio economic and cultural background which is very important as systems should be able to cater to different user groups.

CONCLUSION

This research in progress is from a bigger study being conducted in Global Digital Health which attempts to understand the key factors in AIH for Digital Innovation of Health Data Analytics. Literature review shows that Digital Health Innovation from AIH provides many opportunities to manage digital data for consumers, but it also at the same time faces obstacles such as: consumer's resistance, technical problems, political, digital leadership, data portability, data sharing and use, data security and access, data transfer and ownership, and data authorization. Some of these issues are technically related with digital health systems development whereas other issues relate to trust and consumer confidence, and significance of consumer culture, in data management by health service providers.

From a technical perspective each of the issues that are studied here have an important role to play in digital health innovation to be successful for AIH. The limitation of this study is based on the data being investigated from respondents at universities, and findings of this study needs to be amplified and used with caution, and the conceptual constructs, variables, research instrument scales and validation, hypotheses and the model, further tested on larger population of respondents. This study will focus on the discovery of key factors and provide a deeper insight into successful functioning of Digital Health Innovation.

REFERENCES

ADHA. (2019). What is digital health? *Australian Digital Health Agency*. https://www.digitalhealth.gov.au/get-started-with-digital-health/what-is-digital-health

Agarwal, R., Gao, G., Des Roches, C., & Jha, A. K. (2010). Research commentary—The digital transformation of healthcare: Current status and the road ahead. *Information Systems Research*, *21*(4), 796–809. doi:10.1287/isre.1100.0327

Anderson, M., & Anderson, S. L. (2019). How Should AI Be Developed, Validated, and Implemented in Patient Care? *AMA Journal of Ethics*, *21*(2), E125–E130. doi:10.1001/amajethics.2019.125 PMID:30794121

Australia's National Digital Health Strategy. (2019). https://conversation.digitalhealth.gov.au/sites/default/files/adha-strategy-doc-2ndaug_0_1.pdf

Bonomi, S. (2016). *The Electronic Health Record: A Comparison of Some European Countries*. Available from: https://www.researchgate.net/publication/303364932_The_Electronic_Health_Record_A_Comparison_of_Some_European_Countries

Chin, W. W. (2010). How to Write Up and Report PLS Analyses. In V. E. Vinzi, W. W. Chin, J. Henseler, & H. Wang (Eds.), *Handbook of Partial Least Squares Concepts, Methods and Applications* (pp. 650–690). Berlin: Springer-Verlag. doi:10.1007/978-3-540-32827-8_29

Cripps, H., & Standing, C. (2012). *Building patient trust in electronic health records, Australian eHealth Informatics and Security Conference*. Edith Cowan University Research Online. https://ro.ecu.edu.au/cgi/viewcontent.cgi?referer=https://www.google.com.au/&httpsredir=1&article=1002&context=aeis

Dameri, R. P. (2012). Defining an evaluation framework for digital cities implementation. In *Information Society (i-Society), 2012 International Conference on* (pp. 466-470). IEEE.

Davis, F. D. (1989). Perceived usefulness, perceived ease of use, and user acceptance of information technology. *MIS Quarterly, 13*(3), 319-340. Retrieve from http://www.jstor.org/stable/249008

Dzenowagis, J., Kelley, E., Kluge, H., & Ganesh, V. (2018). *Digital technologies: shaping the future of primary healthcare*. WHO Headquarters. https://www.who.int/docs/default-source/primary-health-care-conference/digital-technologies.pdf?sfvrsn=3efc47e0_2

Fragidis, L., & Chatzoglou, P. (2018). Implementation of a Nationwide Electronic Health Record (EHR): The International Experience in 13 Countries. *International Journal of Health Care Quality Assurance, 31*(2), 116–13. doi:10.1108/IJHCQA-09-2016-0136 PMID:29504871

Ginsburg, P., Loera-Brust, A., Brandt, C., & Durak, A. (2018). *The opportunities and challenges of data analytics in healthcare.* Report Produced by Artificial Intelligence and Emerging Technologies Initiative.

Hambleton, S., & Aloizos, J. (2019). Australia's digital health journey. *The Medical Journal of Australia, 210*(6), S5–S6. doi:10.5694/mja2.50039 PMID:30927473

Jha, A. K., Doolan, D., Grandt, D., Scott, T., & Bates, D. W. (2008). The use of health information technology in seven nations. *International Journal of Medical Informatics, 77*(12), 848–854. doi:10.1016/j.ijmedinf.2008.06.007 PMID:18657471

Jiang, F., Jiang, Y., Zhi, H., Dong, Y., Li, H., Ma, S., ... Wang, Y. (2017). Artificial intelligence in healthcare: Past, present and future. *Stroke and Vascular Neurology, 2*(4), e000101. doi:10.1136vn-2017-000101 PMID:29507784

Krumholz, H. M. (2014). Big data and new knowledge in medicine: The thinking, training, and tools needed for a learning health system. *Health Affairs, 33*(7), 1163–1170. doi:10.1377/hlthaff.2014.0053 PMID:25006142

Mohammed, A., & Yunus, A. (2017). Technology Acceptance in Healthcare Service: A Case of Electronic Medical Records (ERM). *International Journal of Academic Research in Business and Social Sciences, 7*(11).

Patrick, K., Hekler, E.B., Estrin, D., Mohr, D.C., Riper, H., Crane, D., Godino, J., & Riley, W.T., (2016). *The pace of technologic change: implications for digital health behavior intervention research.* Academic Press.

Sandhu, K., & Corbitt, B. (2008). A framework for electronic services system. *International Journal of Electronic Customer Relationship Management*, *2*(1), 50. doi:10.1504/IJECRM.2008.019568

The Brookings Initiative on artificial intelligence and emerging technologies seeks to establish a proper societal framework for the impending "digitalization of everything." (n.d.). https://www.brookings.edu/research/the-opportunities-and-challenges-of-data-analytics-in-health-care/

World Health Organisation. (2019). https://www.who.int/behealthy/digital-health

World Health Organisation. (2019). Retrieved Apr 21, 2019 from https://www.who.int/behealthy/digital-health

Yoo, Y., Henfridsson, O., & Lyytinen, K. (2010). Research commentary—the new organizing logic of digital innovation: An agenda for information systems research. *Information Systems Research*, *21*(4), 724–735. doi:10.1287/isre.1100.0322

Chapter 2
Digital Health Innovation Enhancing Patient Experience in Medical Travel

Anita Medhekar
https://orcid.org/0000-0002-6791-4056
Central Queensland University, Australia

ABSTRACT

Digital health technological innovations are disrupting every sector of the economy, including medical travel/tourism. Global patients as medical tourists are using patient-centric digital health technologies, enhancing patient/medical tourists experience and making it more transparent and engaging with health-care providers and medical tourists. Digital communication tools such as e-mail, online appointments, smartphones, instant messaging applications, social media tools, user-generated content by online patient communities, tele-medicine, tele-radiology, my-Health records, Skype consultation, WhatsApp, health video, electronic health records, health data analytics tools, and artificial intelligence-enabled health technologies enhance the medical travel decision-making process, reduce cost, improve patient care and transparency of communication, and engage the relationship between the patient and the healthcare provider with positive outcomes, medical tourist experience, and empowerment.

INTRODUCTION

Medical travel/tourism (MTm) is a process where people travel within the country or overseas for medical treatment/surgery. Medical travel can be treatment-driven or destination-driven, based on patient's need for treatment, health service quality of the hospital, less waiting time, national and international accreditation, diagnostic expertise, super-surgical speciality and surgeon's reputation (Medhekar, 2014). As determined from the MTm Association site, some of the popular destination-driven treatments are dental (Thailand, India, Mexico and Poland), cosmetic (Thailand, Argentina and Mexico), hair transplant (Turkey), bariatric (Thailand, India and Mexico), sex-realignment (Thailand) and surrogacy/fertility (In-

DOI: 10.4018/978-1-7998-3274-4.ch002

dia and Thailand). Treatment-driven are cosmetic, dental, eye surgery, heart, hip and knee replacement, organ transplant, oncology/cancer, reproductive treatment and stem cell therapy.

According to Shaw et al. (2018) digital health innovation has three goals of reducing costs, enhancing patient experience, and improve healthcare outcomes. Thus, digital innovation in health technologies and its adoption in MTm related services are enhancing medical tourist (MTs) experience and making it more patient-centric, transparent and engaging. Digital communication tools using web 2.0 technologies, e-Health-2.0, and Medicine-2.0, are: e-mail, on-line appointments, smart-phones, instant messaging application, social media tools, user-generated content by online patient communities, tele-medicine, Skype, WhatsApp, messenger, health video, electronic health-records, health-data analytics tools and Artificial Intelligence (AI) enabled technologies (Fisher & Clayton, 2012; Lupton, 2014; Shaw et al., 2018; Thackeray et al., 2008). The use of innovative digital health technologies, e-health records, health-data analytics, improves transparency of communication in real time, enhances medical travel decision making process, improves patient-centered personalised care and relationship between the patient as MTs and medical professionals, with positive MTs engagement, empowerment and experience.

Hospitals and diagnostic clinics involved in treating foreign patients' need to have an online profile to increase market share and communicate information to attract potential foreign patients, receive enquires and book them as actual patients for treatment, via their online medical consultant. Medical consultant establishes direct contact and communicates with the patients to personalise their healthcare needs and provide holistic healthcare solutions as per treatment requirements (McKinsey & Company, 2013). Online digital health technological tools facilitate communication and engagement between the patient/MTs, doctor/healthcare provider and medical-tour facilitators in a timely manner. It helps to communicate information in real-time and engages and empowers the patient to make informed decision regarding their medical travel plans and enhances patient experience and outcomes.

Medical tourism hospitals and popular MTm destinations in developing countries, such as Thailand, India, Dubai, Singapore, Malaysia and Mexico are increasingly adopting innovative patient-centric digital health/e-health technological tools to engage with foreign patients, improve healthcare practices for clinicians/medical professionals, and provide positive MTm experience. It has been a challenge for MTm hospitals as well as patients/MTs to accept, embrace and adopt digital technologies and manage their medical travel journey (Medhekar, 2017). The main aim of embracing digital technologies in MTm is to provide timely access to world class Joint Commission International (JCI) accredited, quality of medical treatment, in state-of-the-art hospitals facilities and positive MTm experience to the MTs, so they can choose the hospital, surgeon's super-speciality and the destination for their medical surgery and improve their physical health and quality of life (Medhekar, Wong & Hall, 2014, 2019).

Digital revolution is disrupting every sector of the economy including healthcare and tourism. Digital revolution is driven by innovators of healthcare technologies, start-up firm, investors/entrepreneurs, medical professionals, healthcare providers and government policy makers to bring about a change in healthcare ecosystems. A human and a patient/MTs centred approach to digital health will enhance patient experience and empower them to make right choices and decision to travel abroad for medical treatment/surgery. MTm hospitals and healthcare providers treating foreign patients need to engage with digital technologies to attract, communicate, maintain transparency and retain foreign MTs for repeat visits with positive healthcare and MTm experience. Medical technologies include a wide range of products and services to treat medical conditions and diseases, for example, medical devises, innovative healthcare services, digital health records tools, social-media tools and smart-phone applications, healthcare transportation, 3D printing of medical products, tele-medicine, patient's health records, information technology, tele-radiology, mobile health technologies, AI, and health informatics.

Literature review indicates publications on digital health innovative technologies adoption by MTs and MTm healthcare providers for their own benefit is increasing market share, hospital branding and provides positive MTm experience to foreign patients, is relatively an emerging new area of research. This exploratory chapter is structured as follows. The Section 1 of the chapter introduces the growing importance and significance of medical travel/tourism and digital health tools used by MTm hospitals in treating patients/MTs in developing countries. Section 2 provides the literature review on social exchange theory, MTm and adoption of digital technologies by MTm sector to attract MTs and enhances MTm experience. Section 3 covers methodology and explores through qualitative content analyse of MTm hospital websites, the various digital health tools adopted to enhance foreign patient's decision to travel abroad for surgery and positive MT experience. Section 4 discusses the benefits from adopting digital e-health platforms to patients/MTs and MTm hospitals. Final sections present recommendations for MTm policy implications, future research directions and conclusions to advance the knowledge in the field of adopting digital e-health tools and MTs enhanced digital experience.

LITERATURE REVIEW

Adoption and use of innovative digital tools such as e-mail, smart-phones, instant messaging application, social media tools, tele-medicine, Skype, WhatsApp, messenger, health video, and electronic my-health-records, and health-data analytics tools and Artificial Intelligence (AI) enabled technologies helps to attract and retain foreign patient, increase market share by private hospitals, health travel agencies but also enhances patients/MTs experience and MTm decision making process. This is an emerging research area in healthcare related MTm and travel research. Having realised the tremendous benefits from adoption and application of digital health innovative tools among potential and actual MTs, healthcare providers, including hospitality and tourism sectors have started using innovative digital tools for promoting and communicating their MTm related products, super-surgical specialities, medical hotels and services to targeted potential MTs/patients. Literature will provide background to the underling theories in context of use of digital technologies in health tourism by the MTm hospitals/providers and the MTs/patients.

Medical Tourism

Medical travel/tourism literature is multidisciplinary as evident from systematic review of literature (Adam et al., 2015; Connell, 2015; Collins et al., 2019; Lunt & Carrera, 2010, 2011; Lunt, et al., 2016; Majeed & Lu, 2017). Medical travel is international economics in action and relates to international trade in healthcare services, where Article 1:2 of General Agreement on Trade in Services (GATS), defines and differentiates between four different modes of delivery of healthcare services (Chanda, 2002; Medhekar, Wong & Hall, 2019). Mode-1 cross border supply, Mode-2 consumption abroad, Mode-3 commercial presence, and Mode-4 movement of healthcare personnel for delivery of healthcare services abroad (Chanda, 2002). Privatisation and globalisation of healthcare, internet technologies, is driving this growth, where global hospitals are competing to promote online their surgical-specialities, and potential patients/MTs are searching the internet to seek treatment abroad (Han & Hwang, 2018; Lunt & Carrera, 2011; Medhekar & Newby, 2012). Developing countries since the Asian Financial Crisis, have increasingly adopted an export-led-growth strategy to gain from trade in healthcare services, having a multiplier effect on the economy (Burns, 2015; Medhekar, 2014; NaRanong & NaRanong, 2011; Pocock & Phua, 2011).

There are health economics related demand and supply side factors that drive people to travel overseas for medical treatment/surgery. Demand-side push factors are: high cost of surgery at home, treatment not available due to regulatory reasons in developed countries, lack of medical expertise in less developed countries, surgery waiting-list, lack of state-of-the-art medical equipment and diagnostic technology, and uninsured or under-insured people for particulate types of surgery (Bookman & Bookman, 2007, Medhekar et al., 2014 & 2019; Medhekar & Newby, 2012; Turner, 2010 & 2011; Yazdanpanah, Parsaei & Jeihooni, 2018). The supply-side pull factors include, affordable cost of surgery, no surgery waiting-list, JCI accredited hospital quality, availability of surgical expertise, patient safety, hospital employees, hospital precision, state-of-the-art medical equipment and technologies, post-surgery care, and tourism/holiday opportunity at an attractive destination (Collins et al., 2019; Khan, et al., 2016; Medhekar et al., 2014 & 2020; Tuner, 2010).

Further, MTm hospitals and medical-tour facilitators have increasingly adopted internet based digital health innovative tools like tele-medicine, to communicate and consult directly in real-time with potential patients/MTs and promote their medical hospital brand and surgical-super- specialities to increase global market share (Burns, 2015; Cormany & Baloglu, 2011; Crooks et al., 2011; Medhekar & Newby, 2012; Speier, 2011). Study by George and Henthorne (2008), with a focus on state of Kerala and Goa in India, concludes that the use of tele-medicine, face-to-face consultation and tele-radiology into medical travel/tourism by MTm hospitals and tour facilitators, improves MTs satisfaction, perception and loyalty, before and after medical travel. However, potential medical travellers are concerned regarding the credibility and trust-worthiness of the information posted on the MTm hospitals and medical-tour facilitators website, before they travel abroad for surgery (Agag & El-Masry, 2017; Han & Hwang, 2018; Mahuire et al., 2016; Mason & Wright, 2011).

Social Exchange Theory

Social exchange theory is borrowed from behavioural psychology, classical economics and sociology (Emerson, 1976) is evolving. Social Exchange is defined as "voluntary actions of individuals that are motivated by the return they are expected to bring" (Blau, 1964, p. 91). Any relationship between individuals, groups, online communities with common interests (human right activist, MTs/patients, and doctors), is motivated by the positive healthcare experience and outcomes that they expect to bring to everyone based on costs and benefits, and group norms may be followed in the use of various digital e-health tools. This theory can be applied to healthcare promotion and communication by MTm hospitals and medical-tour facilitators with patients/MTs by using digital health tools to attract potential MTs, form relationships with stakeholders from demand and supply-side and increase their global competitiveness.

Social exchange is different to economic exchange which is extrinsic, where buyers and sellers meet at a market place, virtual or a shop front where terms of sale are determined in relation to cost, quality and quantity of goods and services exchanged in return of price paid by the buyer- under a legal obligation. Whereas social exchange is intrinsic, where one person may provide good and services to another person in trust and good faith, without any obligation, that it will be reciprocated in terms of payment (Blau, 1964). The exchange of intangible information between the hospital, medical-tourism facilitators and potential patients involves costs and benefits, which can be examined within the context of social exchange theory. In case of adoption and use of digital health technology such as social media and mobile-apps related to sharing user generated content (UGC) about patient data, healthcare information and experiences by actual or potential patients/MTs is more altruistic relative to hospital and MTm facilitators, whose aim is to increase global market share by attracting and retaining medical-tourists for future visits.

Whereas, actual MTs voluntarily share information on digital health tools and post positive and negative experiences of MTm hospital, surgery, country, and medical-tour facilitator which benefits the actual as well as potential MTs/patients. In this case, Homans (1974) three propositions- as outlined in Emerson (1976) (i) action based on success from the chosen action is greater than the alternative, (ii) positive past-stimulus or past actions will be repeated, and (iii) deprivation-satiation related to law of diminishing returns, can be applied to health tourism. The propositions of Homans are applicable from both the demand-side (patient) and the supply-side (hospital and medical-tour facilitator). From supply-side, if (i) use of digital health technologies for promotion and communication by hospitals and MTm facilitators and improving overall healthcare service quality; is rewarded in terms of increased market share, transparency in quality of healthcare services provided to MTs based on success and popularity of their healthcare services, they will continue to use digital health technologies. (ii) Furthermore, if past healthcare service quality, results in positive healthcare outcomes, such actions and advice will be repeated.

Similarly, from the demand-side, patients'/MTs actions of feedback and information sharing are voluntary and altruistic, in terms of communicating their lived experiences on digital health tools such as WhatsApp, messenger, patient-testimonials, social media to hospitals, medical doctors, facilitators, potential patients, friends and strangers, which are rewarded in terms of (i) getting medical value for money by choosing the best hospital, surgeon and surgery overseas, (ii) repeat visits and loyalty due positive MTm experience, and (iii) potential MTs benefit from making informed decisions, saves cost and waiting time to get positive health outcomes which provides intrinsic happiness. Moreover, hospitals will receive real time feedback from patients, to improve their services, as well as potential patients will also be helped through this exchange of positive and negative information from other patient's satisfaction or dissatisfaction experienced in choosing the hospital and surgeon for surgery overseas. Therefore, social exchange through social networking helps to communicate, collect and share information by creating UGC on e-Health-2.0, Medicine-2.0, and e-Healthcare clusters in online healthcare space (Chretien, Azar & Kind, 2011; Eysenbach, 2008; Hawn, 2009; Van de Belt et al., 2012) to promote global healthcare to potential patients/MTs by digital health technologies and produce positive healthcare experience and outcomes. As asserted by Thackeray (2008) digital tools are *"more powerful then agency-based advertising"* (Thackeray et al., 2008, p.340).

Growth of internet, and adoption of e-Health and e-Medicine digital applications is playing a key role in the dissemination and promotion of health travel/tourism information and changing the way patients and medical professionals interact and communicate through its various digital health technologies. Private hospitals and medical travel agencies use digital technologies to promote and communicate global healthcare services to patients, because health tourists search online information by various digital health tools and create health information communities with similar MTm related interest, before they make the decision to travel abroad for treatment. It is important to focus on credible and trustworthy health tourism information to be able to make informed choices regarding host-country of treatment, hospital and surgeon's expertise and success rate.

Digital Health Technologies

Various types of innovative digital health technologies are used for health promotion, marketing healthcare information that has a positive behaviour change in health outcomes. Digital healthcare technological tools help to connect healthcare providers with the patients providing personalised care in terms of diagnosis, consultation, medical treatment, drug test and preventative medicine to enhance MTm experience and improve healthcare outcomes. These technologies according to Joseph (2019) range from: (i) Self-serving online digital tools, which help the patients to take online consulting/appointments with the doctor, auto renewal of prescription, electronic upload of medical records and payments. (ii) Digital wellness tool, such as wearable technology, which helps the patients to have real-time consultation with the physician and maintain their health and wellbeing by monitoring their health through online consultations about diet, exercise, medications and treatment plans. (iii) Digital health clinical transparency tools ensure information asymmetry related to patient's health records, clinical data and graphs, diagnostic reports, treatment and medication plans. It helps the patients to make informed decisions and the clinicians to provide real time information, personalised treatment and improve hospitals performance. (iv) Financial transparency digital tool provides financial information related to costs of first appointment, medication, diagnostic tests, surgery, post-surgery care, and fees charges at various levels of treatment. This guides the patients to compare pricing and quality of treatment offered and make informed decisions. (v) Remote digital health monitoring tool where the doctors monitor the health of the patient and send reminders to the patient and the personal caretaker to improve healthcare outcomes (Joseph, 2019).

Medical travellers extensively search for MTm information via digital health tools before they decide to travel abroad and create travel experience reviews on social-media e-health communities during and post-travel experiences (Parra-López et al., 2012). Potential MTs are accessing the websites and using various digital health tools to search for travel information posted by medical travel agencies and by MTs on digital health platforms, based on their experiences, opinions, pictures and videos and process the information, before, making a decision to travel for surgery (Buhalis & Law, 2008; Chung & Koo, 2015; Kim & Kwon, 2010; Xiang & Gretzel, 2010). Therefore, adoption and use of digital health tools by MTm healthcare providers and patients/MTs, facilitates to create, document, share, evaluate, apply, and communicate health related knowledge, which is dynamic process, in MTm decision making process and enhances patient/MTs experience of surgery abroad (Medhekar, 2017).

Xiang and Gretzel (2010) study found that internet search engines direct travellers to use various social media tools to search for travel related information. This suggest that tourism marketers need to focus on online marketing of tourism related goods and services on social media sites, which has consumer generated experiences posted and shared on YouTube, Facebook, twitter, Flicker, Wikis, and social networking sites. Narangajavana et al. (2017) study added UGC information posted on social media platforms must be from trustworthy source, as potential MTs trust positive content and form positive expectations, before they travel, about a destination based on the information.

A longitudinal exploratory study by Van de Belt et al. (2012) from 2009-2011, found that 873 hospitals in 12 countries of Western Europe increasingly used social media tools to promote their healthcare services overtime such as YouTube (25%-19.7%), LinkedIn (20.5%-31.8%) and Facebook (10%-67.0%) and Twitter, which improved communication with patients and provision of patient-centred care and hospitals reputation. Antheunis, Tates and Nieboer (2013) study concluded that 70.7% of medical professionals used LinkedIn and 51.2% Twitter for communication with colleagues and for marketing their medical services to potential patients. Furthermore, 59.9% of patients used Twitter for exchanging advice and increasing knowledge and 52.3% patients used Facebook for social support and health advice.

Korda and Itani (2013) empirical findings conclude that nearly 57% of generation X (born between 1961 and 1981) and 56% of generation Y (born between 1981 and 2001) searched for health-related information; and in 2010, nearly 80% of the adults searched for health information using the internet search engines. Nearly, 67% of surveyed physician and 65% of nurses according to Deloitte (2010) health report were interested in using digital health and social media applications such as smart- phone for professional networking and marketing their healthcare services. These tools such as Facebook-likes and Yelp-reviews are UGC by patients to rate their healthcare lived experiences with the hospital, healthcare quality, surgeon, patient safety, and provide recommendation to potential patients (Lopez et al., 2012; Timian et al., 2013).

METHODOLOGY

For this study, the source of data collection was from the home page websites of popular private medical-tourism hospitals in India, Thailand and Singapore. These popular hospitals were found from the Google search engine as listed in Table 1. These hospitals are involved in treating domestic and foreign MTs/ patients. Hospital home-page sites and other related to the hospital were studied to find out the various digital health and social media tools used to disseminate information to the professionals, actual and potential MTs/patients. Hospitals are using internet linked digital tools to receive feedback and provide quick source of healthcare information regarding its facility and super-speciality to the MTs, medical-tourism facilitators and all other businesses involved in medical travel/tourism.

Once the hospitals were identified, which were involved in MTm and treating foreign patients, the social research method of content analysis (Creswell, 2014) of the hospital home page website was used. The author personally studied and explored the hospital home page websites and digital health tools to extract relevant information and data. Global patients/MTs search the hospital websites and use the various digital health and social media tools, supported by the internet for specialist treatment and medical travel related information. The home page web-links of eighteen (18) international hospital websites in Table 1, helped to determine the various types of information posted by the MTm hospitals to attract domestic and global MTs as customers, and MTm facilitators, to gather all the information required regarding the healthcare facility. For example: select a city for the location of the hospital, medical facilities, surgical super-specialities, find a doctor/surgeon, make an enquiry/online consultation, hospital accreditation, surgery-cost comparisons, patient experience testimonials, online payments and chat, news and media, health information, plan your visit, seminars and workshops and medical research related information.

On the google map-website, one can find the exact location map and the address for various hospital and their branches at different locations and super-surgical-specialities. Due to the limitation of the time the author decided to choose six (6) popular hospitals in three countries, with multi-super-speciality. Table 2 lists the different types of digital tools used by the wellness resorts and hospital websites in the three countries.

Since the use of innovative digital health, digital social media and smart-phone apps the strategies used for adopting digital e-health tools for creating and sharing healthcare information has changed. Hospitals, healthcare professionals, and medical travel agencies use digital health tools from the supply-side to attract potential wellness and MTs to their healthcare facility. From the demand-side, potential

Table 1. Selected list of international hospitals

Hospital Treating Foreign Patients: India, Thailand & Singapore		
Hospitals in India	Hospitals in Thailand	Hospitals in Singapore
1. Apollo Hospital Group (AHG) http://www.apollohospitals.com/ 2. Asian Heart Institute (AHI) http://www.asianheartinstitute.org/ 3. Fortis Group (FG) http://www.fortishealthcare.com/ 4. Max Healthcare (MX) http://www.maxhealthcare.in/index.php/about-us 5. Narayan Health (NH) http://www.narayanahealth.org/ 6. Wockhardt Hospital (WH) http://www.wockhardthospitals.com/	1. Bangkok Nursing Home https://au.hotels.com/go/thailand/best-bangkok-hospitals (BNH) 2. Bumrungrad International Hospital (BmIH) https://www.bumrungrad.com/en/ 3. Bangkok International Hospital (BIH) https://bangkokinternationalhospital.com 4. Samitiveg Sukhumvit Hospital (SSH) https://www.samitivejhospitals.com/sukhumvit/ 5. The Bangkok Christian Hospital (BCH) https://www.health-tourism.com/medical-centers/bangkok-christian-hospital/ 6. Thantakit International Dental Center (TIDC) https://www.thaidentalcenter.com	1. Mount Elizabeth Hospital (MEH) https://www.mountelizabeth.com.sg/? 2. Gleneagles Hospital (GH) https://www.gleneagles.com.sg/ 3. Parkway East Hospital (PEH) https://www.parkwayeast.com.sg/ 4. National Heart Centre (NHC) https://www.nhcs.com.sg/ 5. Raffles Hospital (RH) https://www.rafflesmedicalgroup.com/hospital 6. John Hopkins Singapore International Medical Centre (JHSIMC) https://www.hopkinsmedicine.org/singapore/

Source: Developed for this paper

Table 2. Types of digital tools used by hospitals and patients

	Types of Digital Health Tools	Example
1	Blog- where authors add content (patient and provider)	Bloggers, Word press
2	Communities of practice-Thematic networking	Telehelp, Discussion forums
3	Collaborative sites for information filtering & sharing	Digg sites, chat rooms
4	Microblog- real-time brief messaging	Twitter, TV-face-face-consulting
5	Mashups-combines data from 2 or more services	Health Maps, Whoissick, Mobile Medical Travel and Health Apps
6	Media sharing sites- videos, images, photos, power-point, the doctors' channel, document, power-point	Flicker, Slide-share, YouTube, Medting, Scribd, telemedicine, tele-radiology
7	Professional networking sites	LinkedIn, Doc2Doc, Drs hangout
8	Social networking sites	Facebook, MySpace, Google+
9	Social Bookmarking site- save, share, discover webpages	Delicious
10	Wiki- information, multimedia sharing	Wikipedia, Fluwiki

Source: Collated from medical tourism hospital websites

and actual wellness and MTs use various social media and e-health tools to search and share information regarding their healthcare lived experience and quality of services provided by accredited MTm hospitals, specialist surgeon, and medical travel facilitator.

For this study 18 MTm international tourism hospital websites were explored. Content was analysed to identify key themes, such as pricing, treatment type, waiting time, accreditation, and YouTube videos, patient experience blogs/testimonials and social media tools. The key components of content analysis as seen from Table 3, home pages of the 18 hospitals provide information that patients seek, before they decide to travel abroad for surgery: (i) General information regarding the hospital/healthcare provider, (ii) on-line patient consultation/enquiry with the hospital-find a doctor, (iii) Patient healthcare information and treatment plan, (iv) International patient information regarding legal requirements, visa and travel arrangements, and (v) information for healthcare professionals, and (vi) Social media and digital health tools and helpline. 'My Health' login receives and stores patient personal data in a secure online environment, so that the patient can access and download their diagnostic test results. Further, it also helps the patient to stay on wellness-program to manage conditions like diabetes and a Live-Care chat for real-time health help-line.

Table 3. Information on medical-tourism hospital internet home page

India Hospitals	**AHG**	**NH**	**WH**	**FH**	**AH**	**MAXH**
1- Vision/Mission	Y	Y	Y	Y	Y	Y
Multi-Speciality	Y	Y	Y	Y	Y	Y
Top Ten Procedures	Y	Y	Y	Y	Y	Y
Healthcare Facilities	Y	Y	Y	Y	Y	Y
National Accreditation	Y	Y	Y	Y	Y	Y
JCI Accreditation	Y	Y	Y	Y	Y	--
2- Find a Doctor	Y	Y	Y	Y	Y	Y
Online Appointment	Y	Y	Y	Y	Y	Y
Online Feedback	Y	Y	Y	Y	Y	Y
Online Payment/bill	Y	Y	Y	Y	Y	Y
3- Patient Care Guide	Y	Y	Y	Y	Y	Y
Health Information	Y	Y	Y	Y	Y	Y
Get Home Care	--	--	--	--	--	Y
Help Line & FAQ	Y	Y	Y	Y	Y	Y
4- International Patient Special Services	Y	Y	Y	Y	Y	Y
5- Careers	Y	Y	Y	Y	Y	Y
Education-Research	Y	Y	Y	Y	Y	Y
Insurance & Partners	Y	Y	Y	Y	Y	Y
6- Help Line & FAQ	Y	Y	Y	Y	Y	Y
Social media tools	Y	Y	Y	Y	Y	Y
News & Media	Y	Y	Y	Y	Y	Y
My Health login	Y	Y	Y	Y	--	--
Thailand Hospital	**BNH**	**BmIH**	**BIH**	**SSH**	**BCH**	**TIDC**
1- Vision/Mission	Y	Y	Y	Y	Y	Y
Multi-Speciality	Y	Y	Y	Y	Y	Y
Top Ten Procedures	Y	Y	Y	Y	Y	Y
Healthcare Facilities	Y	Y	Y	Y	Y	Y
National Accreditation	Y	Y	Y	Y	Y	Y
JCI Accreditation	Y	Y	Y	Y	Y	Y
2- Find a Doctor	Y	Y	Y	Y	Y	Y
Online Appointment	Y	Y	Y	Y	Y	Y
Online Feedback	Y	Y	Y	Y	Y	Y
Online Payment	Y	Y	Y	Y	Y	Y
3- Patient Care Guide	Y	Y	Y	Y	Y	Y
Health Information	Y	Y	Y	Y	Y	Y
Get Home Care	--	Y	Y	Y	Y	Y
Help Line & FAQ	Y	Y	Y	Y	Y	Y

continued on following page

Table 3. Continued

4- International Patient Special Services	Y	Y	Y	Y	Y	Y
5- Careers	Y	Y	Y	Y	Y	Y
Education-Research	Y	Y	Y	Y	Y	Y
Insurance & Partners	Y	Y	Y	Y	Y	Y
6- Help Line & FAQ	Y	Y	Y	Y	Y	Y
Social media tools	Y	Y	Y	Y	Y	Y
News & Media	Y	Y	Y	Y	Y	Y
My Health login	Y	Y	Y	Y	Y	Y
Singapore Hospitals	**MEH**	**GH**	**PEH**	**NHC**	**YRH**	**JHSIM**
1- Vision/Mission	Y	Y	Y	Y	Y	Y
Multi-Speciality	Y	Y	Y	Y	Y	Y
Top Ten Procedures	Y	Y	Y	Y	Y	Y
Healthcare Facilities	Y	Y	Y	Y	Y	Y
National Accreditation	Y	Y	Y	Y	Y	Y
JCI Accreditation	Y	Y	Y	Y	Y	Y
2- Find a Doctor	Y	Y	Y	Y	Y	Y
Online Appointment	Y	Y	Y	Y	Y	Y
Online Feedback	Y	Y	Y	Y	Y	Y
Online Payment	Y	Y	Y	Y	Y	Y
3- Patient Care Guide	Y	Y	Y	Y	Y	Y
Health Information	Y	Y	Y	Y	Y	Y
Get Home Care	Y	Y	Y	Y	Y	Y
Help Line & FAQ	Y	Y	Y	Y	Y	Y
4- International Patient Special Services	Y	Y	Y	Y	Y	Y
5- Careers	Y	Y	Y	Y	Y	Y
Education-Research	Y	Y	Y	Y	Y	Y
Insurance & Partners	Y	Y	Y	Y	Y	Y
6- Live help line & FAQ	Y	Y	Y	Y	Y	Y
Social media tools	Y	Y	Y	Y	Y	Y
News & Media	Y	Y	Y	Y	Y	Y
My Health login	Y	Y	Y	Y	Y	Y

Source: Developed for this paper (Y-Yes, -- No)

Narayana Health in partnership with Hewlett Packard in 2014 launched Cloud-e-Health, to deliver affordable quality of healthcare services, and real time disease surveillance in rural areas (Express News Service, 2014). The 'Follow Us Menu' on the hospital home pages: Facebook, Twitter, Blogs, LinkedIn, Google Plus, Pinterest, Instagram and YouTube testimonials etc, improves communication, information and overall enhances patients experience before and after medical travel abroad. From Table 4 we can examine the various digital health tools adopted by the MT hospitals under study, to communicate with the domestic and international patients/MTs, including the medical facilitators and professionals.

Home pages of international hospitals examined, have well-developed with various digital health tools and e-health social media communication channels and the various ways the patients and medical professionals can communicate; for example: live talk with Hospital consultant (window pops up on the right hand corner of the home page), social media 'Follow-Us Menu' icons pictures such as of Facebook, Twitter, Alexa, YouTube, LinkedIn, tele-medicine, tele-radiology, face-face consulting, Slide-share, Alexa, Blogs, and Google plus. Hospitals without a 'Follow-Us Menu' have LinkedIn or a Facebook accounts for communication. Medical-tourism e-health related social site must be interactive and user friendly, as they promote healthcare services available to the patients. These MTm sites also must be functional based on providing medical and surgical information regarding various forms of treatment, connectivity to related healthcare services, assessment, promotion of related healthcare services, commercial opportunity of the site to gather consumer data, and communication between the patient and the medical consultant (Lunt, Hardey & Mannion, 2010).

Table 4. Digital health applications used by hospitals in India, Singapore, and Thailand

India Hospitals	**AHG**	**NH**	**WHG**	**Fortis**	**AH**	**MAXH**
Website	Y	Y	Y	Y	Y	Y
Virtual tour- Visit	Y	Y	Y	Y	Y	Y
Live chat	Y	Y	Y	Y	--	--
LinkedIn	Y	Y	Y	Y	Y	Y
YouTube Testimonials	Y	Y	Y	Y	Y	Y
YouTube Health Info	Y	Y	Y	Y	Y	Y
On-Twitter	Y	Y	Y	Y	Y	-
Photo/Video Sharing	Y	Y	Y	Y	Y	Y
Blogs	Y	Y	Y	Y	Y	Y
Discussion Forum	Y	Y	Y	Y	Y	--
Health Mobile-App	Y	Y	Y	Y	--	Y
Face Book	Y	Y	Y	Y	Y	Y
Cloud e-Health	-	Y	Y	Y	--	--
Wikipedia	Y	Y	Y	Y	Y	Y
Phone & E-mail	Y	Y	Y	Y	Y	Y
Flickr	Y	Y	Y	Y	--	--
Patient Testimonials	Y	Y	Y	Y	Y	--
Webinar Hospital Channel	--	--	--	Y	--	--
Google Plus	Y	Y	Y	Y	Y	Y
T-tumblr.	--	--	--	Y	--	--
Instagram	Y	--	--	--	--	--
Slide-Share	Y	--	--	--	--	--
Pinterest	--	--	--	--	--	--
Live Bookmark	--	--	--	Y	--	--
Add Line Friends	--	--	--	--	--	--
Thailand Hospitals	**BNH**	**BmIH**	**BIH**	**SSH**	**BCH**	**TIDC**
Website	Y	Y	Y	Y	Y	Y
Virtual tour- Visit	Y	Y	Y	Y	Y	Y
Live chat	Y	Y	Y	Y	Y	Y
LinkedIn	Y	Y	Y	Y	Y	Y
YouTube Testimonials	Y	Y	Y	Y	Y	Y
YouTube Health Info	Y	Y	Y	Y	Y	Y
On-Twitter	Y	Y	Y	Y	Y	Y
Photo/video Sharing	Y	Y	Y	Y	Y	Y
Blogs	Y	Y	Y	Y	Y	Y
Discussion Forum	Y	Y	Y	Y	Y	Y
Health Mobile-App	Y	Y	Y	Y	Y	Y
Face Book	Y	Y	Y	Y	Y	Y
Cloud e-Health	Y	Y	Y	Y	Y	Y
Wikipedia	Y	Y	Y	Y	Y	Y
Phone & E-mail	Y	Y	Y	Y	Y	Y
Flickr	Y	Y	Y	--	Y	Y
Patient Testimonials	Y	Y	Y	Y	Y	Y
WEBINAR- Hospital Channel	Y	Y	Y	Y	Y	Y
Goole Plus	Y	Y	Y	Y	Y	Y
T-tumblr.	--	Y	--	--	--	--
Instagram	Y	Y	Y	Y	Y	Y
Slide-Share	Y	Y	Y	Y	Y	Y
Pinterest	--	--	--	--	--	--
Live Bookmark	Y	Y	Y	Y	Y	Y
Add Line Friends	--	Y	--	--	--	--
Singapore Hospitals	**MEH**	**GH**	**PEH**	**NHC**	**RH**	**JHSIM**
Website	Y	Y	Y	Y	Y	Y
Virtual tour- Visit	Y	Y	Y	Y	Y	Y

continued on following page

Table 4. Continued

Live chat	Y	Y	Y	Y	Y	Y
LinkedIn	Y	Y	Y	Y	Y	Y
YouTube Testimonials	Y	Y	Y	Y	Y	Y
YouTube Health Info	Y	Y	Y	Y	Y	Y
On-Twitter	Y	Y	Y	Y	Y	Y
Photo/Video Sharing	Y	Y	Y	Y	Y	Y
Blogs	Y	Y	Y	Y	Y	Y
Discussion Forum	Y	Y	Y	Y	Y	Y
Health Mobile-App	Y	Y	Y	Y	Y	Y
Face Book	Y	Y	Y	Y	Y	Y
Cloud e-Health	Y	Y	Y	Y	Y	Y
Wikipedia	Y	Y	Y	Y	Y	Y
Phone & E-mail	Y	Y	Y	Y	Y	Y
Flickr	Y	Y	Y	Y	Y	Y
Patient Testimonials	Y	Y	Y	Y	Y	Y
Webinar- Hospital Channel	Y	Y	Y	Y	Y	Y
Goole Plus	Y	Y	Y	Y	Y	Y
T-tumblr	--	--	--	--	--	Y
Instagram	Y	Y	Y	Y	Y	Y
Slide-Share	Y	Y	Y	Y	Y	Y
Pinterest	Y	Y	Y	Y	Y	Y
Live Bookmark	Y	Y	Y	Y	Y	Y
Add Line Friends	--	--	--	--	--	Y

Source: Developed for this paper (Y-Yes, -- No)

Various branded super-speciality hospitals in countries of Asia, are popular amongst foreign tourist. Such as Bumrungrad International and Bangkok Hospital, Asian Heart, Indian Apollo Group, Fortis, Wockhardt, and Raffles Singapore. Most of them are adopting and using digital health and social media tools like LinkedIn, Blogs, Flicker, Facebook, YouTube patient testimonials, virtual photo sharing, to market and disseminate their healthcare service information to potential global patients (Crooks et al., 2011; Medhekar, 2017). Besides, health related communication, patients also share information on tourism, hotel, and their positive and negative experiences or satisfaction and dissatisfaction to inform potential health tourists and provide valuable feedback about cost, waiting-time, and pre-post-surgery care. Usually this content is generated by the users such as hospitals, patients, their families and friends, medical travel agencies, online communities of patients, medical professionals, and other hospitals as competitors in global health tourism industry (Miller & Tucker, 2013).

Following the literature review and the exploratory findings, the following hypothesised Figure 1 model is proposed for future research for digital health innovation adoption by MTm healthcare providers and MTs /patients.

H-1: Digital health innovation will positively improve *digital literacy*.

H-2: Digital health innovation will positively improve medical tourism hospital/healthcare providers *efficiency and outcomes.*

H-3: Digital health innovation will positively improve *communication* between the healthcare providers and MTs/patients' needs and experience.

H-4: Digital health innovation will positively improve *information trust and transparency* between hospital/healthcare providers and MTs/patients.

Figure 1. Hypothesized model for digital health innovation adoption
Source: Proposed conceptual hypothesized model

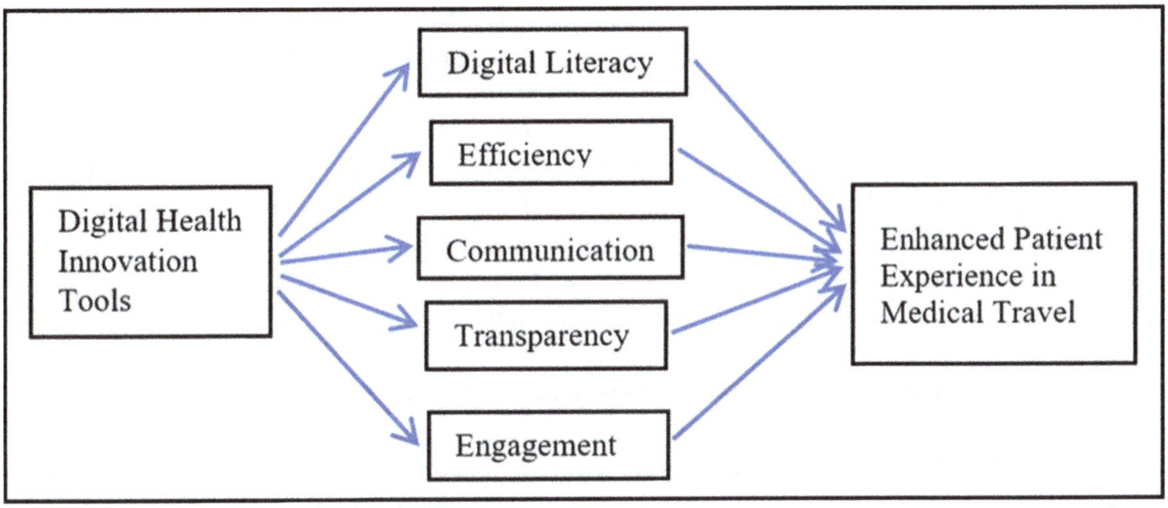

H-5: Digital health innovation will positively improve *engagement* by MTs/patients to make informed decision to travel abroad for surgery.
H-6: Digital health innovation will positively enhance MTs/patients *experience in medical travel/tourism.*

A qualitative cross-sectional study by Moghavvemi et al. (2016) of 51 private hospitals websites promoting medical-tourism in India, Malaysia and Thailand were studied with policy recommendations to improve hospitals online presence and activity. They found differences between the three countries hospital websites that were analysed based on five dimensions: hospital information and facilities, hospital admission and medical services, online interactive services, external activities and technical items related to website functionality. Griffis et al. (2014) cross sectional review of USA hospital related user activity of social media platforms in hospitals varied with 94.41% Facebook page likes, 50.82% having Twitter follower accounts, 99.14% with Yelp reviews, and all hospitals 99.41% having Four-square check-in, concludes that the adoption and utilisation of social media and digital health across US-hospitals varied based on hospital characteristics.

Furthermore, recent empirical study by John et al. (2018) on the application of social media in promoting MTm hospitals, examined using social medial monitoring framework, as how 41 hospitals in Thailand disseminate information, engage with online users on Facebook and Twitter in particular, for marketing MTm, and influence the potential MTs decision to travel abroad for medical treatment. This study used 41 items to measure six key dimensions for Facebook and Twitter/social media tools applying content analysis for online users: involvement, interaction, intimacy, consumer insight, influence and impacts over social media. The results concluded that marketer collected more information regarding user feedback, patient/consumer experience and insight from Facebook users than Twitter, and no significant difference was found in other dimensions, due to lack of engagement and effort to collect customer feedback from healthcare providers' side. Wellness resorts, hospitals, medical travel facilitators and hotels catering to MTs stay are using digital health and various social media network tools for promoting healthcare service, surgical-super-specialities, to potential patients, as well as to know about patient's experiences and testimonials of their MTm healthcare services.

BENEFITS OF DIGITAL HEALTH INNOVATION TO MEDICAL-TOURISM

According to Placidway (2019) there are many benefits to the MTm healthcare provider/hospital as well as to the MTs from adopting patient-centric digital health technologies in MTm, due to increased two-way engagement, communication, digital transparency resulting in positive healthcare outcome. Further, Vas Narasimhan, CEO of Novartis comments "We are on the verge of a digital revolution across every aspect of the healthcare sector, from the lab bench to the patient's bedside" (Sandoz, 2019). According to McKinsey & Company (2013) report, digital health big data analytics uses AI, and improves access to healthcare, predicts and reduces surgery waiting-time, by providing patient-centric personalised treatment, including digital devices which empower the patients taking preventative actions, through reminders to take medicine, exercise, and monitor their own health conditions and save life.

Benefits to Medical-Tourism Healthcare Providers and Medical-Tourists

- **Increased Market Share and Global Presence:** With increased global demand for medical travel/tourism, adopting digital health tools, increases global market share of the MTm hospitals and medical-tour facilitators. Hospitals engaged in treating foreign patients market their healthcare facility and super-speciality of treatment along with JCI accreditation logo, 360-degree virtual video, online skype consultancy, credible and honest patients' testimonial videos, establishing online patient Q&A discussion platform and hospital branding such as Apollo Hospital group in India and Bumrungrad in Thailand and Raffles in Singapore;
- **Improved Access to Healthcare:** Digital health technologies, uses AI, and improves access to healthcare, predicts and reduces waiting time and customising personalised diagnostic tests, treatment, surgery and post-surgery care with positive healthcare outcomes;
- **Patient-centric Treatment:** Medical-tourism hospitals and medical-tour facilitators provide patient-centric information packages, regarding different types of treatment such as dental, bariatric, eye surgery, hip and knee replacement, and reproductive treatment, which covers the overall budget related to the cost of travel, accommodation, treatment, diagnostic tests, personal attendant, including privacy and safety of patient, medical history and diagnostic reports, post-surgery care and other related requirements such as tourism and travel cost of accompanying family member/companion;
- **Reduced Costs:** Operational cost efficiency of the hospital is improved due to online presence, reaching wider domestic and global consumers as MTs/ patients;
- **Digital Literacy:** Innovative digital e-health tools, drives digital literacy among the consumers to use computer, tablets and mobile phone based digital health applications;
- **Patient Education:** Hospitals benefit by providing online information for patient education regarding various treatments, surgery, pre and post-surgery care, health benefits and costs;
- **Hospital Brand Awareness:** Medical-tourism hospitals such as Apollo, Wockhardt, Asian Heart, Raffles, John Hopkins Singapore, Bumrungrad and Bangkok Hospitals are well known global MTm branded hospitals due to their gold class JCI accredited quality, state-of-the-art medical facilities, reputed surgeons, and adopting extensive digital health tools to market, create and distribute health related content, patient testimonials regarding healthcare/MT experience and communicate with global patients;

- **Convenience of Online Health Consulting and Shopping:** Global patients experience the convenience of exploring the hospital websites for availability of medical treatment, hospital, specialist surgeon, cost comparisons, accreditation, and online appointment and consultation via e-mail, skype, Facebook or WhatsApp; before planning to travel abroad for surgery to a super-speciality hospital and a destination of choice;
- **Transparency in Medical Treatment and Travel Processes:** Potential medical-tourists can ensure transparency in communication related to costs of treatment, hospitals accreditation, medical professionals ethics and honesty, surgery waiting time, surgeon's reputation and expertise, treatment plan, surgical outcomes, patient safety, privacy, confidentiality and security related to patient medical history, health data and diagnostic results, date of surgery, diagnostic facilities, and quality of post-surgery care and rehabilitation facility via online consultancy, quotation management tool, surgery appointment and password protected diagnostic reports drop-box pre and post travel;
- **Credibility and Ethical Medical Practice:** Global patients are looking for honesty, medical ethics and credibility in medical practice, hospital employees, cost of surgery, out-of-pocket costs, medical professionals' expertise, success rate for surgery, patient feedback, personalised treatment plan, diagnostic results, pre and post-surgery care and patient satisfaction;
- **Transparency and Trust:** Improves transparency of information, communication and trust between the healthcare providers and the MTs/patients;
- **Establish Long Term Trusting Relationship and Repeat Visits:** Adopting digital e-health technologies makes communication in real time possible, marketing reputed medical hospitals brand to attract foreign patients, increases transparency regarding cost of surgery, accredited quality and patient safety, design patient-centric treatment solutions and provide positive medical-tourism experience to medical travellers, thereby attracting first time medical-tourists and increasing repeat visits, loyalty, and global market share.

SOLUTIONS AND RECOMMENDATIONS

Due to globalisation and privatisation of healthcare travelling to developing countries for medical reasons/ surgery is on the rise. The business of medical travel/tourism involved two sectors of the economy – medical and tourism (Bookman & Bookman, 2007; Medhekar at al., 2019). Internet has revolutionised as to how international consumers as patients/MTs choose MTm hospitals and MTm facilitators and host-country of treatment based on internet advertising, JCI-accreditation, and reviews by actual MTs online. Wellness resorts, private hospitals and medical-tourism facilitators use digital e-health technology for promoting healthcare services directly to patients, and increase market share, profitability, and visibility on the internet and communication transparency to positively enhance health efficiency and patient experience (John, Larke & Kilgour, 2018; Moghavvemi et al., 2016).

Health travel/tourism industry uses innovative digital e-health tools to communicate with domestic and overseas patients/MTs in a competitive global healthcare environment. Potential health travellers use various digital e-health tools to communicate, search, consult, produce, disseminate and share reliable information regarding health and medical travel experience. Potential patients/MTs search for information through various internet based digital health tools before and during medical travel decision-making process, and generate content after medical treatment, about their healthcare experience, and upload testimonials on hospital and medical-tour agency's social-media platforms (John et al., 2018; Medhekar,

2017). In applying the social exchange theory, it is evident that patients as potential health tourists, explore the digital health related platforms to gather information posted by hospitals, health professionals medical travel facilitators and actual medical-tourists regarding surgery waiting time, availability of surgery, hospital accreditation and acquire knowledge to make comparison between home and host-country's healthcare costs and from medical-tourism abroad.

A systematic review by Moorhead, Hazlett and Harrison (2013) over the 2002-2012 period, on use of digital technologies in healthcare such as YouTube, Facebook, Blogs, LinkedIn and Twitter, by hospitals in healthcare communication with the patients, noted numerous benefits, if used in a responsible manner by the hospital, health professionals, and patients. The benefits related to (i) availability and access to health information, (ii) user created shared information on a health topic, (iii) interaction with public, patients and physicians, (iv) patient to patient social and emotional support, (v) monitoring public health on target communities, and (vi) influence health policy and outcomes. The limitations relate to, patients' confidentiality, privacy, data security, information quality, reliability, and credibility posted by the users (Moorhead et al., 2013). The following policy implications for digital e-health innovation and adoption by MTm sector are summarised:

1. **Digital Literacy:** Digital literacy should be encouraged, to use various internet-based tablet and mobile applications related to internet search for hospitals, surgery cost, consulting online with medical doctor, uploading diagnostic reports, registering on health records, posting patient medical travel testimonials on digital e-health applications for efficiency in positive healthcare outcomes;
2. **Professional communication:** Hospitals and patients create and share MTs experience regarding medical treatment overseas via various digital health and social media tools. Hospitals and medical staff are using digital health tools for professional communication and promotion of their MTm business. Professionalism should be maintained at all levels, when communicating and contributing to health-related trustworthy content on digital health, to ensure efficiency and transparency in global healthcare service delivery;
3. **Patient data privacy must be ensured:** Patients/MTs connect in a virtual social setting, receive and give feedback to the hospital and potential MTs as patients. Digital health tools, help the actual MTs to express their experiences about medical travel journey, seeking emotional support for treatment as cancer, or knee replacement on online support communities (Bender et al., 2011) likes and dislikes related to MT hospital and host-country of treatment, specialist surgeon, pre and post-surgery nursing care, and overall enhance their MT experience;
4. **Research incentive for innovative digital health applications must be promoted by the government:** Digital tools help the global MTs to make informed choices using the UGC on social media adopted and used by the hospitals for attracting and communicating health information to the potential and actual MTs and assisting in enhancing their medical-tourism decision-making process and MTs experience;
5. **Digital health, medical legal, ethical issues:** It is essential that medical-tourism service providers such as hospitals, medical travel agencies hotels, ambulance services, airports, pharmacies and policy makers understand the advantage of innovating and adopting digital health technologies the supply-side medical-tourism stakeholders and the demand-side potential and actual MTs/patients. Hospital's digital health platform should be monitored by the hospital's medical web-master, considering accreditation, medical legal and ethical practices, credible, trustworthy, and transparent information is communicated to the MTs/patient.

FUTURE RESEARCH DIRECTIONS

Future research could collect qualitative and quantitative data to explore how adoption of digital health tools and technologies have and could enhance healthcare providers efficiency as well as medical-tourists experience. Whether, seeing a doctor face-to-face verses consulting online by using digital health tools makes MTs/patient enhances their health experience of medical treatment aboard and feel empowered in healthcare decision-making process. Furthermore, hypothysed relationship as shown in Figure 1, regarding adoption of digital health innovation tools can be studied quantitatively, and items developed to operationalise these constructs.

CONCLUSION

This paper explores the use of digital e-health technological innovations in enhancing patient/MTs experience. Innovative digital health tools are used to promote MTm related services to potential global medical-tourists which intensifies competitions and increase market share for hospitals treating foreign patients. Digital e-health technologies such as social media tools help to understand how individuals communicate with one another, how they form relationships and how communities are formed based on the exchange of health communication between actual and potential MTs and healthcare providers in terms of health information search, share, create content, compare treatment cost, provide feedback and organise information related to medical experience and post-surgery care. Healthcare related digital technologies are changing rapidly and news innovative applications and tools on tablets and smart phone mobile apps are developed and adopted by healthcare providers to market their healthcare services and produce user-generated content to communicate transparently in a professional manner and enhance patient experience and healthcare outcomes. There are many opportunities for medical-tourism hospital and medical-tour facilitators to use innovative digital health tools to promote their services globally to attract foreign patients to their hospital and host-country for medical treatment. However, there are also concerns related to digital health literacy, medical legal and ethical practises related to posting credible and trustworthy information by the healthcare providers, medical-tourism facilitators and the patients.

REFERENCES

Adam, K., Snyder, J., Crooks, V. A., & Johnston, R. (2015). Tourism discourse and medical tourists' motivations to travel. *Tourism Review*, *70*(2), 85–96. doi:10.1108/TR-04-2014-0015

Agag, G. M., & El-Masry, A. A. (2017). Why do consumers trust online travel websites? Drivers and outcomes of consumers trust towards online travel websites. *Journal of Travel Research*, *56*(3), 347–36. doi:10.1177/0047287516643185

Antheunis, M. L., Tates, K., & Nieboer, T. E. (2013). Patients' and health professionals' use of social media in healthcare: Motives, barriers and expectations. *Patient Education and Counseling*, *92*(3), 426–431. doi:10.1016/j.pec.2013.06.020 PMID:23899831

Bender, J. L., Jimenez-Marroquin, M., & Jadad, A. R. (2011). Seeking support on Facebook: A content analysis of breast-cancer group. *Journal of Medical Internet Research, 13*(1), e16. doi:10.2196/jmir.1560 PMID:21371990

Blau, P. M. (1964). *Exchange and Power in Social Life*. New York: John Wiley.

Bookman, M. Z., & Bookman, K. R. (2007). *Medical-tourism in Developing Countries*. New York: Palgrave Macmillan. doi:10.1057/9780230605657

Buhalis, D., & Law, R. (2008). Progress in information technology and tourism management: 20 years on and 10 years after the Internet-the state of eTourism research. *Tourism Management, 29*(4), 609–623. doi:10.1016/j.tourman.2008.01.005

Burns, R. L. (2015). Medical-tourism opportunities and challenges: Illustration from US-India trade. *International Journal of Healthcare Management, 8*(1), 15–26. doi:10.1179/2047971914Y.0000000091

Chanda, R. (2002). Trade in Health Services. *Bulletin of the World Health Organization, 80*(2), 158–163. PMID:11953795

Chretien, K. C., Azar, J., & Kind, T. (2011). Physicians on Twitter. *Journal of the American Medical Association, 305*(6), 566–568. doi:10.1001/jama.2011.68 PMID:21304081

Chung, N., & Koo, C. (2015). The use of social media in travel information search. *Telematics and Informatics, 32*(2), 215–229. doi:10.1016/j.tele.2014.08.005

Collins, A., Medhekar, A., Wong, H. Y., & Cobanoglu, C. (2019). Factors influencing outbound medical travel from the USA. *Tourism Review, 74*(3), 463–479. doi:10.1108/TR-06-2018-0083

Connell, J. (2015). From medical-tourism to transnational healthcare? An epilogue for the future. *Social Science & Medicine, 124*, 398–401. doi:10.1016/j.socscimed.2014.11.015 PMID:25467883

Cormany, D., & Baloglu, S. (2011). Medical travel facilitator websites: An exploratory study of web page contents and services offered to the prospective medical-tourist. *Tourism Management, 32*(4), 709–716. doi:10.1016/j.tourman.2010.02.008

Creswell, J. W. (2014). *Research Design: Qualitative, Quantitative, and Mixed Methods Approaches* (4th ed.). Thousand Oaks, CA: SAGE Publications.

Crooks, V. A., Turner, L., Snyder, J., Johnston, R., & Kingsbury, P. (2011). Promoting medical-tourism in India: Messages, images, and the marketing of international patient travel. *Social Science & Medicine, 72*(5), 726–732. doi:10.1016/j.socscimed.2010.12.022 PMID:21310519

Deloitte. (2010). *How digital technologies is transforming health and social care*. Available from https://www2.deloitte.com/content/dam/Deloitte/uk/Documents/life-sciences-health-care/deloitte-uk-connected-health.pdf

Emerson, R. M. (1976). Social exchange theory. *Annual Review of Sociology, 2*(0), 335–362. doi:10.1146/annurev.so.02.080176.002003

Eysenbach, G. (2008). Medicine 2.0. Social networking, collaboration, participation, apomediation, and openness. *Journal of Medical Internet Research, 10*(3), e22. doi:10.2196/jmir.1030 PMID:18725354

Fisher, J., & Clayton, M. (2012, 2Q). Who gives a tweet: assessing patients' interest in the use of social media for healthcare. *World Views on Evidence-Based Nursing,* 100-108.

George, B. P., & Henthorne, T. L. (2009). The incorporation of telemedicine with medical-tourism: A study of consequences. *Journal of Hospitality Marketing & Management, 18*(5), 512–522. doi:10.1080/19368620902950097

Griffis, H. M., Kilaru, A. S., Kilaru, A. S., Werner, R., Asch, D. A., Hershey, J. C., & ... . (2014). Use of Social Media across US Hospitals: Descriptive Analysis of Adoption and Utilization. *Journal of Medical Internet Research, 16*(11), e264. doi:10.2196/jmir.3758 PMID:25431831

Han, H., & Hwang, J. (2018). Growing competition in the healthcare tourism market and customer retention in medical clinics: New and experienced travellers. *Current Issues in Tourism, 21*(6), 680–702. doi:10.1080/13683500.2015.1104292

Hawn, C. (2009). Take two aspirins and tweet me in the morning: How Twitter, Facebook and other social media are reshaping healthcare. *Health Affairs, 28*(2), 361–368. doi:10.1377/hlthaff.28.2.361 PMID:19275991

John, S., Larke, R., & Kilgour, M. (2018). Applications of social media for medical-tourism marketing: An empirical analysis. *Anatolia, 13*(2), 1–13. doi:10.1080/13032917.2018.1473261

Joseph, T. (2019). *Digital Tools for the Future of Healthcare Providers.* Available from https://www.fingent.com/blog/digital-tools-for-the-future-of-healthcare-providers

Khan, M. J., Chelliah, S., & Haron, M. S. (2016). International patients; Travel decision-making process-A conceptual framework. *Iranian Journal of Public Health, 45*(2), 134–145. PMID:27114978

Kim, K., & Kwon, N. (2010). Profile of e-patients: Analysis of their cancer information-seeking from a national survey. *Journal of Health Communication, 15*(7), 712–733. doi:10.1080/10810730.2010.514031 PMID:21104502

Korda, H., & Itani, Z. (2013). Harnessing social media for health pormotion and behaviour change. *Health Promotion Practice, 14*(1), 15–23. doi:10.1177/1524839911405850 PMID:21558472

Lopez, A., Detz, A., Ratanawongsa, N., & Sarkar, U. (2012). What patients say about their doctors online: A qualitative content analysis? *Journal of General Internal Medicine, 27*(6), 685–692. doi:10.100711606-011-1958-4 PMID:22215270

Lunt, N., & Carrera, P. (2010). Medical-tourism: Assessing the evidence on treatment abroad. *Maturitas, 66*(1), 27–32. doi:10.1016/j.maturitas.2010.01.017 PMID:20185254

Lunt, N., & Carrera, P. (2011). Systematic review of web sites for prospective medical tourists. *Tourism Review, 66*(1/2), 57–67. doi:10.1108/16605371111127224

Lunt, N., Hardey, M., & Mannion, R. (2010). Nip, tuck and click- Medical-tourism and the emergence of web-based health information. *The Open Medical Informatics Journal, 4*(1), 1–11. doi:10.2174/1874431101004010001 PMID:20517465

Lunt, N., Horsfall, D., & Hanefeld, J. (2016). MTm: A snapshot of evidence on treatment abroad. *Maturitas*, *88*, 37–44. doi:10.1016/j.maturitas.2016.03.001 PMID:27105695

Lupton, D. (2014). The Commodification of patient opinion: The digital patient experience economy in the age of big data. *Sociology of Health & Illness*, *36*(6), 856–869. doi:10.1111/1467-9566.12109 PMID:24443847

Mahuire, A., Bussmann, S., Kocker, C., Verra, S., Giurgi, L. A., & Ruggeri, K. (2016). Raising concerns about the information provided on medical travel agency websites: A place for policy. *Health Policy and Technology*, *5*(4), 414–422. doi:10.1016/j.hlpt.2016.07.001

Majeed, S., & Lu, C. (2017). *Changing Preferences, Moving Places and Third-Party Administrators: A Scoping Review ofMedical-tourism Trends (1990-2016)*. Almatourism. doi:10.6092/issn.2036-5195/6675

Mason, A., & Wright, K. (2011). Framing medical-tourism: An examination of appeal, risk, convalescence, accreditation, and interactivity in medical-tourism websites. *Journal of Health Communication*, *16*(2), 163–177. doi:10.1080/10810730.2010.535105 PMID:21161812

McKinsey & Company. (2013). *The big-data revolution in US healthcare: Accelerating value and innovation*. Available from https://www.mckinsey.com/industries/healthcare-systems-and-services/our-insights/the-big-data-revolution-in-us-health-care

Medhekar, A. (2014). Government policy initiatives for developing sustainable medical-tourism industry. *Journal on Business Review*, *3*(3), 95–105.

Medhekar, A. (2017). The Role of Social Media for Knowledge Dissemination in Medical-tourism - A Case of India. In R. Chugh (Ed.), *Harnessing Social Media as a Knowledge Management Tool* (pp. 25–54). IGI Global. doi:10.4018/978-1-5225-0495-5.ch002

Medhekar, A., & Newby, L. (2012). Information Search for Medical Treatment Abroad. *Journal of Applied Global Research*, *5*(13), 53–72.

Medhekar, A., Wong, H. Y., & Hall, J. (2014). Medical-tourism: A Conceptual Framework for an Innovation in Global Healthcare Provision. In A. Goyal (Ed.), *Innovations in Services Marketing and Management: Strategies for Emerging Economies* (pp. 148–169). IGI Global. doi:10.4018/978-1-4666-4671-1.ch009

Medhekar, A., Wong, H. Y., & Hall, J. E. (2019). Factors influencing inbound medical travel to India. *Journal of Health Organization and Management*, *33*(2), 155–172. doi:10.1108/JHOM-08-2018-0234 PMID:30950309

Medhekar, A., Wong, H.Y., & Hall, J.E. (2020). Healthcare Providers Perspective on Value in Medical Travel to India. *Tourism Review*. (forthcoming) DOI 10.1108/TR-06-2019-0276

Miller, A. R., & Tucker, C. (2013). Active social media management: The case of healthcare. *Information Systems Research*, *24*(1), 52–70. doi:10.1287/isre.1120.0466

Moghavvemi, S., Ormond, M., Musa, G., Mohamed-Isa, C. R., & Chandy, J. C. (2017). Connecting with prospective medical-tourists online: A cross-sectional analysis of private hospital websites promoting medical-tourism in India, Malaysia and Thailand. *Tourism Management*, *58*(Feb), 154–163. doi:10.1016/j.tourman.2016.10.010

Moorhead, S. A., Hazlett, D. E., Harrison, L., Carroll, J. K., Irwin, A., & Hoving, C. (2013). A New Dimension of Healthcare: Systematic Review of the Uses, Benefits, and Limitations of Social Media for Health Communication. *Journal of Medical Internet Research, 15*(4), e85–e101. doi:10.2196/jmir.1933 PMID:23615206

Narangajavana, Y., Fiol, C. L. J., Tena, M. A., Artola, R.-M., & Sánchez-García, J. (2017). The influence of social media in creating expectations. An empirical study for a tourist destination. *Annals of Tourism Research, 65*(1), 60–70. doi:10.1016/j.annals.2017.05.002

NaRanong, A., & NaRanong, V. (2011). The effects of medical-tourism: Thailand's experience. *Bulletin of the World Health Organization, 89*(5), 336–344. doi:10.2471/BLT.09.072249 PMID:21556301

Parra-López, E., Bulchand-Gidumal, J., Gutiérrez-Taño, D., & Díaz-Armas, R. (2011). Intentions to use social media in organizing and taking vacation trips. *Computers in Human Behavior, 27*(2), 640–654. doi:10.1016/j.chb.2010.05.022

Placidway. (2019). *The Power of digital health in medical-tourism*. Available from http://www.placid-solutions.com/infographics-power-digital-health-medical-tourism/

Pocock, N. S., & Phua, K. H. (2011). Medical-tourism and policy implications for health systems: A conceptual framework from a comparative study of Thailand, Singapore and Malaysia. *Globalization and Health, 7*(1), 12. doi:10.1186/1744-8603-7-12 PMID:21539751

Sandoz. (2019). *How digital tools are improving access to healthcare*. Available from https://www.sandoz.com/stories/access-healthcare/how-digital-tools-are-improving-access-healthcare

Shaw, J., Agarwal, P., Desveaux, L., Palma, D. C., Stamenova, V., Jamieson, T., ... Bhattacharya, O. (2018). Beyond "Implementation": Digital health innovation and service design. *Digital Media, 48*(1), 1–5. doi:10.103841746-018-0059-8 PMID:31304327

Speier, A. R. (2011). Brokers, consumers and the Internet: How North American consumers navigate their infertility journeys. *Reproductive Biomedicine Online, 23*(5), 592–599. doi:10.1016/j.rbmo.2011.07.005 PMID:21955489

Thackeray, R., Neiger, B. L., Hanson, C. L., & Mckenzie, J. F. (2008). Enhancing Promotional Strategies within Social Marketing Programs: Use of Web 2.0 Social Media. *Health Promotion Practice, 9*(4), 338–343. doi:10.1177/1524839908325335 PMID:18936268

Timian, A., Rupcic, S., Kachnowski, S., & Luisi, P. (2013). Do patients "like" good care? Measuring hospital quality via Facebook. *American Journal of Medical Quality, 28*(5), 374–382. doi:10.1177/1062860612474839 PMID:23378059

Turner, L. (2010). Medical-tourism and the global market place in health services: US patients, international hospitals and the search for affordable healthcare. *International Journal of Health Services, 40*(3), 443–467. doi:10.2190/HS.40.3.d PMID:20799670

Turner, L. (2011). Canadian medical-tourism companies that have exited the marketplace: Content analysis of websites used to market transnational medical travel. *Globalization and Health, 7*(40), 1–16. doi:10.1186/1744-8603-7-40 PMID:21995598

Van de Belt, T. H., Berben, A. S., Samsom, M., Engelen, L. P., & Schoonhoven, L. (2012). Use of Social Media by Western European Hospitals: Longitudinal Study. *Journal of Medical Internet Research*, *14*(3), e61–e71. doi:10.2196/jmir.1992 PMID:22549016

Xiang, Z., & Gretzel, U. (2010). Role of social media in online travel information search. *Tourism Management*, *31*(2), 179–188. doi:10.1016/j.tourman.2009.02.016

Yazdanpanah, A., Parsaei, A., & Jeihooni, A. K. (2018). The role of digital marketing in medical-tourism industry in point of view of medical-tourism policy makers of Shiraz in 2017. *Universal Journal of Pharmaceutical Research*, *3*(1), 1–6. doi:10.22270/ujpr.v3i2.128

ADDITIONAL READING

Abubakar, M., & Ilkan, M. (2016). Impact of online WOM on destination trust and intention to travel: A medical-tourism perspective. *Journal of Destination Marketing & Management*, *5*(3), 192–201. doi:10.1016/j.jdmm.2015.12.005

Benyon, D., Quigley, A., O'Keefe, B., & Riva, G. (2014). Presence and digital tourism. *AI & Society*, *29*(4), 521–529. doi:10.100700146-013-0493-8

Cillers, L., Viljoen, K. L.-A., & Chinyamurindi, W. T. (2018). A study on students' acceptance of mobile phone use to seek health information in South Africa. *The HIM Journal*, *47*(2), 59–69. doi:10.1177/1833358317706185 PMID:28537211

Flott, K., Callahan, R., Darzi, A., & Mayer, E. (2016). A Patient-Centered framework for evaluating digital maturity of health services: A systematic review. *Journal of Medical Internet Search*, 18(4), e75, 1-10.

Lupton, D. (2013). The digitally engaged patient: Self- monitoring and selfcare in the digital health era. *Social Theory & Health*, *11*(3), 256–270. doi:10.1057th.2013.10

Morahan-Martin, J. M. (2004). How Internet Users Find, Evaluate, and Use Online Health Information: A Cross-Cultural Review. *Cyberpsychology & Behavior*, *7*(5), 497–510. doi:10.1089/cpb.2004.7.497 PMID:15667044

O'Connor, S., Hanlon, P., O'Donnell, C. A., Garcia, S., Glanville, J., & Mair, F. S. (2016). Understanding factors affecting patient and public engagement and recruitment to digital health interventions: A systematic review of qualitative studies. *Medical Informatics and Decision Making*, *16*(120), 5–15. doi:10.118612911-016-0359-3 PMID:27630020

Otte-Trojel, T., De Bont, A., Rundall, T. G., & van de Klundert, J. (2016). What do we know about developing patient portals? a systematic literature review. *Journal of the American Medical Informatics Association*, *23*(e1), e162–e168. doi:10.1093/jamia/ocv114 PMID:26335985

Smith, B., & Magnani, J. W. (2019). New technologies, new disparities: The intersection of electronic health and digital health literacy. *International Journal of Cardiology*, *292*, 280–282. doi:10.1016/j.ijcard.2019.05.066 PMID:31171391

Sobo, E. J., Herlihy, E., & Bicker, M. (2011). Selling medical travel to US patient-consumers: The cultural appeal of website marketing messages. *Anthropology & Medicine*, *1*(1), 119–136. doi:10.1080/13648470.2010.525877 PMID:21563007

Wagle, S. (2013). Web-based medical facilitators in medical-tourism: The third party in decision-making. *Indian Journal of Medical Ethics*, *10*(1), 28–33. doi:10.20529/IJME.2013.006 PMID:23439194

KEY TERMS AND DEFINITIONS

Digital Health: Digital health also known as e-Health is a system where computer technologies and tele-medicine is used to connect, communicate and manage healthcare information, manage health risk, promote health and wellbeing by the providers/ clinicians and the people/patients. Use of information and communication technologies help to enhance efficient delivery of health information and communication between the physician and the patient and empowers the patient to manage their health and health records.

Digital Health Innovation: Digital health innovation is defined as tools designed to use internet to engage online and reduce healthcare cost, accessible, provide positive healthcare outcomes and enhance patient experience.

Digital Health Literacy: It is defined as the extent to which digital tools are applied and used by the healthcare service providers and the patients to deliver and access affordable quality of healthcare services to the patients. With the diffusions of internet technology, digital/e-Health literacy means peoples knowledge and skills to use innovative internet and communication technologies and devices such as laptop, tablet, and mobile phone apps to search for health information which is appropriate for health decision making process and communicate effectively with the doctor.

Health Information Sources: Medical-tourists gather internal and external information from various sources, before they decide to travel abroad for surgery: for example- friends and family, brochures, television, health insurance, e-health platforms, social media, YouTube, and internet websites of government, medical-tour facilitators, medical-tourism hospitals and international accreditation bodies to make an informed decision and enhance their overseas medical travel experience.

Medical-Tourism: Health-tourism and two branches. Medical-tourism and Wellness tourism. It is a phenomenon where a patient travels domestic/overseas, with/without a companion, for medical treatment. Medical treatment/surgery could be invasive and involve complex surgical procedures with the use of highly specialized medical technology and skilled surgeons, for the improvement of health and quality of life. MTs may combine it with a vacation if health permits at an exotic destination, pre or post-surgery for recuperation.

Medical-Tourist: Medical-tourists is a patient who buys a medical product or healthcare services online using digital technologies. Medical-tourist travels within a country or overseas, for the purposes of receiving medical treatment/surgery if it is not available and affordable in their place or country of residence. Medical-tourists may also engage in some tourism related activity if health permits.

Chapter 3
An Affordance Perspective on the Enabling and Disruptive Effects of Social Media Tools on Self-Management of Chronic Illness

Nwakego Isika
https://orcid.org/0000-0003-1601-2930
The University of Melbourne, Australia

Antonette Mendoza
https://orcid.org/0000-0002-6903-1169
The University of Melbourne, Australia

Rachelle Bosua
https://orcid.org/0000-0003-0218-3018
Open University of the Netherlands, The Netherlands

ABSTRACT

This chapter examines the appropriation of social media tools by chronically ill adults to better understand and manage their illness using an affordance perspective. Despite the continued attention that information systems scholars have directed to studies on affordances and social media, there seems to be limited discussion on the negative, disruptive effects that social media could have on accomplishment of illness management goals. Accordingly, the authors argue that social media affordances could have both positive, enabling effects on illness management outcomes or negative, disruptive effects.

DOI: 10.4018/978-1-7998-3274-4.ch003

INTRODUCTION

Social media technologies have had a considerable impact on society acting as platforms for activism; support for new business models and, to organize people around common causes such as health (McKenna et al. 2017; Rozenblum and Bates 2013; Urquhart and Vaast 2012). Accordingly, today a growing number of chronically ill adults make use of social media technologies to better understand and manage their illness. Digital technologies such as social media and other technological innovations could assist the healthcare sector by empowering people to take control of their illnesses. It is suggested that the use of digital tools such as social media may lead to decreased costs and administrative effort for care delivery, increasing practice efficiency and supporting patient self-management (Agarwal et al. 2010).

It appears that prior studies conducted on social media use for health are focused on motivation mechanisms, i.e. influences on health-related outcomes in these settings and have overlooked the processes of appropriation of Social Media Tools (SMT) within the public context to manage one's health and wellbeing (Agarwal et al. 2010; Fichman et al. 2011; Merolli et al. 2013). To this effect, there has been limited empirical investigation into how SMTs are utilized by these individuals to better understand and manage their chronic illness. Hence, it is necessary to further explore how social media tools are used to gain a more in-depth insight into potential benefits or drawbacks of these tools in the context of chronic illness self-management.

Affordance theory was proposed in the field of ecological psychology to address the "action possibilities" offered to an animal by its environment (Fayard and Weeks 2014; Gibson 1986). This seminal theory has been adopted in several fields including Information Systems (IS) to understand the relationship between an IT artefact and its users within a specified use context (Anderson and Robey 2017; Orlikowski et al. 2006).

Accordingly, the purpose of this chapter is to examine the affordances of social media which enable or deter illness management for chronically ill adults. Consequently, the guiding research question is: *How do social media technology features enable or disrupt chronic illness management practices of chronically ill adults?*

To address the research question, the authors conducted a multiple case study to analyse enabling and disruptive affordances of four different SMTs having a range of features. This study presented in this chapter forms part of a larger research project that investigates the appropriation of social media tools by adults with chronic illness. The larger study applied a multiple case study with mixed methods and also examines influences and processes of appropriation across the selected SMT tools: Reddit (text-based), Instagram (Photo-based/hybrid), Youtube (video-based/hybrid) and Facebook (hybrid).

The remainder of this chapter proceeds as follows: the next section gives an overview of related studies on the use of social media tools, followed by the chosen research approach, data collection protocol, data analysis and findings. Finally, we wrap up by discussing our findings and drawing theoretical and practical implications.

THEORETICAL BACKGROUND

Social Media Tools (SMTs) are commonly defined as: *"a group of Internet-based technologies that allows users to easily create, edit, evaluate and link to content or other creators of content"* (Kaplan and Haenlein 2010; Kietzmann et al. 2011). Several terms are used in the literature to describe SMTs such as social technologies, social computing, Web 2.0 and others. The term "social media" includes technologies such as blogs, video-sharing sites, micro-blogs, forums, websites, virtual worlds or wikis created to facilitate virtual interaction by users and creation of user-generated content (Kane et al. 2014; Kaplan and Haenlein 2010; Kietzmann et al. 2011). Figure 1 illustrates the different levels of immersion provided by the different categories of social media tools.

Figure 1. Social media tools and technologies categorized by level of interaction/immersion (Adapted from Ngai et al. 2015)

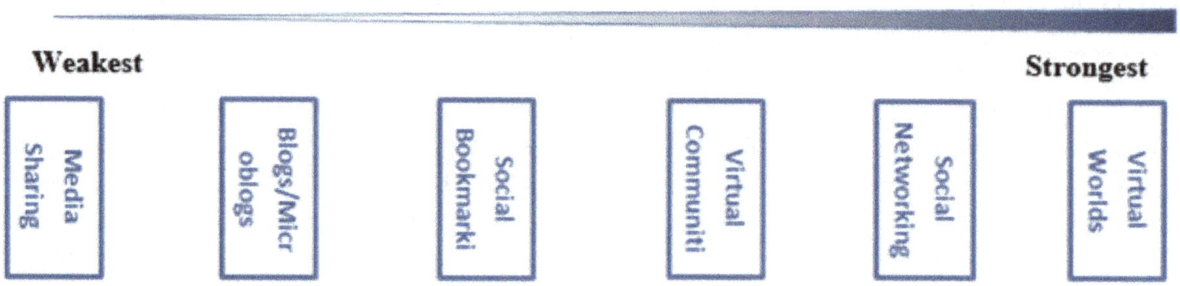

Several characteristics differentiate social media from older technologies: user-generated content, peer-to-peer communication, networking, multimedia-orientation and user-friendliness (Kane et al. 2014; Majchrzak et al. 2013; Panahi et al. 2012). Furthermore, social media systems in the public context are continually evolving around a set of core elements, with emerging features (Alaimo and Kallinikos 2017; Spagnoletti et al. 2015; Yoo 2010). As a result, social support, financial gains, knowledge and innovation are facilitated on a global scale (Agarwal et al. 2008; Choy and Schlagwein 2016; Leong et al. 2016; Orlikowski and Scott 2015; Vaast et al. 2017).

Social Media Use in the Context of Chronic Illness Self-Management

The World Health Organization (WHO) defines chronic illness as an illness that persists for more than three months and could result from infections, injury or emotional distress leading to abnormal mental conditions (Dadgar and Joshi 2018; WHO 2016). Recent studies have highlighted the growing global burden of chronic diseases such as diabetes or cancer due to biological and preventable lifestyle factors such as increased sedentary living and an ageing population (Bodenheimer 2002; Dadgar and Joshi 2018; Georgeff 2014; Ho et al. 2019). Furthermore, a recent report by the World Health Organization (WHO 2016) states that currently 60% of deaths globally are due to chronic disease and these figures are expected to rise to 73% of all deaths regardless of socio-economic class by 2020. In fact, according to that report, the projected increase in chronic illness related to mortality for developing nations is 79% of all deaths (Department of Health & Human Services 2016; WHO 2016).

Several studies have argued that SMTs have a role to play to alleviate some of the challenges involved in managing chronic illness. These challenges include personal repercussions from being chronically ill against the backdrop of struggling healthcare services that are ill-equipped to provide long-term care for individuals with chronic illness. Although scholars in the healthcare sector have been conducting studies into the influences and potential benefits of online community membership, the majority of existing studies have been carried out on the predecessors of social media such as discussion boards, forums and chat rooms (Ho et al. 2019; Merolli et al. 2015; Patel et al. 2015; Samhan et al. 2018). Moreover, healthcare scholars have focused on the mechanisms/personal factors such as emotional support exchanges, and social, supportive exchanges that motivate adoption and use of SMTs by chronically ill adults. As a result, they have overlooked environmental influences from the SMT on adoption and use for chronic illness management. Further, with the notable exception of the study by Chung (2014), the processes of use have been overlooked in these studies. Even so, that study was conducted on an older technology-a discussion board. Because the healthcare sector is better equipped to provide episodic care for chronically ill patients, some scholars argue that SMTs could serve as a valuable source of some aspects involved in self-management of chronic disease (Bernardi 2016; Merolli et al. 2015; Pousti et al. 2014; Wang et al. 2017).

Given the high attrition rates that are ascribed to custom-built health SMTs in the healthcare sector, it is crucial to gain a complete understanding of the technologies that are being appropriated and derive transferable insights to guide the design of illness management SMTs (Dadgar and Joshi 2018).

Social Media Affordances for Chronic Illness Management

According to Gibson (1979), the features (or feature-list) of an object exist/s apart from the people who use them, but those features are infused with meaning *"relative to the posture and behaviour of the animal being considered"* (pp. 127–128). Researchers in the IS field have used the notion of affordances to understand the action possibilities available to users of an IT artefact (Goh et al. 2011; Majchrzak et al. 2013; Majchrzak and Markus 2012; Treem and Leonardi 2012). More recent studies stress the importance of the social environment in influencing users' perception and realization of affordances and scholars suggest that users may perceive the possibilities of actions available in a technology design as either constraining or enabling according to their social norms and beliefs (Bernardi 2016; Vaast et al. 2017). Regarding social media, affordance theory suggests that the features of an SMT could serve as the foundations for affordances based on the action possibilities inherent in the design of such technologies (Faraj and Azad 2012; Karahanna et al. 2018; Vaast et al. 2017).

More recently, scholars have started to examine the affordances of SMTs for chronically ill cohorts. For instance, Merolli et al. (2013; 2015) proposed a set of therapeutic affordances experienced by chronically ill cohorts by applying SMTs to their illness management practices. Among the identified affordances were: narration, self-presentation, identity, flexibility, structure and adaptation (Merolli et al. 2013, 2015). Similarly, Pousti et al. (2013) and Bernardi (2016) examined SMT in the context of chronic illness and collectively found a set of affordances that may influence outcomes and serve to motivate continued engagement with these SMT communities.

With the exception of the study by Pousti et al. (2013) the examined studies on SMT affordances have neglected potential negative affordances, leading to an imbalanced notion that SMT only offers positive, enabling affordances to its users. The study by Pousti applied a sociomaterial perspective that identified four main constraints from SMT appropriation in the chronic illness context which include: emotional discomfort, legal implications, low self-efficacy, poor information quality and social concerns. Yet, that work did not delineate which actors (chronically ill individuals, healthcare providers or the carers in the study) in the SMT context were constrained by the disruptive affordances reported by the study. This distinction is important because affordances are specific to the type of actor who encounters them. Some scholars suggest that affordances should be viewed through a socio-technical lens (Bernardi 2016; Majchrzak et al. 2013; Merolli et al. 2013). A socio-technical view of affordances proposes that they are only partially determined by the features of technology and emerge from the user's task-oriented interactions with an IT artefact (Bernardi 2016). Accordingly, in health-related studies, affordances are conceptualized as potential outcomes from adoption and use of an SMT to manage chronic illness.

Studies on affordances have neglected potential negative affordances, leading to an imbalanced notion that SMT only offers positive, enabling affordances to its users. The one study by Pousti et al (2014) did not delineate the specific constraints that were experienced by chronically ill adults. Accordingly, there is room for further work that examines the enabling and disruptive affordances provided by SMTs to specific groups of users that impact the accomplishment of their specific tasks.

RESEARCH METHODOLOGY

According to Yin (2013), there are three characteristics that should be considered when choosing a research design for a study: (1) The type of research question posed, (2) the extent of control a researcher has over an actual behavioural event and (3) the degree of focus on contemporary events, as opposed to entirely historical events. With these design criteria in mind, this study took an interpretivist perspective to obtain rich insights into the context of social media appropriation by chronically ill adults. Given that the study is driven by 'how' and 'why' type of questions, it was essential to apply a case study methodology to obtain a rich understanding of social media appropriation within the context of chronic illness management. Furthermore, this study used a multiple case study approach to allow for the examination of social media appropriation by chronically ill cohorts within its context - social media tools (Yin 2013). Given that a case study approach is recommended to examine contemporary phenomena and when an issue is not well understood, this approach suits the aim of the study.

The authors applied the framework provided by Ngai et al. (2015) based on Media Richness Theory (MRT), which classified social media tools based on their unique features. Based on this, four social media tools - Facebook, Instagram, YouTube and Reddit were selected as the specific cases for examination in this study (Isika et al. 2016; Ngai et al. 2015; Ngai et al. 2015). Reddit is a text-based SMT, similar in structure to an online bulletin board; YouTube is primarily a video sharing SMT, Instagram is chiefly an image sharing SMT and Facebook a social media site that contains a hybrid of features that include text, images and videos. It is necessary to note that these selected SMTs may also have other features and capabilities; for example, Instagram also allows sharing of short videos called "*stories*" which are available for 24 hours. Moreover, throughout the study, these SMT underwent several updates which expanded their feature-set to include other functionality; for instance, YouTube restricted the messaging feature and added image sharing functionality. Also, these four social media tools are among the most used social media tools globally (Burzler 2018; Fadel 2012; Sareah 2015).

Numerous scholars have argued that social media research in IS could benefit from the application of case studies and similar methods to drive theoretical development about processes and influences facilitated by these tools (McKenna et al. 2017; Urquhart and Vaast 2012). More importantly, the use of a multiple case study will aid in strengthening theoretical development by highlighting the conditions and interrelationships between concepts that are necessary for different appropriation outcomes among these chronically ill cohorts (Miles, Huberman, & Saldaña, 2014). Moreover, through a multiple case study approach, this study can explore unique themes within each case and generalize themes which are found across each research site (Eisenhardt 1989; Miles et al. 2014; Walsham 1995; Yin 2013).

DATA COLLECTION AND ANALYSIS

The researcher searched on Facebook, Instagram, Reddit and YouTube using the keyword: "*fibromyalgia*" or "*fibro*". Once these groups were located, permission was sought from the gatekeepers to these online communities where applicable (Reddit and Facebook) to contact users within these communities and collect data from these communities for use in this research. This was done by sending online messages to these gatekeepers that included the plain language statement and consent forms explaining the study in general and the anticipated activities that would be carried out by the researcher or requested from informants who provided consent. There were 42 key informants in total and these cohorts participated in online interviews with the authors and permitted observation of their activities related to illness management for the duration of the study. Each interview lasted 60-90 minutes, and a schedule had to be carefully negotiated due to the time differences caused by geographical distance. Due to the geographically dispersed nature of the study informants, interviews were conducted through Skype, Gmail chat applications and through social media sites chat features such as Facebook Messenger depending on the preferences of the key informants (Schultze 2011).

For this study, the qualitative data collection involved using semi-structured interviews, observation, physical artefacts and research memos to gain an understanding of SMT appropriation in the chronic illness context. The semi-structured interview used in this study allowed the authors to co-create meanings from the perspective of study informants (Myers and Newman 2007; Schultze and Avital 2011; Yin 2013). According to Yin (2013) applying a casual observation process to a case study allows the researcher to *"assess the occurrence of certain types of behaviours"* which could serve to enrich the insights derived from data collected via interviews (Yin 2013). Online observation was used in this study to allow the study of appropriation behaviours of the research participants on these social media tools (Konijn et al. 2013; MacColl et al. 2005). Some behaviours such as posting, and commenting could be observed, but some other actions such as lurking could not easily be observed. The researcher joined these groups and followed these profiles for the duration of the data collection period to note the activities and norms within these chronic illness communities. To minimize the potential influence on study participants, the researcher was a neutral observer and casually observed the same group of informants who consented to participate in the interviews (Walsham 2006). With the consent of the gatekeepers where relevant (Facebook and Reddit) one researcher casually observed the entire group to gain a general understanding of activities and norms within these types of communities.

Physical artefacts are one of the data collection tools available for evaluation in a qualitative study (Tsang 2013; Yin 2013). At the start of data collection, the researcher examined the features of these social media tools to better understand their material/technical properties which are important to chronically ill users (Alaimo and Kallinikos 2017; Benbasat and Zmud 2003; Kallinikos et al. 2012; Leonardi 2012; Orlikowski et al. 2006). To this effect, the findings allowed the authors to gain familiarity with the digital environments and explore to what extent these environments could offer various affordances or constraints to chronically ill users (Isika et al. 2016). The researcher also kept memos during the data collection and analytic process as an analytic exercise to expand on the researcher's thoughts about emergent themes that were found during analysis and these memos were stored in the case database using NVivo 11 pro (Miles et al., 2014; Miles, Quarterly, & Dec, 1979; Strauss, Corbin, & Strauss, 2008; Yin, 2013).

The authors adopted a two-phased approach using a mix of inductive and deductive approaches to analyse the collected data. The first phase of coding involved an inductive approach that comprised line-by-line review of the interview transcripts open coding, using strategies like 1) descriptive coding; 2) emotion coding; 3) attribute coding; 4) process coding and; 5) in vivo coding (Charmaz 2008; Gioia et al. 2013; Miles et al. 2014; Saldana 2009). These strategies allowed labels to be assigned to each line of interview data based on the meaning interpreted by the researcher from these data. The next phase first involved axial coding to cluster similar themes from the collection of codes generated in the initial coding step (Miles et al. 1979, 2014; Saldana 2009). Axial coding allowed the researcher to understand the relationship between concepts from the interview data better while remaining sensitive to new findings from the dataset (Charmaz, 2006; Gioia et al., 2013; Strauss et al., 2008). A benefit of this approach was that it allowed the voices of key informants to be preserved in the derived themes that emerged from the analysis activities, which is in keeping with the interpretive stance of this study. Finally, interpretive coding was applied to abstract themes to more aggregate dimensions to account for the main concepts that were found in collected data (Charmaz, 2006; Gioia et al., 2013; Strauss & Corbin, 2008).

FINDINGS

Cross-Case Background

Based on that classification strategy, the key characteristics of each case are described below to provide a background to the following sections:

- **Facebook:** Facebook was found to provide a mix of capabilities that supported the key informants' *need for presence, connection, entertainment and conversations* through technical features such as groups, contacts tab and the activity stream (news feed) that served as mechanisms that support these needs. The key informants of the Facebook case were all members of fibromyalgia groups and followed fibromyalgia pages which gave them access to others in similar circumstances with whom they could interact;
- **Instagram:** At first glance, image sharing sites such as Instagram present functionality to the user that supports the *display of a public self* with a lower emphasis on connections and *a higher focus on reputation and building of a public image/identity with a high emphasis on image*. The popular technological mechanisms used by key informants seemed to be the sharing images, searching, hashtagging these images and creating sub-profiles for illness management purposes. Key informants indicated that these mechanisms served to support ad-hoc community formation around their posts, giving access to a community of similar others;
- **YouTube:** Overall, key informants shared that YouTube *enables a high level of self-disclosure* through the video blogging activities that users carry out on the SMT. The study key informants were all YouTubers who considered themselves central parts of the chronic illness community of YouTube and the structure of the site allowed ad-hoc community formation around video uploads. Further, users could interact with a video upload through features such as like or dislike of a video clip, subscribing and viewing;

- **Reddit:** Reddit appeared to focus on *emphasizing conversations, groups and reputation* through mechanisms such as subreddits, posts and a Karma point system which is allocated to the user based on her/his posts and comments on the SMT. Key informants indicated that the Reddit SMT allowed for greater anonymity within these groups because the profiles did not require a high level of personalization and in some cases did not require a link with other social technologies the user may have adopted, for example, Reddit did not require a verified email account prior to adoption.

Each SMT had a range of technical capabilities built in to support the needs of their user base; but there were a few features that were similarly implemented across all SMTs such as: newsfeed; content recommendation; content publication; integration with other sites through social plugins; discussion capabilities through comments and postings; and gamification mechanisms. Yet the extent to which of these capabilities are supported for each site differs, based on the central vision of the social media tool.

Reddit

Because of the interactions between the individual incentives to adopt and use Reddit for illness management and the influences exerted on these cohorts by the community and technology of the Reddit site, the following eight key affordances which served to enable illness management were observed:

- **Belonging:** Reddit affords these cohorts the ability to belong in a community of others who are connected by a shared condition, as a consequence of the community provided by the SMT, these cohorts are able to feel connected to others in the community through sharing experiences or subscribing to the subreddit;
- **Compartmentalization:** This affordance allowed key informants to operate in each subreddit as a separate space, with the option of customizing taglines, making use of throw-away accounts and other options which enabled separation of their activities on Reddit SMT;
- **Considered Participation:** The text-based nature of Reddit allowed thoughtful communication by chronically ill individuals. Key informants indicated that they appreciated the lack of immediacy that the text-based nature of Reddit provided;
- **Storytelling:** Chronically ill cohorts could share their stories with others in the Reddit SMT through the posting feature provided by the tool. Through posting, key informants could narrate their experiences and share with others in the same community;
- **Presence:** The Reddit SMT provided a sticker on the side of the subreddit which indicated how many members of the community were online at any time;
- **Reputation:** Reddit affords this through a point system called karma which is allocated to the user as a result of his/her posts and comments on the platform. Karma is finally determined by the community through the number of likes they give to a specific post;
- **Sensemaking:** The sensemaking affordance refers to the extent to which the user is able to utilize the tool in making sense of their symptoms through collaborating with others or reading the experiences of others. This affordance may be realized before or after the official medical diagnosis by healthcare professionals. Through activities like lurking or participating in these subreddits, these informants could learn about their illness and collectively make sense of symptoms and problems presented to the community.

Additionally, there was a key constraint which acted as a disruptor which was:

- **Emotional Overload:** Due to the constant deluge of notifications and updates of members posts on the group feed, this served as a constraint. Some key informants noted the emotional overload they experienced as a consequence of participation on Reddit.

YouTube

- **Self-Presentation:** The process of sharing experiences with similar others in an immediate video format allows these cohorts to enjoy a therapeutic release. This is partially influenced by the sense of anonymous sharing because there is no initial knowledge of who will view these videos and so these cohorts are able to freely present themselves in a controlled context to similar, understanding others without fear of judgment or ridicule. The sense of therapeutic release is supported by the technology features and protected by the community that ensure that these self-disclosure episodes are not subject to trolling or similar negative behaviour;
- **Identity:** YouTube allows these informants and their subscribers to develop a shared sense of identity. This emerges through shared terms and identification signals, such as spoonie, fibro-warrior and identifying with celebrities who are said to have the same illness. Similar to some previous studies, in the YouTube case, the identity affordance allowed some key informants to take on a central position in the chronic illness network and assume the identity of a knowledgeable, empowered patient;
- **A Creative Outlet:** As most informants reported, the YouTube SMT serves as an outlet for creative expression through the different processes involved in creating a channel, creating and editing content;
- **Sensemaking:** The sensemaking affordance for chronically ill users refers to the extent to which the user is able to utilize the tool in making sense of their symptoms. This affordance may be realized before or after the official medical diagnosis by healthcare professionals;
- **Storytelling:** YouTube allowed these cohorts the opportunity to share their daily lived experiences with others in the same condition online.

Instagram

- **Therapeutic Self-Expression:** The process of sharing experiences with similar others in and through specialized profiles allows these cohorts to enjoy self-presentation. This is partially influenced by the sense of private sharing because cohorts are able to freely express their illness management needs to similar, understanding others without fear of judgment or ridicule;
- **Ad-Hoc Community Affiliation:** Instagram affords these cohorts the ability to affiliate with a community of others who are connected by a shared condition, as a consequence of the hashtagging community formation feature provided by the SMT;
- **Compartmentalization:** This affordance allowed key informants to operate in their illness management profiles, separate from the profiles followed by other members of their offline network;
- **Identity:** Users could make multiple profiles to engage in different activities across the site, allowing a sense of fluidity based on their intended interaction on the SMT;

- **A Creative Outlet:** Instagram SMT serves as an outlet for creative expression through the different processes involved in creating a channel, creating and editing content;
- **Identity:** Identity was seen to allows chronically ill users to craft identities around their illness such as spoonie and through the use of the fibromyalgia butterfly.

Facebook

Identified affordances which enable appropriation of Facebook by chronically ill adults:

- **Compartmentalization:** This affordance allowed key informants to operate in each privacy in groups of other chronically ill cohorts;
- **Reputation:** Enables the user to know the standing of other users due to the tags attached by the Facebook SMT to each member in the groups based on how long they have been in the group;
- **Storytelling:** It was observed that these cohorts were able to share detailed stories about issues of concern with others in the group;
- **Considered Participation:** This allowed members to remain in the SMT environment without any pressure to interact with others;
- **Persistence:** This allows new users to interact with and benefit from content long after it has been discussed by other members of the online community. Sometimes, this content may be discussing rules and community guidelines or information resources;
- **Sensemaking:** The sensemaking affordance refers to the extent to which the user is able to utilize the tool in making sense of their symptoms. This affordance may be realized before or after the official medical diagnosis by healthcare professionals.

Identified constraint which disrupts appropriation of Facebook by chronically ill adults:

- **Emotional Overload:** Due to the constant deluge of notifications and updates of members posts on the group feed, this served as a constraint. Some key informants noted the emotional overload they experienced as a consequence of participation on Facebook.

SOLUTIONS AND RECOMMENDATIONS

The enabling affordances found in the present study which agree with previous work include narration/storytelling, identity, triggered attendance/considered participation, sensemaking and metavoicing (Majchrzak et al. 2013; Merolli et al. 2015; Treem and Leonardi 2012). Two unique affordances in the present study include creative outlet and compartmentalization. Disruptors to chronic illness management found in this study include emotional overload/metavoicing and misinformation. Accordingly, this section discusses the illness management possibilities offered to study informants by the examined SMT features and so these affordances are termed: enablers (affordances) and disruptors (constraints). Findings support current theory which suggests that social media allows users to *act-through* these SMTs and by-pass the limitations imposed on key informants due to their chronic illness or geographical location. The next section discusses these enabling or disruptive affordances identified from this study and Table 1 provides a summary of these across all cases.

Table 1. Affordances which enable or disrupt appropriation for illness management purposes

Affordances	Concept	Reddit	YouTube	Instagram	Facebook
Enabler	Belonging	High	High	High	High
	Compartmentalization	High	Medium	High	High
	Storytelling	High	High	Low	High
	Sensemaking	High	Low	Medium	High
	A creative outlet	Low	High	High	Medium
	Considered Participation	High	High	High	High
Disruptor	Emotional overload	High	Low	Medium	High
	Misinformation	Medium	High	High	Low

Enablers to Appropriation for Better Chronic Illness Management Outcomes

The first affordance concerns the sense of belonging these key informants derived through association with others having the same fibromyalgia condition. Because fibromyalgia is a debilitating chronic condition, study informants found it necessary to associate with similar others who could relate to their challenges through SMTs. The *sense of belonging affordance* is in line with previous studies which had found similar affordances termed as: association (Treem and Leonardi 2012), connecting like-minded people to each other (Majchrzak and Markus 2012) or building a support network (Bernardi 2016) proposed by previous scholars (Kietzmann et al. 2011; Majchrzak et al. 2013). This affordance occurs because of the SMT capability to connect like-minded individuals to create and exchange content around illness management. To enjoy a sense of belonging, study informants joined communities on the examined SMTs which were identifiable using similar descriptive terms such as fibro-warriors or spoonies. On community-based SMTs, these terms were explicitly disclosed in the name and description of the group or subreddit. Similarly, study informants in the Instagram and YouTube case had descriptive terms in their profiles to serve as calling cards for others with fibromyalgia.

The study at hand also suggests compartmentalization affordance. Compartmentalization was viewed by these individuals as a means to conduct illness management activities separate from their other online activities. Compartmentalization was evident on these SMTs to varying degrees (see Table 1). Our findings suggest compartmentalization was essential to study informants because of the stigma associated with having an invisible chronic illness such as fibromyalgia. Through compartmentalization, informants were able to enjoy privacy in a safe environment occupied only by others who could relate to their daily struggles with fibromyalgia. For instance, concerning the *compartmentalization* affordance: on the Reddit SMT, users were able to create throw-away accounts to post private content that they may not necessarily want to be associated with their main profile. If not, every post made in every subreddit using an account could be seen and viewed by anyone with internet access. While on the Instagram SMT, users could create a separate account for carrying out their illness management needs. This finding further unpacks the visibility affordance (Treem and Leonardi 2012) noted by previous scholars because compartmentalization allowed these users to apply selective visibility for different audiences based on their level of comfort in discussing illness-related issues. Moreover, the compartmentalization affordance extends the notion of structure proposed by previous scholars who suggest that SMTs could guide chronically ill users to a pre-filtered set of illness-specific information (Merolli et al. 2015). Taking this idea further, compartmentalization affordance allows users to carry out and engage in illness management practices in a separate space from their other activities on the examined SMTs.

Thirdly, our study demonstrates that the examined SMTs afforded storytelling to varying degrees and findings show that these informants could openly discuss all aspects of their lives to varying degrees of support (see Table 1) based on the material features of the SMT. Of course, the extent of a user's storytelling depends on their decisions concerning anonymity, privacy and their health condition. Nonetheless, the study informants could narrate their experiences through images, texts, videos using SMTs to share their positive or negative experiences with understanding others in the same community. Storytelling in this study supports narration affordances (Bernardi 2016; Merolli et al. 2015) reported in previous studies. Those studies had suggested that narration/storytelling served to foster a shared experience of illness and offer opportunities for chronically ill users to learn from the experiences of others in the same community. Further, the present study suggests that narration/storytelling is influenced by the features of the technology artefact under consideration. For instance, storytelling on YouTube was quite immediate and personal due to the intimate nature of video-based communication; Reddit supported storytelling by allowing users to create text-based posts. Conversely, it was observed that Instagram appeared to be applied more playfully through posting of memes to illustrate the humorous aspects of life with fibromyalgia.

The next affordance found in this present study relates to sensemaking, another shared affordance that allowed members of these communities to collaboratively solve illness-related challenges through conversations on these SMTs. In YouTube, affordance relied on the capabilities of video creation and commenting, while on Facebook, key informants could make a post, others in the community would comment, and as a community this allowed them to make sense of their illness. This finding adds to previous research that suggested that SMTs afford users meta-voicing (Majchrzak et al. 2013), the sensemaking affordance is a result of the consolidation of multiple users opinions pooled together to solve a problem. (Treem and Leonardi 2012). The last two identified affordances concern: creative outlet affordance and considered participation affordance. In the present study, SMTs offer chronically ill users a creative outlet, supporting supports creative expression for its users through meme creation and videos. The creative outlet affordance was identified in three cases: YouTube, Instagram and Facebook. Those three SMTs support study informants hedonic needs to engage in creative activities to communicate information support and raise awareness about fibromyalgia. Our study suggests that the examined SMTs enable their creative expression to different extents (see Table 1) this affordance helps maintain a sense of well-being despite the physical and mental toll that Fibromyalgia takes on sufferers.

Our findings also point to the notion of considered participation affordance. The examined SMTs allows its users to interact to different extents based on their current needs. As discussed earlier, study informants could engage in tentative, reactive or proactive appropriation pattern; the examined SMTs did not enforce interaction with others on its users. Instead, considered participation enabled members to remain in the SMT environment without the pressure to interact with others. This affordance was especially crucial because it allowed informants control over their activities on the examined SMTs while allowing access to information and emotional resources to help their personal illness management practices. This affordance agrees with the concept of adaptation proposed by previous scholars who noted that SMTs allow chronically ill users to adapt their interactions with others based on their personal circumstances (Merolli et al. 2015).

SMT Features That Disrupt Appropriation for Chronic Illness Management Practices

The present study also identified two constraints which could disrupt illness management practices for the study informants which were: emotional overload and misinformation. First, emotional overload constraint refers to the bombardment with negative content that was experienced by some key informants on the community-oriented SMTs (Reddit and Facebook). Our findings suggest an imbalance between positive and negative posts on the community-based SMTs (Reddit and Facebook). Due to the mental repercussions of suffering from a stigmatized chronic illness, some key informants on the Reddit and Facebook were negatively affected by the constant need for emotional support from others on these SMTs. For example, there were many posts about potential suicides or to rant and vent to others in the safe space provided by SMTs. Accordingly, some informants in the Reddit and Facebook case study reported feeling overwhelmed, hopeless and depressed by the constant barrage of depressive posts. A reason for this lies in the design of Reddit and Facebook. These SMTs serve notifications to community members about every new post submitted in the community and could serve to create a negative atmosphere.

During the study, the researcher witnessed some incidents where community members exit the group because they were unable to continue to remain in such negative spaces. This finding unpacks the triggered attendance affordance (Majchrzak et al. 2013) from previous studies to show that the constant notifications and updates from the group served to disrupt the achievement of positive illness management outcomes. This study shows that the triggered attendance afforded by the notifications and newsfeed features of SMTs like Reddit and Facebook may disrupt appropriation because of the overwhelmingly negative streams of content these individuals are exposed to. Moreover, emotional overload was also a consequence of trolling behaviour as noted during the observation phase of the study, where individuals in the community may witness or get into arguments with others in the community which could result in disappropriation.

Finally, the present study suggests that misinformation constraint could disrupt positive illness management outcomes. While these SMTs could serve as a safe place to collectively make sense with others about illness-related concerns, the present study also suggests that the examined SMTs may also constrain illness management through misinformation. In the present study, misinformation was found to derive from scammers/spammers trying to take advantage of the desperation of these individuals. Further, despite the good intentions of other chronically ill adults in the community, there was a potential to receive bad/dangerous advice because the experience of fibromyalgia is highly individual. However, study informants shared that they were aware of this potential for harm and made sure to discuss each piece of advice received from others in the community with the GPs, especially if it concerned medication. The appearance of this constraint varied significantly between the examined SMTs. First, participants on community-based SMTs like Reddit and Facebook appeared to manage misinformation through the involvement of other chronically ill users in the community. Reddit and Facebook chronically ill users seemed to be vigilant to dubious content posted in the online group concerning bad advice, miracle cures and spam. As a result, the incidents of misinformation were minimized although spammers and scammers worked around the group by sending private messages to intended victims. Although misinformation was not directly observed or discussed by informants from the YouTube and Instagram studies, our observations reveal the existence of several accounts about fibromyalgia cures by others in the community. Those posts ranged from accounts selling cures to accounts proposing untested holistic medical aids to relieve symptoms.

Furthermore, this chapter provided a set of six enabling affordances identified within the case studies; the chapter also identified two constraints which serve to disrupt positive appropriation outcomes among the study informants. Finally, each of the outlined sections in the discussion culminated in a set of ten propositions that address the study questions. The next section concludes this chapter by providing a summary of the research findings, study implications and directions for future research.

FUTURE RESEARCH DIRECTIONS

This study contributes to the growing interest on affordance theory and its role in IS, particularly in the social media context. The present study exposes the underlying affordances which act to enable or disrupt chronic illness management. This work examines how different social media tools are appropriated by chronically ill adults. By so doing, our findings showcase needs that may drive adoption and use of diverse SMTs, the influential factors on different types of SMTs and; the different affordances which may enable or disrupt appropriation across different types of SMTs. Our study also presents useful information for chronically ill adults.

SMTs are powerful tools which could provide illness management resources such as supportive social relationships or information support about coping with illness and medications. There is a potential for harm through spam, misinformation and emotional overload because of the constant need for help from others in the community. Therefore, chronically ill adults are advised to consider the risks carefully and involve their primary care physician in this practice to evaluate advice received from the SMTs. It may serve these individuals to select an SMT based on their illness management needs. Those individuals who need information support resources may benefit from community-based SMTs like Reddit and Facebook because of the significant community membership. Those large communities offer chronically ill adults the opportunity to access a plethora of treatment plans which may assist their education, empowerment and self-advocacy. On the other hand, individuals with severe mental health issues may benefit more from SMTs such as Instagram or YouTube, where there is a more positive atmosphere filled with emotionally uplifting content. Ad-hoc communities such as YouTube Instagram may offer more positive emotional outcomes than the community-based SMTs like Reddit and Facebook which showcase a barrage of emotionally charged content which could be detrimental for mental health. Our study is limited in the following ways: the number of participants recruited for the interviews and qualitative portion of the study. A possible direction for future research would be to conduct a long-term study to evaluate how social media affordances are encountered by chronically ill adults and how these affordances enable or disrupt positive illness management outcomes. An area that deserves further study lies in the effects of SMT community dynamics on information use by chronically ill adults. As found in the present study community-based SMTs such as Reddit or Facebook were constantly filtering through misinformation or spam to prevent dissemination of dangerous advice which could have dangerous repercussions on others in the community. Future work could investigate the occurrence of misinformation on community-based and ad-hoc SMTs to develop guidelines on how best to protect against these incidents for vulnerable chronically ill adults. Further, a study on that aspect could include the trajectory on how information received for illness management are verified, applied or discarded and to what extent primary care physicians are informed on/included in this process.

CONCLUSION

Our work suggests several ways that SMT appropriation may affect chronically ill adults in terms of affordances which may enable or disrupt illness management outcomes. To reiterate, this present study views affordances as opportunities for goal-oriented action (Gibson 1986; Merolli et al. 2015; Treem and Leonardi 2012). This work suggests that social media allows users to *act-through* these SMTs for illness management needs and affords a sense of belonging. Belonging to a community of similar others allows users to feel validated, accepted, understood. This finding supports previous studies which had coined the terms association, connection, or building a support network (Bernardi 2016; Majchrzak et al. 2013; Treem and Leonardi 2012). The present work goes further to suggest that belonging is essential to combat the isolation and stigma of chronic illness. Belonging enables emotional well-being especially in terms of a challenging illness like fibromyalgia. The sense of belonging may be enjoyed through tentative, reactive or proactive appropriation patterns. Other affordances which align with previous studies include storytelling, sensemaking, identity and considered participation (Bernardi 2016; Majchrzak et al. 2013; Merolli et al. 2015; Treem and Leonardi 2012).

This work also suggests that SMTs afford compartmentalization. Through compartmentalization, users could freely vent and discuss the ramifications of their illness in a safe space free from the view of others in their online or offline community who may not relate to their experiences. Compartmentalization was offered to varying degrees on the examined SMTs. For instance, Reddit provided throwaway accounts, while Instagram provided multiple profiles for users. Compartmentalization is crucial to chronically ill adults because it allows private discussions in a judgement-free virtual space. The present work extends SMT and affordance studies to demonstrate additional affordances which may lead to positive illness management outcomes.

Taking this further, the present work extends this line of research to show dangerous outcomes that may arise from SMT appropriation. In contrast to previous studies which have only discussed enabling affordances from SMT use, this study suggests that SMTs may have negative impacts on chronically ill adults through disruptive constraints like emotional overload and misinformation. Emotional overload is a consequence of constant bombardment with emotionally charged posts seeking emotional support or discussing suicide. The technology features of SMTs serve users with notifications based on the topics or groups they follow. Fibromyalgia is a challenging progressive condition, and the majority of posts made by sufferers could be depressing and discouraging for chronically ill adults. Another notable constraint is misinformation. Users on SMTs receive advice from other chronically ill adults and may rely on that illness management resource. Yet, there should be concerns about the credibility of some information received because other users on the SMT are not medical professionals. Moreover, there is a significant risk of falling victim to bad advice (fibromyalgia is highly individual), scammer or spam.

REFERENCES

Agarwal, R., Guodong, G., DesRoches, C., & Jha, A. K. (2010). The Digital Transformation of Healthcare: Current Status and the Road Ahead. *Information Systems Research, 21*(4), 796–809.

Agarwal, R., Gupta, A. K., & Kraut, R. (2008). The Interplay between Digital and Social Networks. *Information Systems Research, 19*(3), 243–252.

Alaimo, C., & Kallinikos, J. (2017). Computing the Everyday: Social Media as Data Platforms. *Information Society, 33*(4), 175–191.

Anderson, C., & Robey, D. (2017). Affordance Potency: Explaining the Actualization of Technology Affordances. *Information and Organization, 27*(2), 100–115.

Benbasat, I., & Zmud, R. W. (2003). The Identity Crisis within the Is Discipline: Defining and Communicating the Discipline's Core Properties. *MIS Quarterly, 27*(2), 183–194.

Bernardi, R. (2016). How Do Online Communities of Patients Aggregate on Twitter? An Affordance Perspective. Icis, 1–19.

Bodenheimer, T. (2002). Patient Self-Management of Chronic Disease in Primary Care. *Jama, 288*(19), 2469.

Burzler, N. (2018). *Most Popular Social Networks Worldwide 2018*. Academic Press.

Charmaz, K. (2006). *Constructing Grounded Theory: A Practical Guide through Qualitative Analysis* (Vol. 10). Academic Press.

Charmaz, K. (2008). Grounded Theory as an Emergent Method. Handbook of Emergent Methods, (3), 155–170.

Choy, K., & Schlagwein, D. (2016). Crowdsourcing for a Better World: On the Relation between IT Affordances and Donor Motivations in Charitable Crowdfunding. *Information Technology and People, 29*(1), 221–247.

Dadgar, M., & Joshi, K. D. (2018). The Role of Information and Communication Technology in Self-Management of Chronic Diseases: An Empirical Investigation through Value Sensitive Design. *Journal of the Association for Information Systems, 19*(2), 86–112.

Department of Health. (2012). *Integrated Chronic Disease Prevention*. World Health Organization.

Department of Health & Human Services. (2016). *Care for People with Chronic Conditions: Guide for the Community Health*. Author.

Eisenhardt, K. M. (1989). Building Theories from Case Study Research. *Academy of Management Review, 14*(4), 532–550.

Fadel, K. J. (2012). User Adaptation and Infusion of Information Systems. *Journal of Computer Information Systems, 52*(3), 1–10.

Faraj, S., & Azad, B. (2012). The Materiality of Technology: An Affordance Perspective. Materiality and Organizing: Social Interaction in a Technological World, 237–258.

Fayard, A.-L., & Weeks, J. (2014). Affordances for Practice. *Information and Organization*, *24*(4), 236–249.

Fichman, R. G., Kohli, R., & Krishnan, R. (2011). The Role of Information Systems in Healthcare: Current Research and Future Trends. *Information Systems Research*, *22*(3), 419–428.

Georgeff, M. (2014). RACGP - Digital Technologies and Chronic Disease Management. Australian Family Physician, 842–6.

Gibson, J. J. (1986). 04-JJ Gibson-Ch8-Affordances. Chapter Eight The Theory of Affordances, 127–136.

Gioia, D. A., Corley, K. G., & Hamilton, A. L. (2013). Seeking Qualitative Rigor in Inductive Research: Notes on the Gioia Methodology. *Organizational Research Methods*, *16*(1), 15–31.

Goh, J. M., Gao, G. G., & Agarwal, R. (2011). Evolving Work Routines : Adaptive Routinization of Information Technology in Healthcare. *Information Systems Research*.

Greenhalgh, T. (2009). Chronic Illness: Beyond the Expert Patient. BMJ, 338, 629–631.

Ho, S. Y., Guo, X., & Vogel, D. (2019). Opportunities and Challenges in Healthcare Information Systems Research: Caring for Patients with Chronic Conditions. *Communications of the Association for Information Systems*, (44), 852–873. doi:10.17705/1CAIS.04439

Househ, M., Borycki, E., & Kushniruk, A. (2014). Empowering Patients through Social Media: The Benefits and Challenges. *Health Informatics Journal*, *20*(1), 50–58.

Isika, N. U., Mendoza, A., & Bosua, R. (2016). The Use of Social Media by Adults with Chronic Illness: Analysing the Support Mechanisms of Four Social Media Platforms. In *The 27th Australasian Conference on Information Systems* (Vol. 1). Academic Press.

Kallinikos, J. (2002). Reopening the Black Box of Technology. ICIS, 287–294.

Kallinikos, J. (2012). Form, Function, and Matter: Crossing the Border of Materiality. In Materiality and Organizing: Social Interaction in a Technological World (Vol. 1, pp. 45–66). doi:10.1093/acprof:oso/9780199664054.003.0004

Kallinikos, J., Leonardi, P. M., & Nardi, B. A. (2012). The Challenge of Materiality: Origins, Scope, and Prospects. *Materiality and Organizing: Social Interaction in a Technological World.*

Kane, G. C., Alavi, M., Labianca, Giuseppe, J., & Borgatti, S. P. (2014). What's Different about Social Media Networks? A Framework and Research Agenda. MIS Quarterly, 38(1), 274–304.

Kaplan, A. M., & Haenlein, M. (2010). Users of the World, Unite! The Challenges and Opportunities of Social Media. *Business Horizons*, *53*(1), 59–68.

Karahanna, E., Xu, S. X., Xu, Y., & Zhang, N. (2018). The needs–affordances–features perspective for the use of social media. *MIS Quarterly*, *42*(3), 737–756. doi:10.25300/MISQ/2018/11492

Kietzmann, J. H., Hermkens, K., McCarthy, I. P., & Silvestre, B. S. (2011). Social Media? Get Serious! Understanding the Functional Building Blocks of Social Media. *Business Horizons*, *54*(3), 241–251.

Konijn, E. A., Veldhuis, J., & Plaisier, X. S. (2013). YouTube as a Research Tool: Three Approaches. *Cyberpsychology, Behavior and Social Networking*, *16*(9), 695–701.

Leonardi, P. M. (2012). Materiality, Sociomateriality, and Socio-Technical Systems: What Do These Terms Mean? How Are They Different? Do We Need Them? *Materiality and Organizing: Social Interaction in a Technological World.*

Leong, C., Pan, S. L., Newell, S., & Cui, L. (2016). The Emergence of Self-Organizing E-Commerce Ecosystems in Remote Villages of China: A Tale of Digital Empowerment for Rural Development. *MIS Quarterly*, *40*(2), 475-A8.

MacColl, I., Cooper, R., Rittenbruch, M., & Viller, S. (2005). Watching Ourselves Watching: Ethical Issues in Ethnographic Action Research. OZCHI 2005 Proceedings, 1–4.

Majchrzak, A., Faraj, S., Kane, G. C., & Azad, B. (2013). The Contradictory Influence of Social Media Affordances on Online Communal Knowledge Sharing. *Journal of Computer-Mediated Communication*, *19*(1), 38–55.

Majchrzak, A., & Markus, M. L. (2012). Technology Affordances and Constraints in Management Information Systems (Mis). Encyclopedia of Management Theory, 5.

McKenna, B., Myers, M. D., & Newman, M. (2017). Social Media in Qualitative Research: Challenges and Recommendations. *Information and Organization*, *27*(2), 87–99.

Mendoza, A., Carroll, J., Stern, L., & Linda, S. (2010, Mar.). Software Appropriation Over Time : From Adoption to Stabilization and Beyond. *Australasian Journal of Information Systems*, 5–23.

Merolli, M., Gray, K., & Martin-Sanchez, F. (2013). Health Outcomes and Related Effects of Using Social Media in Chronic Disease Management: A Literature Review and Analysis of Affordances. *Journal of Biomedical Informatics*, *46*(6), 957–969.

Merolli, M., Gray, K., Martin-Sanchez, F., & Lopez-Campos, G. (2015). Patient-Reported Outcomes and Therapeutic Affordances of Social Media: Findings from a Global Online Survey of People with Chronic Pain. *Journal of Medical Internet Research*, *17*(1), e20.

Miles, M. B., Huberman, M. A., & Saldaña, J. (2014). *Qualitative Data Analysis: A Methods Sourcebook.* SAGE Publications, Inc.

Miles, M. B., Quarterly, A. S., & Dec, Q. M. (1979). Qualitative Data as an Attractive Nuisance. *The Problem of Analysis*, *24*(4), 590–601.

Myers, M. D., & Newman, M. (2007). The Qualitative Interview in IS Research: Examining the Craft. *Information and Organization*, *17*(1), 2–26.

Ngai, E., Moon, K. L. K., Lam, S. S., Chin, E. S. K., & Tao, S. S. C. (2015). Social Media Models, Technologies, and Applications: An Academic Review and Case Study. *Industrial Management and Data Systems*, *115*(5), 769–802.

Ngai, E. W. T., Tao, S. S. C., & Moon, K. K. L. (2015). Social Media Research: Theories, Constructs, and Conceptual Frameworks. *International Journal of Information Management*, *35*(1), 33–44.

Orlikowski, W. J., & Iacono, C. S. (2001). Research Commentary: Desperately Seeking the 'IT' in IT Research - A Call to Theorizing the IT Artifact. *Information Systems Research*, *12*(2), 121–134.

Orlikowski, W. J., Iacono, S., & Iacono, C. S. (2006). Desperately Seeking the 'IT'in IT Research: A Call to Theorizing the IT Artifact. *Information Systems: The State of the Field*, *34*(2), 19.

Orlikowski, W. J., & Scott, S. V. (2015). The Algorithm and the Crowd: Considering the Materiality of Service Innovation. *MIS Quarterly*, *39*(1), 201–216.

Panahi, S., Watson, J., & Partridge, H. (2012). Social Media and Tacit Knowledge Sharing : Developing a Conceptual Model. Academic Press.

Patel, R., Chang, T., Greysen, S. R., & Chopra, V. (2015). Social Media Use in Chronic Disease: A Systematic Review and Novel Taxonomy. *American Journal of Medicine*, *128*(12), 1335–1350.

Pousti, H., Urquhart, C., & Linger, H. (2014). Exploring the Role of Social Media in Chronic Care Management. IFIP Advances in Information and Communication Technology, 446, 163–185. doi:10.1007/978-3-662-45708-5_11

Romanow, D., Cho, S., & Straub, D. W. (2012). Riding the Wave: Past Trends and Future Directions for Health IT Research. *MIS Quarterly*, *36*(3). doi:10.2307/41703474

Rozenblum, R., & Bates, D. W. (2013). Patient-Centred Healthcare, Social Media and the Internet: The Perfect Storm? *BMJ Quality & Safety*, *22*(3), 183–6.

Saldana, J. (2009). *The Coding Manual for Qualitative Researchers*. Academic Press.

Saldana, J. (2009). An Introduction to Codes and Coding. The Coding Manual for Qualitative Researchers, 1–31.

Samhan, B., Crampton, T., & Ruane, R. (2018). The Trajectory of IT in Healthcare at HICSS: A Literature Review, Analysis, and Future Directions. *Communications of the Association for Information Systems*, *43*, 1. doi:10.17705/1CAIS.04341

Sareah, F. (2015). *Interesting Statistics for the Top 10 Social Media Sites*. Academic Press.

Schultze, U. (2011). *The Avatar as Sociomaterial Entanglement: A Performative Perspective on Identity, Agency and World-Making in Virtual Worlds*. ICIS.

Schultze, U., & Avital, M. (2011). Designing Interviews to Generate Rich Data for Information Systems Research. *Information and Organization*, *21*(1), 1–16.

Spagnoletti, P., Resca, A., & Sæbø, Ø. (2015). Design for Social Media Engagement: Insights from Elderly Care Assistance. *The Journal of Strategic Information Systems*, *24*(2), 128–145.

Strauss, A., & Corbin, J. (2008). Basics of Qualitative Research: Techniques and Procedures for Developing Grounded Theory. In *Basics of Qualitative Research Grounded Theory Procedures and Techniques* (Vol. 3). Academic Press.

Strauss, A. L., Corbin, J. M., & Strauss, A. L. (2008). Basics of Qualitative Research. Academic Press.

Treem, J. W., & Leonardi, P. M. (2012). Social Media Use in Organizations: Exploring the Affordances of Visibility, Editability, Persistence, and Association. *Annals of the International Communication Association*, (36), 143–189.

Tsang, E. W. K. (2013). Case Study Methodology: Causal Explanation, Contextualization, and Theorizing. *Journal of International Management*, *19*(2), 195–202.

Urquhart, C., & Vaast, E. (2012). *Building Social Media Theory from Case Studies: A New Frontier for IS Research*. ICIS.

Vaast, E., Safadi, H., Lapointe, L., & Negoita, B. (2017). Social Media Affordances for Connective Action: An Examination of Microblogging Use During the Gulf of Mexico Oil Spill. *MIS Quarterly*, *41*(4), 1179–1205.

Walsh, I., Gettler-Summa, M., & Kalika, M. (2016). Expectable Use: An Important Facet of IT Usage. *The Journal of Strategic Information Systems*, *25*(3), 177–210. doi:10.1016/j.jsis.2016.01.003

Walsham, G. (1995, May). Interpretive Case Studies in IS Research: Nature and Method. *European Journal of Information Systems*, 74–81.

Walsham, G. (2006). Doing Interpretive Research. *European Journal of Information Systems*, *15*(3), 320–330.

Wang, X., Parameswaran, S., Bagul, D. M., & Kishore, R. (2017). Does Online Social Support Work in Stigmatized Chronic Diseases? A Study of the Impacts of Different Facets of Informational and Emotional Support on Self-Care Behavior in an HIV Online Forum. ICIS'2017.

WHO. (2016). *Integrated Care Models: An Overview*. Health Services Delivery Programme.

Yin, R. K. (2013). *Case Study Research: Design and Methods* (Vol. 5). Academic Press.

Yoo, Y. (2010). Computing in Everyday Life: A Call for Research on Experiential Computing. *MIS Quarterly*, *34*(2), 213.

KEY TERMS AND DEFINITIONS

Adoption: Adoption refers to a user's decision to either accept or reject a given technology; adoption studies have two dominant perspectives: either from the perspective of acceptance in a generalized sense or from the perspective of acceptance and integration into a technology use context.

Affordances/Constraints: The concept of affordances was posited by Giddens (1976) in the perceptual psychology field, in his seminal work on how an organism adapts to and understands their environment in terms of form, function and perceptions of goal-oriented actions. In information systems, this theory has been adapted to conceptualize the action potential the features of a technology offer to a user to enable (afford) or disrupt (constrain) achievement of their goals.

Appropriation: The word appropriation derives from the Latin word *'appropriare'* or *'appropriationem'* and is defined in Meriam Webster's dictionary as *"setting apart or taking for one's use"*. It is also defined as *"making something one's own"*. Appropriation has also been defined as the processes or adjustments that occur between system adoption and adaptation over time (Mendoza et al., 2010).

Chronic Diseases/Illness: Chronic illness refers to health conditions that last longer than three months in duration and these often persist for an entire lifetime (Dadgar and Joshi 2018; Department of Health 2012; Romanow et al. 2012). According to a recent report by the World Health Organization (WHO), chronic diseases are the leading cause of mortality worldwide. WHO estimates that by 2020 the deaths resulting from chronic illness will account for 73% of all deaths in developed nations and 79% of all deaths for developing nations (Department of Health & Human Services 2016; WHO 2016).

IT Artefact: The application of technology to enable some tasks within a context/structure (Benbasat and Zmud 2003). Some studies have defined IT artefacts as configurations or bundles of hardware and software features that constitute an information technology (Orlikowski and Iacono 2001).

Materiality: The physical constitution of technological objects (or lack of it) and the implications (social and technical) that these have for creating, design, and use of such objects (Kallinikos 2002, 2012). The notion of materiality also refers to the arrangement of an artefact's physical and digital materials into particular forms that endure across differences in place and time and are essential to users (Alaimo and Kallinikos 2017; Kallinikos et al. 2012; Leonardi 2012).

Online Communities/Online Social Networks: The terms online communities and online social networks are used interchangeably in the literature to refer to digitally-enabled virtual communities comprised of individuals connecting for a common cause or sharing the same practices.

Self-Management/Illness Management: Self-management is a daily, dynamic, interactive practice carried out with the involvement of family, friends, healthcare professionals and other concerned members of the community. Self-management addresses a patient-centred care approach that shares responsibility for ongoing management of chronic conditions with the ill individual (Bodenheimer 2002; Dadgar and Joshi 2018; Greenhalgh 2009; Househ et al. 2014).

Social Media: Synonymous with the term Web 2.0, social media are commonly defined as a set of internet-based, interactive computer-mediated technologies or tools that facilitate the creation and exchange of user-generated content (Kaplan and Haenlein 2010; Kietzmann et al. 2011; Ngai et al. 2015). This term comprises several types of technologies ranging from bookmarking sites such as digg.com to rich media sites such as SecondLife which offer a fully immersive virtual experience to users.

Technology Use: In this study 'use' is defined as the behaviours a user employs in order to make use of an IT artefact for their practices (Walsh et al. 2016).

Chapter 4
Supporting a Value-Based Healthcare Paradigm With Digital Health and Wellness Personalised Monitoring Solutions

Nilmini Wickramasinghe
https://orcid.org/0000-0002-1314-8843
Swinburne University, Australia & Epworth HealthCare, Australia

Steve Goldberg
Inet International Inc., Canada

ABSTRACT

Especially in the US, many are advocating for the incorporation of a value-based system for healthcare delivery including bundled payments for services in an attempt to address escalating healthcare costs. The following proffers the role for digital health solutions to support health and wellness management and the need to develop suitable sustainable business models. However, this approach brings a focus onto comorbidities and chronic conditions, which often need to be addressed or at least better managed before surgery can take place. This opens up the opportunity to examine the potential for digital health solutions such as mobile apps and serious games to provide an enabling or support role for individuals to better manage their chronic conditions. It also brings up the need for better, flexible models to assist health and wellness solution development.

DOI: 10.4018/978-1-7998-3274-4.ch004

INTRODUCTION

In the US, there is a move towards a value-based system (Lynn, 2016; Zuvekas and Cohen, 2016; Rauh et al., 2013; Bozic, 2016;), in which critical components include bundled payments and clearly defined care paths which in turn dictate care processes (Rauh et al., 2013; Bozic, 2016; Kaplan and Porter, 2011; Porter and Tiesberg, 2009; Porter and Lee, 2013; Porter, 2010; Betbeze, 2016; Bracy, 2016). This perspective is also being embraced in other OECD countries such as the UK, throughout Europe and Australia (Gray, 2018; Elf et al., 2017; Wickramasinghe et al., 2019). This is interesting and significant because US, UK, western Europe and Australia all have very different structured healthcare delivery systems and consequent payment mechanisms, thus, for all these countries/regions to be seriously evaluating and incorporating some or all aspects of a value-based care paradigm suggests that this paradigm will have a significant and far reaching impact on healthcare delivery moving forward.

Such a value-based model of care has been enabled by the introduction, adoption and increased penetration of electronic medical records (EMRs) into the care process. These digital health solutions serve to provide essential data and information necessary to facilitate the design of appropriate care paths and the calculation of bundled payments for specific care processes (Hero et al, 2016; Porter and Lee, 2013). However, the system is not without its own challenges, because it tends to take specific data on outcomes and cost and then apply them to general cohorts which can prove problematic and troubling especially for individuals with chronic conditions (Wickramasinghe et al., 2019; Elf et al.,2017). Moreover, some believe that the term value is being confused with efficient, and while the approach suggested by a value-base paradigm typically leads to the realization of greater efficiencies this does not necessarily translate into greater value for all healthcare stakeholders, most especially the patient (Gray, 2018). In this chapter, it is not possible to unpack all the issues of value-based care; however, the focus is on greater equity for patients i.e., subscribing to the WHO directive healthcare delivery for all (WHO, 2019). In particular how technology solutions can be used to support individuals with chronic disease such as diabetes within a value-based paradigm.

What is the Issue?

Assisted largely by federal policies and initiative such as President George W. Bush's 2004 Executive Order enabling eHealth, and the subsequent ARRA/HITECH legislation and Meaningful Use program (Hsu et al, 2005), over the last 10 years in the U.S. the adoption, and use of EMR has significantly increased. This in turn has resulted in the availability and use of significant amounts of captured and generated clinical data. This data is being used by clinicians to provide appropriate care to their patients, which is expected to lead to optimal clinical outcomes. A key aspect of this approach is centred around minimising complications and adverse events as these typically lead to expensive healthcare interventions and unplanned readmissions.

Hence, these data are being used to scrutinise cost, quality and calculate risk assessments at a specific point in time (Lynn, 2016; Zuvekas and Cohen, 2016; Porter and Lee, 2013; Bracy, 2016). In the context of a healthcare system that is facing substantially increasing costs, many encourage the move from a focus on volume to value (Porter and Tiesberg, 2009; Porter and Lee, 2013; Porter, 2010; Betbeze, 2016). This shift in focus is defining appropriate care paths and narrow definitions of risk and then applying them broadly to patients presenting for specific treatments, such as a knee arthroplasty (Porter, 2010; Betbeze, 2016; Bracyc, 2016). Specifically, such an approach often translates into patients being told that their proposed knee surgery is not appropriate at this time and should be delayed until such time it is safer such as when their haemoglobin A1c within a specific acceptable range, or when their body mass index is below a specific level or they have completed smoking cessation. However, this often leaves the patient in a conundrum; how can they address their chronic condition effective so they can then proceed with the needed surgery. This appears to be an opportunity for digital health solutions.

BACKGROUND

The major challenges facing healthcare delivery include: increasing costs, an aging population, and the rapid rise of chronic diseases. Taken together, these challenges are impacting the sustainability of the traditional fee for service systemin the US (Kaplan and Porter, 2012; Moghimi et al, 2013; Haddad et al., 2015). In such a fee for service model, financial incentives are typically structured to reward providers for the quantity and complexity of services, regardless of outcome (2). From the 1990s, many countries including the US, shifted to diagnostic related group (DRG) reimbursements to try to control payments on each patient's most serious diagnosis, but this unintentionally has led to treating patients' illnesses sequentially rather than simultaneously which has the final effect of impacting the cost of care significantly (2). Recognizing this dilemma by 2016 we have seen changes to the traditional volume based approach.

From 2016, CMS has begun to shift payment from volume to value, resulting in aligning 85% of all payments it makes to quality or value while 30% of payments are tied to quality or value through Alternate Payment Models (APM). Contemporaneously, the US is shifting to "value-based reimbursement" in the MACRA1 and MIPS2 programs with the goals to overcome waste, benchmark all providers' Medicare payments and adjust them based on comparison with peers' clinical outcomes for the same procedures. In addition, the US government is shifting to fixed-price "bundling" for many known treatments, e.g. knee and hip replacements (Bracy, 2016; Bumpass et al., 2016). Such reimbursement changes serve to guide providers towards evidence-based medical decisions and procedures. Further, they are supposed to be unbiased and scientifically optimized formulations that describe the best way to treat patients for the best overall outcomes.

In addition, the US Veterans Administration continuously publishes and updates a compilation of best practice guidelines for many chronic diseases3. Most hospitals and payers either adopt or create similar guidelines for their own decisions, and those formulas are typically embedded in hospital/physician EMRs and financials software to reinforce "positive" behaviors, compliance and, ultimately, outcomes.

Similarly, any clinical "centre of excellence" (CoE) also tends to apply the best evidence-based guidelines with its own expertise, with the expectation and intention that such decisions will result in their outcomes and reimbursement being among the most highly ranked, respected, and, hopefully, profitable. Hospitals or physicians who deliver care at lower levels then, may have to settle for average outcomes reimbursement, and poor-performers may be motivated to abandon services they cannot deliver well.

In general, it is well recognized that multiple co-morbidities or chronic conditions such as diabetes tend to lead to poor outcomes and thus, especially in the context of elective surgery many healthcare organisations defer surgery until an appropriate HbA1C is attained.

Sadly, the healthcare delivery dilemma grows. Many scholars, such as Porter (Porter and Tiesberg, 2009; Porter and Lee, 2013; Porter, 2010; Kaplan and Porter, 2011), have proffered that the appropriate strategy is to focus on value not volume. Specifically, Porter and colleagues contend that a key contributor to the current state of escalating costs is that healthcare delivery has been incorrectly defined (ibid).

Specifically, they proffer a model focused on value creation around the customer (Porter and Tiesberg, 2009; Porter and Lee, 2013); i.e., the patient (Porter and Tiesberg, 2009; Porter and Lee, 2013; Porter, 2010; Kaplan and Porter, 2011).

A major contributor to this has been the general embracement of EMRs, which, in turn, enables generation of significant data now being used by healthcare administrators and clinicians to analyse care delivery, and then design and develop appropriate care delivery paths to standardise care delivery, streamline processes and ensure best practice patterns ensue. Connected with this is the ability to use the generated data to identify key risk factors (Porter and Lee, 2013) (e.g. BMI, Haemoglobin A1C and smoking) developed very narrowly, but may be applied more generally and broadly.

However, an equally important component that appears to be being forgotten in this conceptualization is the patient experience. It is the contention of this chapter that by incorporating digital health solutions it becomes possible to not only address the value dilemma but also provide a better patient experience.

Mobile Health

With the current globalization, smartphones have become an integral part of people's lives with their use being applied in many industries. Healthcare system is certainly not left behind in adopting mobile technology in their treatment approaches. Mobile health is enough proof of mobile technology's importance in the healthcare system. MHealth applications have dominated the healthcare landscape due to their capability to simplify access to care and deliver greater care experience from both the health professionals' and the patient's perspectives. The mobile health applications have not only developed into a vibrant ecosystem or a market that is not only dynamic but also provides massive potential. With the adoption of smartphones in the medical care sector proliferating, the business opportunity for MHealth is great.

The fast-growing digital sector, as well as the slow, paced healthcare sector continues to collide thus bringing disruptive alterations to the market. However, the MHealth applications market has been increasing steadily over the last few years with the emergence of the novel technologies, novel business models as well as novel workflows that are revolutionizing the healthcare industry (Stephanie et al, 2017). Shareholders within the healthcare sector are giving life to these revolutionary MHealth solutions. The innovation of the mobile technologies is accelerating fast and maintains a great promise with evidence of these tools playing a positive role in costs of care as well as patient outcomes.

Statistics on Mobile Health

The number of mobile health applications in the present market has proliferated substantially. There are now more than 318,000 health applications available on the top app stores across the globe, approximately double the number of apps which were available in 2015 with more than 200 apps being added in every single day (Källander et al, 2013). The worldwide MHealth apps market is estimated to be valued at 28.320 billion dollars as of 2018 and is postulated to reach 102.35 billion dollars by 2023 (Källander et al, 2013). The core driving aspects motivating the growth of the MHealth market is the up surged adoption of mobile phones and the continued heavy investments into the digital medical market. Källander et al (2013) assert that healthcare consumers continue to show a robust use of digital technology, with numbers increasing annually. Actually, nearly 75% of users surveyed stated that technology is essential to managing their health. This study also recorded increases across the board in the use of smartphones, social media, online communities, electronic health records, and wearable devices. Particularly, approximately half of the healthy population (48%) is consuming MHealth apps compared to 16% consumption in 2014 (Källander et al, 2013).

Healthcare users are taking advantage of the fact that they can use their smartphones anytime and anywhere to access care. In actual fact, nearly 79% of respondents are more likely to identify a caregiver who enhances them to conduct healthcare interactions whether online or on smartphones. Moreover, 50% of consumers are promising to leave their current providers for one that undertakes better technology (Robbins et al, 2017). With this constant and widespread adoption of mobile technologies, mobile technology has evolved as a novel subfield of health. As the eHealth is widely focused on information and communication technologies, mhealth looks forward to discovering more into mobile devices as well as wireless communication. Up to this time, no standardized definitions for MHealth have been recognized. However, WHO defines MHealth as the use of smartphones, personal digital assistants, other wireless communications, and monitoring devices to aid health and public health practice. It was postulated that 50% of persons in remote areas across the world would own mobile phones by 2012 while 500 million individuals would have access to these mobile phones MHealth applications by the year 2015 (Carroll et al, 2017). Accordingly, MHealth is likely to carry all the promises of Electronic Health.

From 2015, approximately 64%, which amounts to about two-thirds of the United States citizens owned smartphones. This is a proliferation from a 35% recorded in 2011 and it is estimated that 90% of the global population will own a smartphone by 2020 (Carroll et al, 2017). According to the current UK data, it is revealed that smartphone usage is up-surging as 66% of the adult population had possession of a mobile phone in the year 2015. This is an upsurge from 61% in the year 2014. Smartphone possession is higher among younger individuals with about 77% possession for those within the 16-24 age brackets (Carroll et al, 2017). Although smartphones possession is particularly higher among young people and those with higher educational achievement and income, those that have a lower income, as well as educational success, is presently probable to be smartphones dependent. This is to mean that they fail to have broadband access at home and have few other options for web-based access other than through smartphones.

Notably, the upsurge of smartphone ownership has led to an increase in the percent of mobile phone apps in the marketplace. Most of these applications are designed to promote health with more than 100,000 health applications available in the Google store as well as iTunes (Carroll et al, 2017). This massive number speaks to both the vast market as well as the ongoing demand for novel tools to assist the public to manage their limitations of the current medical care system to offer such resources. It also helps the public to manage weight-related aims, diet, and fitness. According to a recent study by Carroll et al (2017), about 53% of mobile phones owners possess a smartphone which translates to nearly 45% of all US adults and half of this population has used their phones for looking up on their medical information. While America leads the market in the MHelth growth, other markets are illustrating growth too. For instance, the Asian-Pacific is estimated to develop at a higher rate of more than 35% thus making it the fastest growing MHealth market. According to Carroll et al (2017) research, it is estimated that the United Kingdom, Germany as well as France accounts for 45% share in the Europe mobile health device market as of the year 2014. Thus, it is okay to conclude that MHealth technologies are increasing in popularity worldwide and as a result revolutionizing the face of healthcare. Additionally, there is proliferating usage of health apps among caregivers, patients, as well as the general public. It is good to note that, these apps can only play a role in creating awareness, remote monitoring of individuals, illness self-management, and collection of dietary information (Carroll et al, 2017).

Approximately two-thirds of all adults in America own smartphones or powerful personal computers and tablets that are portable and always connected to the internet. These devices have the capacity to run sophisticated mobile applications which can help the health professionals and caregivers to understand where the patients are and what they are doing in regards to maintaining their health through following keenly on the prescribed activities. Notably, these applications are powerful as they are connected to an extensive array of other devices from wearable sensors to other health systems. The growth of smartphones has wide-ranging implications for the entire healthcare system. In simpler terms, smartphones, as well as other mobile technologies, seem to be the single most promising avenue health professionals have to assist individuals to manage their health and to do so at a certain measure. From encouraging patients to do physical activity to aiding cancer patients with the management of chemotherapy side effects, MHealth is progressively becoming a core platform for delivering medical interventions.

Using technologies such as the text messaging and personal digital assistants as well as smartphones apps, mobile health has a boundless perspective to reduce health problems and advance healthcare delivery, especially in the low and middle-income communities. Abaza & Marschollek (2017) contends that the texting programs have been carried out to create awareness to patients and educate patients, promoting reporting and communication, aiding in data collection of health records, and offering adherence and appointment reminders. Moreover, SMS has also helped to advance maternal as well as children medical health by taking women through the various levels of pregnancy. In addition, personal digital assistants have been used to offer home-based counseling and gathering important medical data that is necessary for identifying some illnesses such as HIV and TB (Abaza & Marschollek, 2017).

Recent applications in the healthcare industry offer consumers with several functions similar to those offered by computers applications. Anshari & Almunawar (2016) claims that most of the healthcare-related apps are available and are easily downloadable from some of the well-known download sites. These apps in the healthcare system can be designed to aid healthcare providers to better their services and work products such as offering online access to health data, health imaging as well as laboratory outcomes. There are several mobile applications that will allow patients to use their mobile phones to track their medical states such as monitoring their heart rate, emergency unit control, and their heart rate.

Health and fitness mobile applications usage has grown by more than 330% in recent years. Advances in artificial intelligence presently enhance apps to comprehend patient cases and respond to questions from consumers with appropriate follow-up inquiries. Fitness, as well as nutrition apps, follow caloric consumption. Integration with some sensors such as the wearable devices expands their capacities dramatically. In fact, health and fitness applications illustrate very high retention rates. As stated in a study by Flurry Analytics, more than 75% of active consumers access their fitness apps at least twice per week and more than 25% of consumers access their health apps over ten times weekly (Anshari & Almunawar, 2016). The great rate of recurrence of usage pushes up involvement, which for app developers offers an attractive chance to upsurge monetization.

Focus Areas

Clearly, the recent explosion in the mobile health invention has come from both the development of research in health sciences, human-computer interactions, and growth in the commercial industry. Commercial fitness mobile technologies such as Nike Fuelband and Fitbit have brought the mobile health into the conventional path, while the health research is making efforts towards developing novel ways to aid patient's efforts to manage their health and to test the effectiveness of the resulting interventions (Klasnja & Pratt, 2014).

A key focus of mobile health research and development in the recent past has been on assisting patients to adopt and maintain healthy lifestyles. Poor diets, behavior risk factors, physical inactivity as well as smoking conducts are core contributors to a prevalent of chronic conditions including chronic illness with high expenses in relation to the human suffering as well as healthcare costs. Until now, these conditions are largely preventable and many recent mobile health technologies have focused on helping patients to improve their health by adopting healthier behaviors (Klasnja & Pratt, 2014). Mobile health technology applications use four major approaches to encourage healthy habits such as social influence, goal setting, gamification, tracking, and feedback.

Interestingly, the main features of almost all MHealth applications are currently being used in tracking health-related habits and offering feedback on those habits. This process is mainly referred to as self-monitoring and has been largely used to support healthy habits change ever since the 1970s and can be efficient for changing an extensive array of habits, from obsessive cogitation to physical activities (Klasnja & Pratt, 2014). Mobile health applications are building a strong and practical self-monitoring practice by simplifying the collection of habit data and by offering individuals with real-time feedback on how they are operating with respect to their behavior change objectives.

In addition, MHealth is a promising and insightful tool for timely and scalable aid of wellness activities and continuity of users care outside the healthcare center. According to Klasnja & Pratt (2014), physical activity trackers such as the Fitbit technology, Bluetooth equipped devices for monitoring the heart rate among other emerging sensors are driving the mHealth applications to track data about users' habits and gives feedback that places a minimal burden thus greatly easing the self-monitoring process. Almost all the wellness applications offer feedback often in the daily or weekly data of tracked activities. Some applications even go to an extra mile of providing the user with charts of more than one type of activity, allowing users to look for patterns in their information and formulate hypotheses in regards to how their activities are connected to each other (Klasnja & Pratt, 2014). This feedback does not only offer the charts but also encourage physical activities. Applications such as the UbiFit offers patients with feedback in the flower garden format on the phone's wallpaper, allowing them to view how active they have been that period of monitoring every time they use their smartphones. Notably, nearly all sensing mobile technologies offer feedback directly on the sensing device allowing users to quickly view how they are progressing without reaching for their smartphones (Klasnja & Pratt, 2014). Such advancements to tracking and receiving feedback are assisting patients to monitor their health activities more efficiently, more easily, and over long periods of time.

The ability to track progress allows MHealth applications to apply a number of other approaches for inspiring healthy activities. One common approach is goal setting. In most of the mobile health applications, patients are able to set goals and to monitor how they are progressing towards those goals. Recent mobile applications discover how to set such medical behavioral goals most efficiently. For instance, such applications such as GoalPost allow patients to set two physical activity aims, the main aim, and a backup aim. Including the backup aim can aid patients to stay inspired and active even during times when they are too busy to attain their primary aim (Klasnja & Pratt, 2014). Such inventions can assist individuals to deal with the chaos of everyday life that result in perfectly regular routines which are hard even for those with the best of intentions.

Along with inspiring healthier behaviors, mobile health applications have a remarkable potential to help patient care outside the healthcare center, where, in due course, users manage their health conditions. Much of the efforts in this area have paid attention to three strategies including, automated decision support, symptom monitoring, as well as self-management training. MHealth applications thus help the care providers to coach patients on how to effectively manage their health conditions. According to Klasnja & Pratt (2014), management of numerous conditions necessitates that patient's symptoms are constantly tracked so that worsening in the individual's state is at the appointed time sensed and treated. MHealth applications make continuous tracking of conditions through the use of sensors or regular self-report possible. This increases the possibility of timely attention and treatment to the worsening of health conditions. By monitoring patient's data such as blood pressure, heart rate, and weight management, health professionals are capable of reducing the rate of patient's hospitalization significantly. Also, the length of hospitalization is reduced at cases when the individuals are hospitalized. Symptom monitoring technologies can assist users to gain care when the necessity first arises, offering them peace of mind and aiding in preventing grave or even fatal health occurrences (Klasnja & Pratt, 2014).

Furthermore, MHealth applications can contain medical knowledge and offer patients with immediate decision support anytime that they need irrespective of whether a caregiver is available. For instance, a health application for management of chemotherapy side effects offers individuals tailored management plans for their reported symptoms. Depending on the reported severity of the patient, they are advised to take different measures such as drinking a lot of fluids, taking certain medication, and rehydration sachets (Klasnja & Pratt, 2014). Such applications help in detecting when the user's condition is worsening and offers immediate advice on what the patient ought to do, increasing the likelihood that the symptoms are dealt with a suitable and timely manner.

In light of the above discussion, it is evident that the MHealth applications offer a great promise for outpatient care as it goes beyond monitoring of symptoms and training. The emergence of the portable sensors that connect to smartphones, such as the electrocardiograms makes it probable for the healthcare system to considerably increase access to high-quality care even in the rural as well as in the under-privileged societies. Equipped with mobile phones and several pocket-size devices, and linked to the regional health center through a video call, community caregivers can act as the observers for the high health professionals in areas where access to the health specialty care is limited. When implemented at a scale, mobile health models could aid in closing the divide in access to care faced by numerous communities across the state and globally.

RESEARCH METHODOLOGY

In the design and development of DiaMonD, a longitudinal research methodology was adopted. This methodology included qualitative and quantitative components, moreover, it subscribed to a user-centred design approach with co-creation following key principles of a design science research methodology Goldberg 2002a-d, Wickramasinghe et al., 2019). The developed DiaMonD solution was then tested in a clinical trial setting using a two arm strategy (Wickramasinghe et al, 2019).

DiaMonD (Diabetes Monitoring Device)

Recognising that, early detection and proactive management of diabetes is essential (Wickramasinghe et al., 2011; Wickramasinghe et al., 2014), DiaMonD (Diabetes monitoring device) was developed to provide patients with diabetes appropriate monitoring to enable better assessment and control of blood

Figure 1.
(adapted from Wickramasinghe et al 2019)

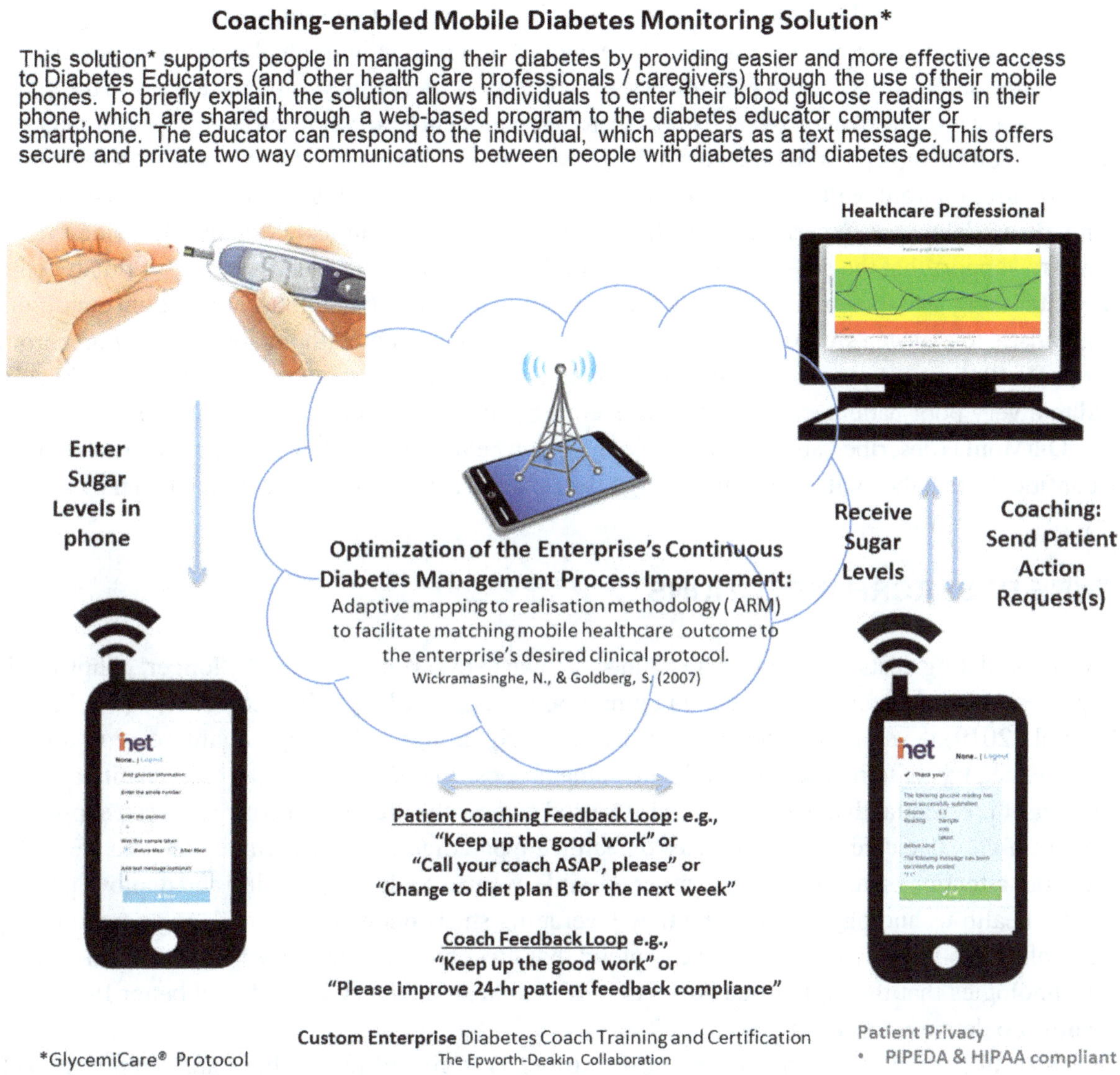

glucose and thus also prevent further complications (Goldberg 2002a-d). Basically, the solution utilizes pervasive mobile technology to transfer critical information between patient and providers so that superior monitoring may ensue. This solution has proved successful in assisting to lower HbA1C (the universally recognised marker for diabetes) in trials in Canada and the US (ibid). Critical success factors around the design of this solution include the use of a user-centred design approach, co-creation and subscribing to a design science research methodology which ensured high useability, usefulness and desirability.

SOLUTIONS AND RECOMMENDATIONS

Solutions such as DiaMonD enable the patient to continually monitor and self-manage to a large extent their diabetes (or other chronic condition). This means that when an individual who has a pre-existing chronic condition or co-morbidity presents for an acute care intervention such as a knew arthroplasty they can already provide evidence that their diabetes (or other chronic condition) is being well managed and they are following a prescribed care plan. This will in turn enable healthcare providers to be comfortable to move forward with the presenting issue that requires surgical intervention and hence form the patient side no delays are experienced and from the provider and healthcare organisation side there is evidence to support that the pre-existing chronic condition is being managed. In today's climate where we are witnessing an exponential growth in the incidents of at least one if not more chronic conditions, it is unrealistic to expect a significant percentage of patients to present without any pre-existing chronic condition. If all these patients are to wait until their HbA1C is at an appropriate level, this is surely going to lead to a very poor patient experience. However, if by utilising digital health and wellness solutions such as DiaMonD (described above) patients not only can better manage their chronic condition but also have confidence that they will be able to undergo the required acute care intervention when they present.

FUTURE RESEACRH DIRECTIONS

Given the escalating costs in most OECD countries to keep everyone stronger for longer, coupled with the rapid rise of chronic conditions and an aging population with longer life expectancy (Wickramasinghe et al., 2019) developing superior approaches to deliver high value, high quality care to all is an imperative; i.e., trying to realise the healthcare value proposition of better access, high quality and high value. Thus it is essential that more research is focused on how the digital transformation can support the delivery of high value care and a value-based healthcare paradigm. This is certainly an area we will be focusing our attention on and looking for other possible avenues to design, develop and deploy appropriate digital health technology solutions be they leveraging smart phone technology, augmented reality/virtual reality, bio-printing or sensors. We contend that it is only through the responsible harnessing of such technologies that the digital transformation of healthcare delivery can effect a better future state for healthcare delivery for us all.

One area in particular we will be exploring further is in regard to coaching and supporting self-management skills.

Coaching and Self-Management Skills in Chronic Diseases

Health coaching and self-management initiatives have attracted an increasing interest in the recent past, driven partially by the growing share of nearly 60% of American adults who have acute conditions (Horton, 2016). These skills are quite useful especially when an individual's condition can be improved through a change in lifestyle or when it necessitates that a patient ought to learn novel methods for monitoring and managing their daily healthcare. Health coaching and self-empowerment, therefore, focus majorly on people with chronic but manageable acute illnesses such as diabetes.

According to Bennett et al (2010), self-management refers to the behaviors that a patient engages in with the aim of advancing their health and actively managing illness Francis et al (2007) in their research found that controlling acute conditions is a hard task and produces a set of difficulties for the patient and their kindred. Therefore, advancing the patient's self-empowerment pertaining to the acute conditions has the potential to progress outcomes such as optimizing quality healthcare, minimizing blood glucose and pressure levels, reducing hemoglobin, and lessening the care service use. Self-management is thus considered to be an important motivating element that helps individuals to take up the roles of the primary caregiver and the healthcare practitioners support and inspires the individual to assume full charge for their personal health. According to Horton (2016), self-management is based on the idea of medical practitioners resolving concerns crucial to the patient with acute conditions.

Wong-Rieger & Rieger (2013) indicates that the most important driving force pertaining to the interest in self-management is the potential to come up with considerable contributions to effective healthcare delivery, as proven by the growing patient engagement in healthcare; advancing application of preventive measures, and lessening reliance on formal care services by improved management of the existing chronic conditions. A report from a number of studies indicates that providing better-quality healthcare necessitates an all-inclusive system approach, which includes increasing health literacy and building productive relations between the dynamically informed individuals and the appropriately prepared healthcare professionals (Francis et al, 2007). Therefore, restructuring primary care to foster better-quality, incorporated, and constant care services that center on the patient and the society is needed to respond to the challenge of acute conditions. Additionally, it is very crucial for acutely ill patients to identify symptoms early and to actively take suitable self-care strategies to possibly mitigate the hospital readmissions and emergency departments (Dye et al, 2018). Health reform programs have a great necessity for accessibility to affordable primary healthcare, advancements in wellness and prevention, and proficiency in healthcare management.

A similar concept to self-management is health coaching. According to the international coaching federation, this approach involves engaging individuals in a thought-provoking and creative practice that motivates them to optimize their own and professional potential. Hospitals are now more responsible for acutely ill patient outcomes due to the transformation of the healthcare systems to value-based initiatives that lead to a decline in the use of preventable emergency department as well as readmissions to health centers (Wong-Rieger & Rieger, 2013). As a result, varying functions have arisen to accolade provision of acute services and advance results of the acutely ill individuals. For instance, patient guides help individuals by reducing hindrances to timely diagnosis as well as therapy. Healthcare delivery administrators and clinical health coaches assist in post-discharge development and treatment synchronization to minimize readmissions. Health coaching is thus defined as a health education technique that advocates for lifestyle changes through a coaching framework that has supported the advance of acute situation self-care. Trainers or coaches have thus been used in a number of situations including the care system, private and social settings.

According to Francis et al (2007), most of these self-management and health coaching inventiveness have been implemented in recognition that treating acute illness needs a novel model of healthcare. These initiatives are intended to mitigate the pricey health crises, for instance, numerous visits to the emergency room, that result from pitiable management of acute conditions and to advance long-term results for patients. Recently, studies have shown that self-empowerment and coaching programs are the only platforms where there is available capacity within the present-day healthcare system for developing better-quality care and minimizing healthcare costs (Hourton, 2016).

According to Dye et al (2018) self-management mediations are often tailored specifically to the needs, life situations, current activation level or involvement of individuals, characteristics such as health literacy, and competence in monitoring their health. Having a dynamic role in self-care of a long-term health situation can enable patients to act for themselves and grow their confidence as it helps them to develop self-efficacy skills to control the multidimensional consequences of chronic illness such as cancer and its treatment. In this case, therefore, self-empowerment and health coaching aids patients to become active partners in their daily healthcare. Well-organized self-care education promotes effective communication with primary caregivers and efficient use of resources such as system navigation (BSpPath, 2012). Similarly, successful self-care initiatives include personalized assessment to enable each individual's apprehension of and confidence in taking care of their acute disease. Teaching and health coaching by a specialist in both self-management knowledge and skills for promoting behavior change, and assistance from the corporation and guidance of a group of health professionals, are critical components to active self-management initiatives. Furthermore, facilitating the adoption of health behaviors by means of coaching individuals in goal setting and action formation and aiding patients' development of problem-solving competence are also critical aspects of efficient self-empowerment education mediations.

CONCLUSION

Use of EHRs/EMRs has led to actual availability and use of data by clinicians to provide high quality and cost-effective care of their patients, hopefully leading to optimal outcomes and minimal complications and adverse events. Specific examples of patient selection based on projected impact to provider quality and outcomes that can lead to withholding of care are cited. The potential for denial or diminution of care for high risk populations, including socioeconomic and marginalized groups, may lead to a new digital divide and digital disparity if not accounted for in operationalizing new payment models. This chapter suggests that this conundrum can be resolved by turning to digital health solutions to provide on-going real time self-management support for chronic conditions such as diabetes so that patients can present to the acute care demonstrating prudent management of their chronic condition so that they can move forward with their required surgical intervention. This means that not only is a value-based care model support but in addition so is a better patient experience. Technology holds the key to this in the form of smart, person centred solutions such as DiaMonD that assist individuals to follow and adhere to an appropriate health and wellness trajectory. The impact of precision health and wellness is still at its infancy but we believe that if correctly and responsibly designed, developed and deployed we can witness not only high value care but also healthier populations and finally a decrease to the growth of chronic conditions.

REFERENCES

Betbeze, P. (2016). *Get comfortable with bundles.* www.healthleadersmedia.com

Bozic, K. (2016). *Transition to value based healthcare*. The Knee Society.

Bracy, C. (2016). *The healthcare value creation equation.* https://www.aaos.org/AAOSNow/2016/Apr/Managing/managing5/

Bumpass, D., & Samora, J. (2016). *Price transparency in healthcare: the other half of the value equation.* https://www.aaos.org/AAOSNow/2015/Jan/advocay/advocay1/?ssopc=1

Chang, B., Bakken, S., Brown, S., Houston, T., Kreps, G., Kukafka, R., . . . Stavri, Z. (2004). Bridging the digital divide: reaching vulnerable populations. *JAMIA, 11*, 448-457.

Economist. (2005). *Cherry picking profitable operations from general service hospitals.* https://economistsview.typepad.com/economistsview/2005/06/cherrypicking_p.html

Elf, M., Flink, M., Nilsson, M., Tistad, M., von Koch, L., & Ytterberg, C. (2017). The care of value-based healthcare for people living with complex long-term conditions. *BMC Health Services Research, 17*(24), 1-6.

Goldberg, S. (2002a). *Building the Evidence for a standardized Mobile Internet (wireless) Environment.* Internal Inet Documentation. Ontario, Canada: Inet.

Goldberg, S. (2002b). *HTA Presentation Rendering Component Summary.* Internal Inet documentation. Ontario, Canada: Inet.

Goldberg, S. (2002c). *HTA Quality Assurance Component Summary.* Internal Inet documentation. Ontario, Canada: Inet.

Goldberg, S. (2002d). *Wireless POC Device Component Summary.* Internal Inet documentation. Ontario, Canada: Inet.

Gray, M. (2018). Value based Healthcare. *BMJ, 356*, 1-2.

Haddad, P., Schaffer, J. L., & Wickramasinghe, N. (2015). Evaluating Business Value of IT in Healthcare: Three Clinical Practices from Australia and the US. In *EHealth-enabled Health: Proceedings of the 15th World Congress on Health and Biomedical Informatics* (*Vol. 216*, p. 183). IOS Press.

Hero, J., Blendon, R., Zaslavsky, A., & Campbell, A. (2016). Understanding what makes Americans Dissatisfied with their healthcare system: an international comparison. *Health Affairs, 35*(3), 502-509.

Hsu, J., Huang, J., Kinsman, J., Fireman, B., Miller, R., Selby, J., & Ortiz, E. (2005). Use of e-health services between 1999 and 2002 a growing digital divide. *Journal of the American Medical Informatics Association, 12*(2), 164–171. doi:10.1197/jamia.M1672 PMID:15561786

Kaplan, R., & Porter, E. (2011). *How to solve the cost crisis in healthcare.* Harvard Business Review Reprint R1109B.

Lynn, J. (2016). *Value based care hurting most vulnerable hospitals.* http://www.hospitalemrandehr.com/2016/03/25/value-based-care hurting-most-vulnerable-hospitals/

Moghimi, H., de Steiger, R., Schaffer, J., & Wickramasinghe, N. (2013). The benefits of adopting e performance Management Techniques. *Health & Technology, 3*(3), 237-247.

Pearlstein, S. (2005, June 8). Free Market Philosophy doesn't always work for healthcare. *Washington Post.*

Porter, M. (2010). What is value in healthcare? *The New England Journal of Medicine, 2010*(26), 2477–2481. doi:10.1056/NEJMp1011024 PMID:21142528

Porter, M., & Lee, T. (2013). *The strategy that will fix healthcare.* Harvard Business Review Reprint R1310B.

Porter, M., & Teisberg, E. (2009). *Redefining Healthcare.* Harvard Business Review Press.

Rauh, S., Wadsworth, E., & Weinstein, H. (2013). The Unintended consequences of Bundled Payments By weeks. *Annals of Internal Medicine, 158*(1), 62–64. doi:10.7326/0003-4819-158-1-201301010-00012 PMID:23277901

Sarkar, U., Karter, A., Liu, J., Adler, E., Nguyen, R., Lopez, A., & Schilling, D. J. (2011). Social disparities in internet patient portal use in diabetes: Evidence that the digital divide extends beyond access. *J. Am Med Infrom Assoc, 2011*(18), 318–321. doi:10.1136/jamia.2010.006015

Walker, D., Mora, A., Demosthenidy, M., Menachemi, N., & Diana, M. (2009). Meaningful Use of EHRs among Hospitals Ineligible for Incentives Lags Behind that of other hospitals, 2009-13. *Health Affairs, 35*(3), 495-501.

WHO. (2019). *Healthcare Service Delivery.* Available at https://www.who.int/healthsystems/topics/delivery/en/

Wickramasinghe, N., John, B., George, J., & Vogel, D. (2019). Achieving Value-Based Care in Chronic Disease Management. *Intervention Study JMIR Diabetes, 4*(2), e10368. doi:10.2196/10368 PMID:31066699

Wickramasinghe, N., Troshani, I., Hill SR., Hague W., & Goldberg, S. (2011). A transaction cost assessment of a pervasive technology solution for gestational diabetes. *International Journal of Healthcare Information Systems and Informatics, 6*(4), 60-76.

Wickramasinghe, S., Kliman, L., Vogel, D., & Goldberg, S. (2014). *Exploring the Possibility for a Pervasive Technology Solution to Facilitate Effective Diabetes Selfcare for Patients with GDM.* Paper presented at 2014 ECIS, Tel Aviv, Israel.

Yamin, C., Emani, S., Williams, D., Lipsitz, S., Karson, A., Wald, J., & Bates, D. (2011). The digital divide in adoption and use of a personal health record. *Intern Med, 171*(6), 568-574

Zuvekas, S., & Cohen, J. (2016). Fee-for-service, while much maligned, remains the dominant payment method for physician visits. *Health Affairs, 35*(3), 411-414.

ADDITIONAL READING

Abaza, H., & Marschollek, M. (2017). mHealth Application Areas and Technology Combinations. Methods of information in medicine, 56(S 01), e105-e122.

Anshari, M., & Almunawar, M. N. (2016). Mobile health (mhealth) services and Online health educators. Biomedical informatics insights, 8, BII-S35388.

Bennett, H. D., Coleman, E. A., Parry, C., Bodenheimer, T., & Chen, E. H. (2010). Health coaching for patients with chronic illness. *Family Practice Management, 17*(5), 24. PMID:21121566

BSpPath, A. H. B. H. (2012). Health coaching and motivational interviewing: Evaluating the chronic disease self-management toolbox as a resource for person-centered healthcare. *International Journal of Person Centered Medicine*, *2*(3), 520–530.

Dye, C., Willoughby, D., Aybar-Damali, B., Grady, C., Oran, R., & Knudson, A. (2018). Improving chronic disease self-management by older home health patients through community health coaching. *International Journal of Environmental Research and Public Health*, *15*(4), 660. doi:10.3390/ijerph15040660 PMID:29614803

Francis, C. F., Feyer, A. M., & Smith, B. J. (2007). Implementing chronic disease self-management in community settings: Lessons from Australian demonstration projects. *Australian Health Review*, *31*(4), 499–509. doi:10.1071/AH070499 PMID:17973606

Hillebregt, C. F., Vlonk, A. J., Bruijnzeels, M. A., van Schayck, O. C., & Chavannes, N. H. (2017). Barriers and facilitators influencing self-management among COPD patients: A mixed methods exploration in primary and affiliated specialist care. *International Journal of Chronic Obstructive Pulmonary Disease*, *12*, 123–133. doi:10.2147/COPD.S103998 PMID:28096666

Källander, K., Tibenderana, J. K., Akpogheneta, O. J., Strachan, D. L., Hill, Z., ten Asbroek, A. H., ... Meek, S. R. (2013). Mobile health (mHealth) approaches and lessons for increased performance and retention of community health workers in low-and-middle-income countries: A review. *Journal of Medical Internet Research*, *15*(1), e17. doi:10.2196/jmir.2130 PMID:23353680

Liddy, C., Johnston, S., Nash, K., Irving, H., & Davidson, R. (2016). Implementation and evolution of a regional chronic disease self-management program. *Canadian Journal of Public Health*, *107*(2), e194–e201. doi:10.17269/cjph.107.5126 PMID:27526218

Lovell, M. R., Luckett, T., Boyle, F. M., Phillips, J., Agar, M., & Davidson, P. M. (2014). Patient education, coaching, and self-management for cancer pain. *Journal of Clinical Oncology*, *32*(16), 1712–1720. doi:10.1200/JCO.2013.52.4850 PMID:24799486

Robbins, R., Krebs, P., Jagannathan, R., Jean-Louis, G., & Duncan, D. T. (2017). Health app use among US mobile phone users: Analysis of trends by chronic disease status. *JMIR mHealth and uHealth*, *5*(12), e197. doi:10.2196/mhealth.7832 PMID:29258981

Stephanie, W. Y., Hill, C., Ricks, M. L., Bennet, J., & Oriol, N. E. (2017). The scope and impact of mobile health clinics in the United States: A literature review. *International Journal for Equity in Health*, *16*(1), 178. doi:10.118612939-017-0671-2 PMID:28982362

Wong-Rieger, D., & Rieger, F. P. (2013). Health coaching in diabetes: Empowering patients to self-manage. *Canadian Journal of Diabetes*, *37*(1), 41–44. doi:10.1016/j.jcjd.2013.01.001 PMID:24070747

ENDNOTES

1. Medicare Access and CHIP Reauthorization Bct of 2015
2. Merit-based Incentive Payment System
3. https://www.healthquality.va.gov/guidelines/

Chapter 5
Digital Transformation Leadership for Smart Healthcare Organizations:
House of Success Model

Dina Ziadlou
https://orcid.org/0000-0002-7000-6462
Colorado Technical University, USA

ABSTRACT

The digital transformation has revolutionized the contexts of healthcare organizations in all aspects, and those hospitals that tend to create a smart digital environment are require to perceive vital factors of digital transformation. The author has created a framework called "House of Success" Model to elaborate on the significant organizational factors contributing to developing a smart healthcare organization in the digital era. This model consists of digital transformation, as the foundation of the house; quadruple aims, as the roof of the house and the ultimate goal of the transformation; and leadership and management, as the pillars of the house. Moreover, the house of success model has four rooms including change management and change leadership, people leadership, digital technology leadership, and the global partnership that resulted in building up a prosperous digital transformation outlook toward sustainable effectiveness development.

INTRODUCTION

The digital era generated by cutting-edge technologies and manifested in Artificial Intelligence (AI), Big Data, IoT, Cloud Computing, robotics, wearables, mobile computing, and virtual reality. The internet revolution has opened new doors for networking, decision making, human-human communication, and human-machine interaction that result in fundamental changes in many aspects such as lifestyle, businesses, trading, and healthcare. All industries, as well as the healthcare industry, have experienced new challenges and opportunities to adopt digital services and adapt to fast pacing changes.

DOI: 10.4018/978-1-7998-3274-4.ch005

In healthcare, digital technologies have changed the approaches of healthcare services, healthcare deliveries, disease management, and population health. The statistical reports have revealed that the digital market is dramatically increasing in the medical field. Dow Jones Institutional News (2016) reported that 77% of executive leaders put digital transformation in the top of their organizations priorities; they have broken down the budget to invest in Big Data and analytical technologies (58%), mobile and digital computing (36%), and SAAS (Software As A Service) (29%). Moreover, Faddis (2018) stated that the Internet of Things would exceed $136 billion in the medical field, and spending in digital transformation will reach $2.1 trillion by 2021. The global digital transformation valued $150.50 billion in 2015, and it will reach approximately $431.71 billion by 2021, and also, the hospital Artificial Intelligence market was evaluated at around $19 billion in 2016, and it is expected to reach $50.23 billion worldwide by 2023 (NewsRx, 2019b; Newswire, 2016).

Expectingly, digital technologies create productivity and dynamic in operation and process of healthcare, including quality improvement, accessibility, and cost-effectiveness as well as medical error reduction, performance improvement, and decision support development (Bowersox, Closs, & Drayer, 2005; Kane, 2015; Schwarzmüller, Brosi, Duman, & Welpe, 2018). The University College London Hospital (2019a) reports that utilizing the artificial intelligence and computer aid diagnosis systems in colonoscopy have reduced the variation in performance and improve decision supports services to detect polyps. Massachusetts General Hospital (2019b) defined AI applications as a potential solution in surgical practice and medical complex problems. Moreover, Royal Adelaide Hospital (2019) states, "The neural network was trained on images of 900 skulls virtually reconstructed from hospital CT scans. When tested on previously unseen images of skulls, the artificial neural network showed 95% accuracy at sex determination" [para1].

Despite all advancements, healthcare organizations are still in the primary stage of transforming into full smart healthcare. In the transformation journey, many hospitals have challenges to maximize the use of digital services due to the high cost of technologies, employees' resistance to change, regulations, complex processes, lack of leadership support, and disparities in healthcare deliveries (Agarwal, DesRoches, & Jha, 2010; Buvat et al., 2018; Faddis, 2018). Therefore, the transition from the traditional model of hospitals to modern medical centers is a sophisticated journey that must be structured in a conceptual model. This transition recalls a beautiful metaphor of caterpillar's journey toward turning into a beautiful butterfly shown in Figure 1 that takes time and many efforts to obtain successful outcomes. For elaborating significant parts of healthcare transformation, the author has structured a model called "*House of Success*."

BACKGROUND

Digital transformation phenomena in healthcare have created favorable and unfavorable consequences for healthcare organizations. Many hospitals are endeavoring to establish digital health technologies to stay competitive in the digital arena. However, there is a lack of a guide that enlightens the road map of hospitals toward uncovering the essential organizational factors in establishing smart healthcare. This research is attempting to elaborate on the significant factors contributing to digital transformation, including people, change, technology, leadership, and partnership to achieve Quadruple Aims of healthcare. This research is an in-depth literature review, monitoring the medical centers' approaches in embracing the digital changes, exploration of healthcare strategies in establishing digital health, and

Figure 1. The digital transformation as a metaphor for the butterfly journey
Permission for using the picture was obtained. The photo is credited to Minch Lewis.

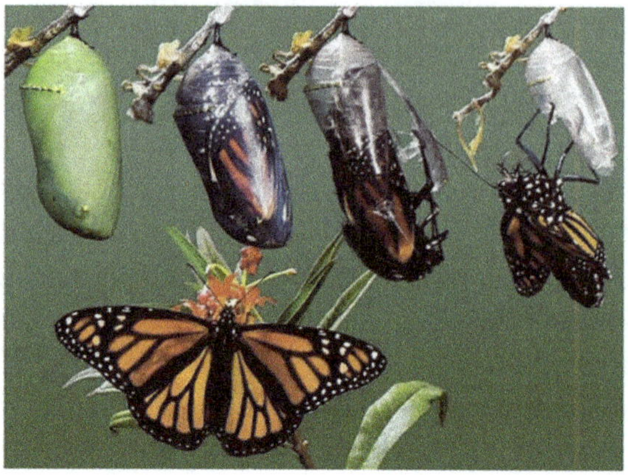

also the experience of the author in practicing the digital health establishment. The author has created a framework with the name of "*House of Success*" to elaborate on the essential factors in digital transformation leadership, contributing to creating smart healthcare organizations.

MAIN FOCUS OF THIS CHAPTER

The focus of the chapter is to introduce the significant factors in digital transformation for creating smart healthcare organizations. To do so, the author has created a model called *House of Success* to introduce the components of digital transformation leadership. Also, the author conducted an in-depth exploration of each component of House of Success to create a comprehensive framework for healthcare organizations. The factors are contributing to digital transformation (DT) leadership for the smart healthcare organizations shown in Figure 2 as the House of Success Model.

The *House of Success Model* consists of essential components in digital transformation leadership, including (1) foundation, which is digital technologies, as the basement of the house, (2) Quadruple Aims, as the roof of the house, (3) leadership and management, as the pillars of the house, and (4) human capital leadership, digital technology leadership, change leadership, and globalization, as the four rooms and body of the house. Therefore, this chapter has been allocated exclusively to delineate these critical components of the house as the critical success factors in the digital transformation leadership to improve the healthcare continuum.

Foundation of House of Success

The foundation of the house of success is digital technologies, as the root causes of changes in many modern businesses that create digital transformation (DT) concept. DT refers to the integration of digital technologies in all dimensions of a business; the digital transformation flow is revolutionizing the business context from infrastructure, process, technology, financial, and operational services to cultural, behavioral, and climate of the organization(Roth & Keller, 2019; Schwarzmüller et al., 2018).

Figure 2. The house of success

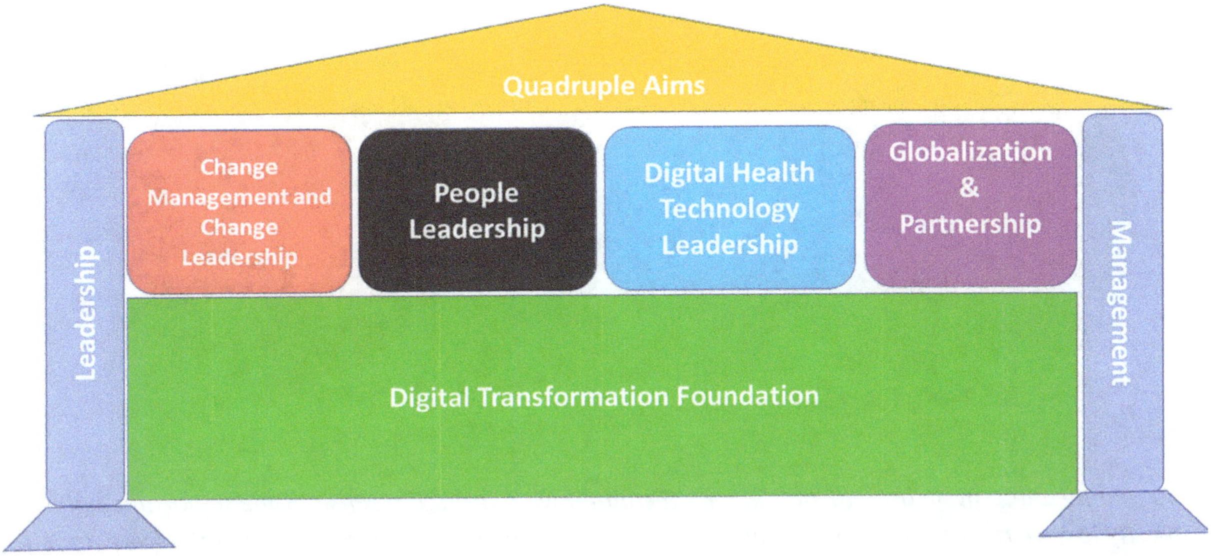

The digitalization via the Artificial Intelligence (AI), Big Data, Cloud Computing, and the Internet of Things (IoT) has shaped the digital medical systems, such as robotic surgery, wearable sensors, real-time location system (RTLS), Clinical Decision Support Systems (DSS), Electronic Medical Records (EMR), telehealth, m-Health, and virtual nursing in order to improve quality, develop access, and reduce cost of healthcare (Bauer, 2002; Coile Jr, 2000; McCullough, Casey, Moscovice, & Prasad, 2010). For instance, the hospitals establish paperless systems such as PACS (Picture Archiving and Communication Systems), as one of the revolutions of digital services, to (1) minimize papers waste; (2) improve access of radiologists' network nationwide; (3) develop telecommunication systems (4) facilitate communication among patients, providers, nurses, and staff; and (5) improve automated systems to provide patient privacy and medical data security (Wang & Alexander, 2013).

Quadruple Aims

In 2014, Bodenheimer & Sinsky introduced the Quadruple Aims and stated it is time to shift from Triple Aims to Quadruple Aims. In Triple Aim, as shown in Figure 3 (1) increase Cost-effectiveness, (2) promote population health, (3) enhance patient experience is the tope bottom line of healthcare, and Quadruple Aim added the fourth element in healthcare goals, which is employees' work-life balance improvement (Bodenheimer & Sinsky, 2014). In quadruple aims, improving work-life balance among the healthcare workforce is highlighted because the healthcare system realized that a value-based system must not only improve the patient experience, but also it must increase the employees' joyfulness, happiness, and satisfaction in order to receive best patients experience (Bodenheimer & Sinsky, 2014). Sikka, Morath, and Leape (2015) stated:

The core of workforce engagement is the experience of joy and meaning in the work of healthcare. This is not synonymous with happiness, rather than all members of the workforce have a sense of accomplish-

Figure 3. The transition from triple aims to Quadruple Aims

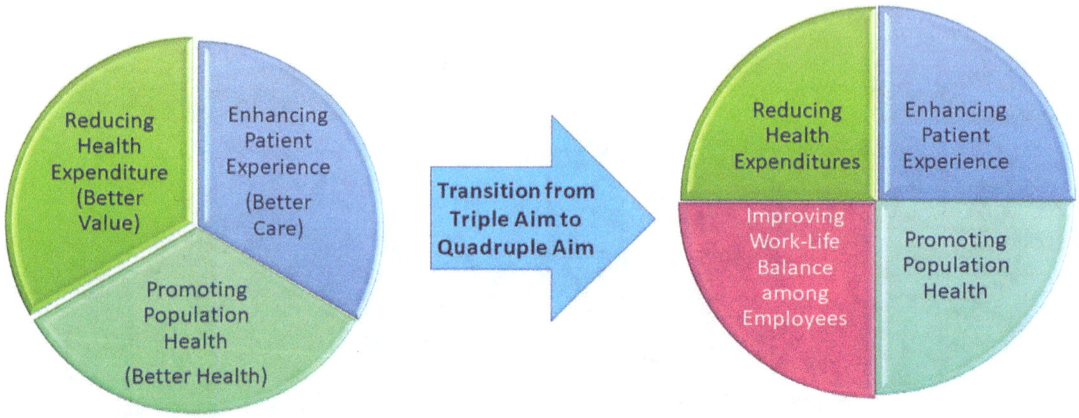

ment and meaning in their contributions. By meaning, we refer to the sense of the importance of daily work. By joy, we refer to the feeling of success and fulfillment that results from meaningful work. (p. 608)

Accordingly, the Institue for Healthcare Improvement (IHI) (2012) discussed that there is a meaningful correlation between healthcare providers' engagement and patient engagement; the staffs who feel respected, valued, and supported are likely more productive than unsatisfied employees. According to Quadruple Aim, a healthy work environment is a place where the workforce has a sense of contribution and accomplishment.

Management and Leadership

The leadership and management are the pillars of the *House of Success* in digital transformation; the organizations need both management and leadership to stay alive and make progress. However, there is a difference between these two concepts. According to Gill (2003), Mintzberg (2009), and Nahavandi (2015), the leadership is an art of human resource empowerment, inspiration, and motivation toward accomplishing goals, values, integrity, trust, and dignity, and the management refers to maintain the existing structure through delegating, communicating, controlling, and monitoring the subordinates to perform their assigned tasks. The leaders endeavor to lead organizations to attain goals, whereas managers. Indeed, leadership is relationship-oriented to create shared value and influencing followers to achieve the desired future, and it is about people's leadership; on the other hand, management is task-oriented, and it is about processes improvement and task management. Nahavandi (2015) stated that leadership focuses on the future to create change based on shared values and emotional connection, but management focuses on the present and to maintain policies and procedures and stabilize the status quo.

The postmodern and modern organizations are endeavoring to inject the leadership skills not only in top leaders but also among directors and managers to combine task-oriented activities and technical skills with relationship-oriented skills. The managers who motivate the employees to accomplish goals, discover talents, and create harmony between employees' performance and organizational goals are the managers who are stepping toward leadership skills (Bennis, Sample, & Asghar, 2015; Nahavandi, 2015).

In digital transformation, the healthcare organizations require the managers filling the gap between employees and leadership level; the managers can perceive the emergence of change in the system and facilitate the process of cultivating the change agents in the system. According to Lipinski (2013), “Organization Development (OD) is the process of creating a model of influence based on the vision and goals of an organization that, when implemented, attempt to obtain a successful outcome for that organization” (p. 64).

Change Management and Change Leadership

We talked about digital technologies, as the basement of House of Success, Quadruple Aim as an umbrella term for achieving healthcare goals, and leaders and managers as pillars of the house. Now, the body of the House of Success consists of four rooms. The first room is about change management and change leadership. The definitions of change management and change leadership are used interchangeably in the management context. However, in digital transformation, the distinction between these two concepts boosts a better understanding of change aspects and constructing organizational development. Change management is defined as the set of processes and activities for preparing, planning, handling, and evaluating the status quo to shift from the current situation to the desired situation (Atchison, 1999; Kotter, 2012; Shafran, 2017). On the other hand, change leadership has referred the art of leadership to create a shared vision, inspire and motivate people, and empower the followers for transformation (Allman, 2009; Arbab Kash, Spaulding, Johnson, & Gamm, 2014; Gill, 2003; Kotter, 1995).

Although change management and change leadership differ in concept, they complete each other. According to Kotter (2012), change management focuses on processes to make the organization profitable and efficient; whereas, the change leadership focuses on the human capacities and their capabilities to nurture them as the change agents. Gardner (2009) stated that the root cause of most of the failures in organizational development is people, not systems; and the most significant constraint for organizational transformation is related to human behavior, action, and relation derived from employees' resistance, poor leadership, and cultural issues, not the complexity of technologies. From Gardner's perspective, the human-related factors in the change process are: (1) before change: resistance to change, poor developed strategy, no established plan, fear of change, poor leadership, and lack of knowledge and awareness of change; (2) during the change: lack of effective communication to share expectation about changes, inadequate support of management, and poor training; (3) after change: no culture development for institutionalize change (Gardner, 2009).

Adeyemi (2017) and Sheri-Lynne & Singh (2007) stated that although government regulations and competitive advantage are two main reasons for the change in the healthcare organizations, the leadership role, as a human-related factor, is one of the vital factors to attain successful changes in the digital transformation of healthcare systems. However, the focus is shifting from leadership-centric role to human value factors to attain successful transformation (Arbab Kash et al., 2014; Hartnell, 2012; PMP, 2018; ValueCenter, n.d.; Van Fleet & Peterson, 2016). Therefore, an in-depth study of human-related factors helps researchers to understand how to lead transformation in postmodern healthcare organizations. In this regard, the first step of digital transformation in smart healthcare organizations must address how to lead people and how to connect them with digital culture.

People Leadership

Comparatively speaking, the shift from traditional hospitals to modern healthcare organization was the revolution of the 21st century. The digital transformation has developed employees-leaders connections via Big Data. It has created a decision making support via artificial intelligence. It has expanded accessibility and convenience to care services through telemedicine. It has engaged patients with their health via mobile health. Moreover, it has increased the efficiency of performance via Electronic Medical Records. However, the role of human capital in embracing change and implementing transformation is the critical part. The human capital is defined as "individual capabilities, knowledge, skills, and experience of the company's employees and managers" (Dess, McNamara, Eisner, & Hyun, 2019, p. 106).

In people leadership category, the three significant factors impacted on leading people in digital transformation have been discussed as the first room of our House of success: (1) stakeholders' engagement, (2) human resource empowerment, and (3) culture development as it is displayed in Figure 4 (Adeyemi, 2017; Herscovitch, 2004; Kelly, 2016; Shuck, Twyford, Reio, & Shuck, 2014; Thomas, 2014; Walsh & Rumsfeld, 2017; Weinstein et al., 2008; Weston, 2017).

Figure 4. Three pivotal factors of leading people in digital transformation

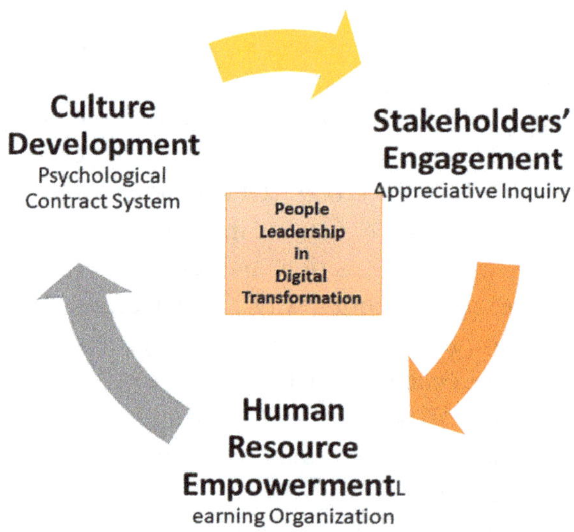

Digital Engagement Development

In modern and postmodern organizations, the attention of leaders must be on human-related factors in order to influence and transform the mindset and behavior of employees (Marshak & Grant, 2008). Nowadays, human capital is the core value of all organizations, and the cooperation of human resources delineates the success of the organization for achieving the desired future.

The employees' engagement is a process of promoting emotional and behavioral energy to attain organizational outcomes. In order to engage the employees in the change process, the leaders of the hospitals must contemplate how to empower and engage different types of stakeholders to create a healthy environment and develop a collective level of engagement (Olden, 2003; Shuck et al., 2014). Olden (2003) pointed out that three capabilities of stakeholders management consist of (1) identifying the type of stakeholders and their stakes, (2) developing organizational policies and procedure based on stakeholders' interest, (3) establishing workflow and bargaining to achieve missions. Accordingly, in the modern healthcare system, involving the physicians and employees in decision making, appreciating the employees, building trust, communicating effectively, and nurturing innovative thinking are the most policies toward cultivating a healthy organization (Adeyemi, 2017; Herscovitch, 2004; Scheer, 2016).

Thanks to technology, healthcare leaders can collect excellent resources to build strategic initiatives upon the employees' experiences and feedback through electronic survey systems during digital health adoption and implementation. The Electronic Medical Record (EMR) has been one of the achievements of the digital transformation, and an example of significant change initiatives in the hospitals, that has brought up the immense lesson learned for the hospitals (Stensaker & Meyer, 2011). Establishing the EMR has indicated that involving physicians, nurses, and employees in all phases of project (planning, implementation, post-implementation) as well as ensuring their adaption and adoption of digital technology, providing appropriate training, creating transparent processes, and providing financial incentives can improve engagement of employees in the process of change and reduce the resistance to change (Adeyemi, 2017; Aziz, 2007; K. H. Cohn, 2015; McCabe & Timmins, 2016).

Physicians and Nurses' Engagement

Notably, physicians and nurses have a critical role in the tangible and intangible outcomes of a hospital. Their engagement in digital transformation can impact on the profitability of the hospital. Cohn (2015) represented a study by Healthcare Consultancy Vital Work-Life and Physician Recruiting Firm Cejka Search among 1,600 physicians and indicated the top critical factor of physicians' engagement in the process of change is, "feeling that my opinions and ideas are valued and have a voice in how my time is structured and used" (p. 60). Furthermore, technology sustains healthcare outcomes. In this regard, McCabe and Timmins (2016) asserted, "Healthcare technology has the power to transform the nursing profession through collecting, synthesizing, and analyzing data about nursing care in a way that demonstrates its impact on the provision of quality outcomes in healthcare" (pp. 105-106).

Patients' Engagement

The horizon scanning of healthcare indicates that full patients' engagement in their health and self-management tools are the inevitable future for healthcare services. The digital technologies have enabled the patients to measure their body weight, heart rate (HR), blood pressure (BP), SPO2, respiratory rate (RR), monitor vital signs, collect all these data as well as blood glaucous and diet, and aggregate all health information in a database for sending to the providers electronically. Through digital technologies, the information can send real-time and with passing the waiting time in doctors' office, transportation, and time and location dependency concerns. However, conceptualizing the digital health and engaging the patients to stay connected and be committed to self-care management are still the challenging points of the digitalization of healthcare.

Human Resource Empowerment

According to World Health Organization (WHO), the human resource empowerment is "a process through which people gain greater control over decisions and actions affecting their health, which signifies a process on both the individual and the community level" (Meskó, Radó, & Győrffy, 2019, p. 2). In people leadership, human resources are the most valuable capital in all organizations. Similarly, in healthcare organizations that serve the health and wellbeing of individuals, communities, and society, the employees are the source of productivity and growth of healthcare. Faddis (2018) argued that forecasting the hospitals' future clarifies that " management at the smart hospital can enhance its operational efficiencies by having a clear picture of asset and labor use based on productivity efficiencies, labor accountability, and the ability to identify solutions to low-performance metrics" (p. 37).

The digital era has significantly impacted the patient's-physicians' relationship and tied them to digital technologies. Nowadays, physicians and nurses utilize digital health from simple techniques such as patients' data entry to sophisticated systems such as robotic surgeries. Also, the patients become more informed and involved in their health through internet and m-Health services. They participate in their treatment and decision-making processes toward self-care management.

Physicians and Nurses Empowerment

Commins (2014) and Weiner (2016) conducted interviews among healthcare leaders and C-suites and cited physicians engagement as the most challenging part of hospital management. Moreover, physicians' involvement in transformation requires creating transparency, involving them in decision making, creating work-life balance, improving processes, and assigning decision-making authority (Commins, 2014; Ommaya et al., 2018; Weiner, 2016). According to Physicians Practice Perspective (2017), 85% of physicians stated that digital health could promote the outcome of healthcare, 45% of them were keen on using digital technologies such as telemedicine and remote patient monitoring, but only 14% of them have been experienced to utilize these technologies.

Furthermore, Wade, Taylor, Kidd, and Carati (2016) conducted a qualitative study to identify impact factors of shifting from the small scale of digital health projects (home telehealthcare) to large-scale projects; the results indicated that clinicians' technology acceptance and leadership support are first fundamental factors in starting establishing digital health projects. Hence, the hospitals must ensure the full acceptance of clinicians and professionals in digital transformation before diving to establish massive digital health changes. Moreover, Lloyd & Ferguson (2017) stated that educating nurses in health informatics and nurturing nursing workforce as informatics specialists may make a bridge between nursing and IT concepts toward creating a universal language of digital transformation; it would help to embrace digital health changes smoothly in healthcare organizations and accelerate the adoption and adaption of digital technologies.

Patients Empowerment

From the patients' perspective, Meskó et al. (2019) describe the patient's empowerment based on four factors: (1) patient roles clarification, (2) knowledge acquisition development, (3) patient skills development, and (4) relationship improvement. Through empowerment, the patients can control their health progression and plan for their future health. Educating, engaging, and motivating the patients are the keys to empowerment, and each hospital, clinic, the medical office is responsible for empowering the patients and promoting their knowledge in proactive collaboration in health-related resources (Carman et al., 2013; Mace, 2015; Nelson, 2014). Carmen et al. (2013) stated that patients' role in designing quality improvement projects in the hospitals and their decision-making authority as citizen involvement programs might foster the response of hospitals to patients' needs and patients' perspectives.

In 2011, the World Health Organization (WHO) reported the new horizon for mobile health. The report had evaluated factors such as awareness, communication, treatment compliance, and accountability of m-Health services for HIV/AIDS and H1N1 in American, European, African, and Eastern Mediterranean countries. According to this report, mobilization increases the participation and engagement of patients in their health monitoring and treatment (World Health Organization, 2011). About 50% of these countries adopt digital health in primary methods of m-health such as SMS-based initiatives, and 28% of Eastern Meditation, 28% of Europeans, and 25% of American regions announced that the m-Health was improved coordination of patients (World Health Organization, 2011).

Moreover, digital technologies such as telemedicine were reported as growing services by Americas (75%), South East Asia (62%), and European regions (64%). Respectively, African countries with 41% and South-East Asia, with 38%, showed the highest rate of health surveys and surveillance (World Health Organization, 2011). However, the lesson learned from all studies strongly emphasized the existence of a comprehensive program for knowledge development in digital health, while lack of knowledge was the main barrier to adopt digital health services. Also, the lack of prioritizing the financial resources allocated for digital health was the main obstacle in adopting the technology (World Health Organization, 2011).

Role of Healthcare Leaders in Human Capital Empowerment

The healthcare organizations must involve healthcare consumers in the decision-making processes, empowered consumers with tools such as Shared Decision Making (SDM) and Decision Aids (DAs) systems, they must develop internet-based communications such as personal health record (PHI), online peer support systems, and self-management tools with an attached survey to increase engagement and obtain feedback. Also, conducting the patients' interview, focus group, case management, and community involvement surveys in qualitative and quantitative methods to collect and analyze consumers' perspectives are the ways of society engagement(Sarrami, Travaglia, Debono, & Braithwaite, 2014). In the US, the Hospital Consumer Assessment of Healthcare Providers and Systems (HCAHPS) survey is one of the efficient tools to evaluate the patient's experience before, during, and aftercare (Moriarty, 2014). Calvillo, Román, and Roa (2015) state:

For real empowerment of patients, all citizens must be capable of accessing systems empowering them, no matter their digital literacy, economic level, education, or disabilities. Therefore, if obstacles and gaps are successfully addressed, at medium-term technology will ease the emergence of a new patient fully equipped for the health-care challenging scenarios of the 21st century. (p. 650)

Culture Development

The digital technology phenomenon was a fortuitous consequence of academic research that converted to the snowball effect and affected all aspects of our lives, including our culture. The culture encompasses all tangible and intangible behavioral aspects of people, including shared beliefs, values, feelings, thoughts, and behaviors in groups, which shape the organizational behavior (Robbins & Judge, 2017).

Buvat et al. (2018) stated that digital culture is the set of seven components: "customer-centricity, innovation, collaboration, digital-first mindset, agility and flexibility, open-culture, and data-driven decision making" (p. 3).

Although the organizational culture change is difficult and takes a long time, it is possible to happen if shared values agree with organizational effectiveness, and organizational climate aligns with the physiological atmospher. In 2017, Capgemini Digital Transformation Institute conducted a study across France, Italy, Germany, Spine, Netherland, Sweden, UK, and the US in 1700,340 organizations to evaluate top barriers in digital transformation. The results indicated that culture (62%) is the top roadblock in organizations. Kluge (2008) stated that the most challenging task in the digital evolution of healthcare is not technical or legal issues, it is about how to identify and create a cultural bridge between the present and future that validate the change. Thimbleby (2013) stated that technology is improving things and making the profit for organizations, whereas human culture does not make a tangible return on investment. It might be the reason for more incentive in technology development rather than culture development (Thimbleby, 2013). Likewise, Edgar Schein (2004) in his book *Organizational Culture, and Leadership* stated that culture is created by shared experience, but it is the leader who initiates this process by imposing his or her beliefs, values, and assumptions at the outset.

Gardenswartz, Rowe, Digh, & Bennett (2003) divided culture into three dimensions. First, the personal culture defined as the integration of personality, skills, interests, and value. Second, organizational culture referred to shared values, knowledge, morals, and believes that shape organizational practice. The third one is the national culture, which is the collection of behaviors, attitudes, norms, and customs of people that derive from their country's history and their origins. Springer, Clark, Faan, Strohfus, and Belcheir (2012) and Smollan and Sayers (2009) argued that the sustainable organizational culture is an intangible factor derived from attitude and reflection of employees, and it can make transformational actions. Bayan (2018) indicated that culture drives continuous knowledge development and talent empowerment to accelerate this process. However, the digital transformation will happen if the employees believe that digital technologies can help them toward their desired, positive future; investment in nurturing digital culture is one of the primary keys to attaining this aim.

Needs of Embracing Multicultural Environment

The economic indicators of global markets, as well as in the US healthcare market, indicate that not only global healthcare trade is increasing but also other indicators such as multiculturality is elevating due to demographic change, globalization, and digitalization. According to the Pew Research Center report, the US demographic trend is projected to be more diverse (59 million immigrants); 43 percent of the millennial generation is not white, and also, the women's roles in leadership are increasing (D. Cohn & Caumont, 2016). Moreover, digital technologies are crossing the borders and connecting all people around the globe with different cultures and values. Digital technologies such as telehealth have been dramatically expanded, and it is going to create a healthcare system without a wall in the future. Therefore, healthcare leaders must figure out how to lead multicultural environments and how to meet patients' and stakeholders' expectations beyond geographical borders. Also, physicians must understand the sociocultural background of patients who are affected by processes of care services via technologies such as telehealth and video conferencing examinations.

Patients Digital Culture Development

In addition to organizational culture development in digital transformation among the workforce, another essential point is to disseminate the culture of digital technologies among patients and healthcare users. However, it is essential to promote health literacy firstly, and afterward develop digital health technology literacy among the patients. In 2013, the WHO report revealed that health literacy is a stronger predictor of the formation of the state of health than income, education, or belonging to various ethnic groups" (Meskó, Drobni, Bényei, Gergely, & Győrffy, 2017, p. 5). Manganello et al. (2017) conducted a study to examine the association of health literacy and digital health; the result indicated that people with low health literacy have limited access and knowledge to use technologies for their healthcare services. Therefore, healthcare industries must apply artificial intelligence technologies, data processing, and data mining to detect and analyze the specifications of patients as well as the culture of the population to simulate and predict their response, behaviors, and health literacy in using of digital health services. In this regard, Manganello et al. (2017) and Meskó et al. (2017) reported that public health has a plan to disseminate preventive medicine via channels of health technologies, it will start with health literacy development and culture development of using digital technology to improve the culture of digital health among the patients.

Digital Health Technology Leadership

The third room of House of Success is digital health technology leadership. The transformation is manifested in shifting from traditional models to modern and post-modern organizations, from analog systems to digital world, from work-oriented employees to work-life balance-oriented workforce, from organizational hierarchy to holacracy organizations, and from linear thinking to nonlinear thinking. Agarwal, DesRoches, and Jha (2010) stated, "There is a substantial consensus that the digital transformation of healthcare through broad and deep use of health information technology (HIT) across the health-care ecosystem, in conjunction with other complementary changes, can reduce costs and improve quality" (p. 796).

According to the Center for Medicare and Medicaid Services' report, the US healthcare spending had increased from $256 billion in 1980 to $2.6 trillion in 2010, and the root cause analysis of this large tolerance was the establishment of digital transformation (Pinkney, 2013). Digital technology is penetrating the entire life cycle of organizations. Hence, the healthcare leaders and managers need to establish comprehensive plans in eight pivotal sections in the life cycle of health technology management shown in Figure 5 as follows:

- Horizon Scanning of Digital Healthcare
- Strategic Planning
- Digital Health Technology Assessment
- Digital Health Project Management
- Digital Health Process Improvement
- Seamless Digital Health Expansion
- Privacy And Security Development
- Continuous Improvement Institutionalization

Figure 5. Eight major elements of digital technology management

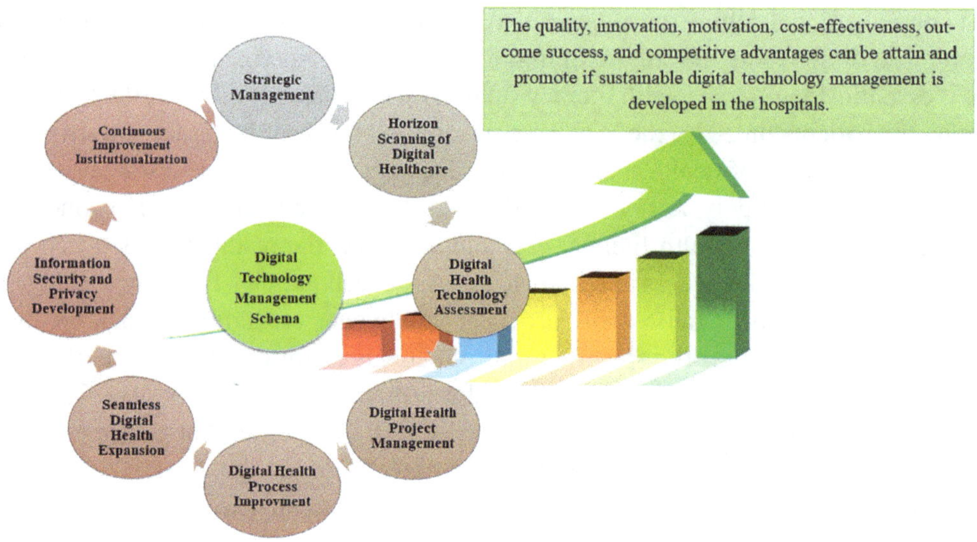

Strategic Planning

The promise of IoT, AI, telemedicine, wearable sensors, remote patient monitoring, and all digital health technologies are real. Notwithstanding, to keep up with the digital revolution, the hospitals must either launch comprehensive digital health strategies or reinvigorate the existing digital health strategies. Dess, McNamara, Eisner, & Hyun (2019) describe, "strategic management of an organization entitled three ongoing processes: analyses, decisions, and actions" (p. 6). The leaders and senior managers need analytics integration skills to produce actionable solutions through forecasting the future of health technologies and to align the digital health strategies continuously. Despite developing sustainable strategies to promote EMR and telehealth as efficient and practical ideas in healthcare organizations, these technologies created challenges in many medical centers due to the lack of a trade-off between present technologies and upcoming digital systems. Furthermore, given the reports, these technologies caused nurses' and physicians' burnout and harm interaction of physicians and patients in their operation (Kuza, 2017; Mary Norine & Rumsfeld, 2017; Morse, 2018; Ommaya et al., 2018). Reifsteck and Reese (2016) recommend the hospitals to establish a committee for oversight of digital health technologies as well as inviting community advisors with digital technology and business strategy experience to work closely with the committee before establishing many technologies.

Digital Health Technology Assessment (HTA)

Gutiérrez-Ibarluzea, Chiumente, and Dauben (2017) described the HTA as "the systematic evaluation of the properties and effects of health technology, addressing the direct and intended effects of this technology as well as its direct and indirect consequences, and aimed mainly at informing decision making regarding health technologies" (p. 1). The HTA can generate valuable information about the efficiency, effectiveness, and efficacy of digital technologies, which is useful for healthcare leaders and policymakers in decision making and strategic planning. Moreover, the HTA fills the gap between evidence and policy-making by providing legal, ethical, technical, economic, social, and organizational aspects (Vukovic, Favaretti, Ricciardi, & de Waure, 2018, p. 93).

Digital Health Technology Project Management

The healthcare organizations are cumbersome and complicated environments; establishing technologies, managing stakeholders, accommodating financial resources, managing risks, creating sustainable outcomes, and providing a balance between quality, cost, and access are sophisticated processes. For implementing the changes, the project management and project coordination are the approaches of healthcare facilities to ensure the scope of projects are being done by specified time with minimum risk and maximum success in initiating, planning, executing, controlling, and closing phases (Scheer, 2016; Tait, 2013). Given the reports, between 35% to 75% of projects change are failed, and most of HIT projects' failures are derived from lack of well-developed planning phase, 50% of failures are due to managerial issues, and 20% of failures come from a lack of effective communication (Scheer, 2016; Tait, 2013). Indeed, the project managers are the hands of leaders that translate and construct the strategies to tangible outcomes.

Digital Health Technology Process Improvement

While healthcare organizations embark sophisticated digital technologies, they must pay specific attention to processes, workflows, value-added, and non-value-added activities. Bourgeois and Stacy (2007) stated, "One of the most important critical success factors towards added value is the facilitation of efficient and effective information sharing in order to establish integrated process methods that improve decision making and balance demands and costs" (p. 8). The digital technologies implementation should not disrupt the clinical processes and clinicians' workflows. Otherwise, not only does it create quality but also waste million dollars, undermine efficiency, and diminish motivation of the workforce, Dyrda (2018, February) quoted from Jeff Swearingen's interview in Baker's Hospital review [para.9]. The process improvement is one of the critical parts of digital technology development because it can be the root of resistance to change, workforce burnout, dissatisfaction, and cost increment in healthcare organizations (Kelly, 2016; Scheer, 2016). Scheer (2016), based on Pricewaterhouse Coopers' Health Research Institute, stated, healthcare waste accounts for $1.2 trillion or more than 50% of the $2.2 trillion spent annually on healthcare. Likewise, the Center for Medicare and Medicaid Service (CMS) (2015) reported overall healthcare spending in 2010 as $2.6 trillion with waste accounting for 40% over the overall expenditures. Hence, the hospitals need to reduce wastes, including transportation, overproduction, waiting time, workflow, reproduction, inventory, human potential, and defect (Jiju, Snee, & Hoerl, 2017; Scheer, 2016). The solutions such as PDCA, Lean Management, Lean Six Sigma, and Kisen have been effective and efficient approaches to manage the processes and eliminate non-value-added activities in hospitals.

Seamless and Interoperable System Expansion

While the digital transformation of healthcare organizations is creating a healthcare system without a wall, the strategic decision-makers and healthcare leaders need to redefine healthcare deliveries, patients' experience, and employees' experience in order to develop a seamless healthcare system. A seamless, integrated system is a system that can aggregate all medical information of patients, public health, mental health, disaster response, and surveillance diseases as well as all information of stakeholders and healthcare plans in a universal database (ONC, 2014, p. x). The universal medical database is a system with the capability of interoperability with EMR, telehealth, m-Health, biometrics, remote patient monitoring, wearable sensors, public health information, and all health-related data to analyze and interpret the information into the actionable strategies. The goal of creating an interoperable healthcare system is to develop a learning health system that patients, patients 'families, providers, nurses, and all healthcare members securely exchange the information and actively collaborate in generating new knowledge and promoting healthcare outcomes (ONC, 2014).

Data Privacy and Security Information Development

One of the most significant challengings in health information management is to secure patient health information(PHI) and assure patients' rights. The proliferation of digital technologies resulted in the enacting of the Health Insurance Portability and Accountability Act (HIPAA) to address entitlements and disclosure of individuals' health data and to assure health information of all patients is protected (Office for Civil Rights, 2013).

According to the HIPAA Privacy Rule, while the cyber breach is a significant threat for healthcare organizations, the medical safeguard for patient privacy and information security must be implemented in all healthcare systems. Likewise, establishing standards and privacy regulations for storing, processing, and exchanging medical records, including the provisions for users and professionals, are the significant parts of the digitalization of healthcare organizations (Center for Control Diseases and Prevention, 2016). Therefore, healthcare leaders must proactively consider cybersecurity as an essential part of digital technology management.

Horizon Scanning of Digital Healthcare

While understanding the threats and risk is essential to manage non-linear changes, the techniques such as horizon scanning help organizations to recognize potential risks and opportunities, to prepare for responding to change, and to improve innovation (Brown, 2007). The horizon scanning of digital health technologies provides a systematic process for healthcare organizations; it provides techniques to monitor the future of digital technologies and to identify the progress of digitalization and mobilization of healthcare services in order to seize the innovations opportunities as well as create/align short term and long-term strategies for the highest quality in patients experience, workforce experience, clinical processes, and costs of care.

The ECRI Institute (2011) presented a protocol and operations manual of horizon scanning of healthcare to the order of Agency for Healthcare Research and Quality (AHRQ) to screen, diagnose, treat, monitor, manage, and follow up on healthcare deliveries, interventions, innovations, and procedures. The horizon scanning analysis illuminates disparities, paradigm shifts, and population health outcomes; afterward, the results can enlighten the strategic initiatives' road map (ECRI, 2011). Moreover, Morris (2013) in Becker's Hospital Review anticipated that in the future, the hospitals would be the places for extremely sick patients, and most of the other patients will be receiving healthcare services remotely by 2035.

Continues Improvement Institutionalization

The USAID Healthcare Improvement Project (HCI) defines "institutionalization as the establishment and maintenance of continuous improvement activities as integral and sustainable within the health system or other organization"(Smith & Saleem, 2013, p. iii). While creating a value-based healthcare system rather than volume-based services (quality rather than quantity) is the central goal of healthcare, a comprehensive plan to cultivate and measure the value continuously must encompass hospitals' operations, performance, and productivity(Kelly, 2016). To do so, the overarching factors in this journey are (1) knowledge and skill development (learning organization), (2) effective communication development, (3) trust and transparency improvement, (3) sense of triumph and worthiness establishment, (4) data collection and evidence-based analysis in addition to applying best practices and benchmarking(Brandrud et al., 2011; Halvorson, 2013; Smith & Saleem, 2013).

Globalization and Partnership

The fourth room of the House of Success is the globalization and partnership. The digital services have removed barriers such as distance, language, and time zone, and increased the interaction between people, governments, and industries (Friedman, 2007; Hill & Hult, 2018). The technology is going to open a door for globalizing individuals rather than globalizing companies, and in the meantime, sustainability creation has vital roles in new modern organizations (Friedman, 2007). Christopher Boone, Dean of Sustainability School of Arizona State University, described sustainability as, "Sustainability is improving human well-being and ensuring social equity for present and future generations while safeguarding the planet's life-supporting ecosystems" (Boone, 2018).

The global goals such as Sustainable Development Goals in the United Nation Agenda shown in Figure 6 is the sample of endeavoring for sustainability development to reduce global inequities in health, education, and human development, to save the planet, human, prosperity, peace, and partnership (Dugani, Duke, & Kissoon, 2016, p. E213). Sustainable Development Goals (SDGs) shown in Figure 6 came to the strategic action of 138 countries with 17 goals to attain them by 2030:

End of poverty (SDG1), Zero Hunger (SDG2), Health and well-being (SDG3), Education growth (SDG4), Gender Equality (SDG5), Water and sanitation (SDG6), Access to energy (SDG7), Economic growth (SDG8), Infrastructural development and industrialization (SDG9), Inequality (SDG10), Sustainable consumption and production (SDG12), Combating climate change (SDG13), Conserve and sustainable use of underwater resources (SDG14), Halting biodiversity loss (SDG15), Peaceful and inclusive societies (SDG16), and Revitalize the global partnership (SDG17). (Brolan et al., 2017; Langlois, Campbell, Prieur-Richard, Karesh, & Daszak, 2012)

Furthermore, the shift explicitly in the nature of businesses due to digital technologies and global trading has led the organizations to redesign their strategies, leadership, human resource, and performance toward the sustainable effectiveness model. The sustainable effectiveness organizations are value-creation organizations, and they consider not only an economic and competitive advantage but also value growth in organizational, ecological, social, and environmental goals (Lawler Iii, 2014).

Friedman (2007), in his book, *The World is Flat*, stated the world is getting flatter. In Globalization 1.0, the key agent of change was human power and his creativity to use wind, steam, and horsepower.

Figure 6. Sustainable development goals of the United Nations
Permission to use this color wheel has been taken from UNs' guidelines for the use of the SDGs logo and 17 icons through SDGpermissions@un.org (UN, September 2018).

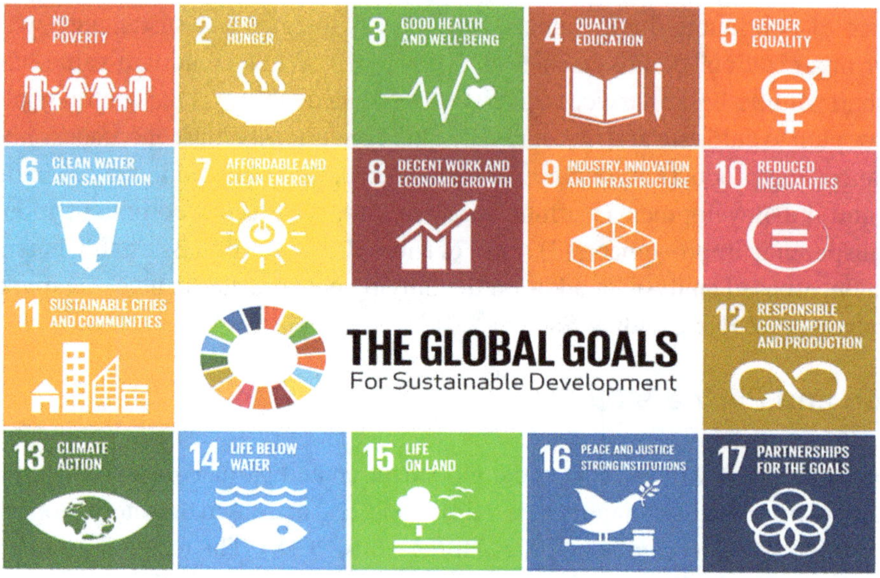
1 NO POVERTY
2 ZERO HUNGER
3 GOOD HEALTH AND WELL-BEING
4 QUALITY EDUCATION
5 GENDER EQUALITY
6 CLEAN WATER AND SANITATION
7 AFFORDABLE AND CLEAN ENERGY
8 DECENT WORK AND ECONOMIC GROWTH
9 INDUSTRY, INNOVATION AND INFRASTRUCTURE
10 REDUCED INEQUALITIES
11 SUSTAINABLE CITIES AND COMMUNITIES
THE GLOBAL GOALS
For Sustainable Development
12 RESPONSIBLE CONSUMPTION AND PRODUCTION
13 CLIMATE ACTION
14 LIFE BELOW WATER
15 LIFE ON LAND
16 PEACE AND JUSTICE STRONG INSTITUTIONS
17 PARTNERSHIPS FOR THE GOALS

The Globalization 1.0 converted the massive world to a common word. The Globalization 2.0 era was the industrial revolution with the manifestation of multinational markets and smaller world. Moreover, now the Globalization 3.0 has flattened the world by developing individualization and empowering people to contribute to global markets individually (pp. 9-10). Jerry Rao stated, "cultures and willing to change have a huge advantage in this world," and "you have to have a strong culture, but also openness to adopt and adapt from others" (as cited in Friedman, 2007, p. 422).

SOLUTIONS AND RECOMMENDATIONS

This research indicated that healthcare organizations strive to have the champions of transformation. They need to develop cross-function interrelationships among digitalization, leadership, individuals, globalization, and change leadership. The healthcare organizations must put globalization in their strategic plans to create sustainable effectiveness organizations and to make a difference in the lives of all people of all ages around the globe. The digital technologies like telemedicine and m-Health can mitigate the borders and increase accessibility to healthcare as well as promote the awareness and knowledge of populations. Moreover, establishing learning systems to empower employees and engaging them in decision making and creating the desired future are important factors that healthcare leaders must develop their strategies based on them. Technology development needs process development and workflow improvement while employee satisfaction is one of the goals of Quadruple Aims. Moreover, patients' empowerment to engage them in their health and well-being lead the healthcare organizations toward the smart organization that embraces sustainable effectiveness that creates not only profit and competitive advantage but also creates value for society and the environment.

FUTURE RESEARCH DIRECTIONS

The opportunities for future research can be to explore the organizational factors to engaging individuals in the process of change, investigating in change leadership models to make progress in global healthcare goals, and understanding the needs of healthcare to achieve quadruple aims. Moreover, the qualitative and quantitative research to explore and investigate the stakeholder's perspective and health leaders' strategies to embrace digital health technologies can enlighten the road map of future healthcare and improve innovative approaches. Also, examining the House of Success model through different research methods to identify the opinion of scholars is an opportunity for future research.

CONCLUSION

For successful digital transformation, smart healthcare organizations require to set their framework based on people, technology, change, leadership, and partnership. In Figure 7, the author has illuminated the final roadmap of creating the desired future based on the House of Success model. This model has conceptualized the road map of digital transformation. Understanding the foundation of digital transformation that is the starting phase and perceiving the quadruple aims that are the ultimate goal can enlighten the road of transformation. Moreover, leaders and managers are responsible for creating the vision for the digital transformation roadmap. Through change leadership, the organization can increases engagement, and through change management, reduces resistance to change. While people leadership is one of the most significant parts of digital transformation, institutionalizing the culture of digital change, empowerment people, and engaging them in the process of transformation maximize the successful outcome. The eight significant components introduced in the digital technology leadership section are the essential keys in a fast-pacing change environment. Moreover, global strategies such as Sustainable Development Goals

Figure 7. The road map of smart healthcare organizations

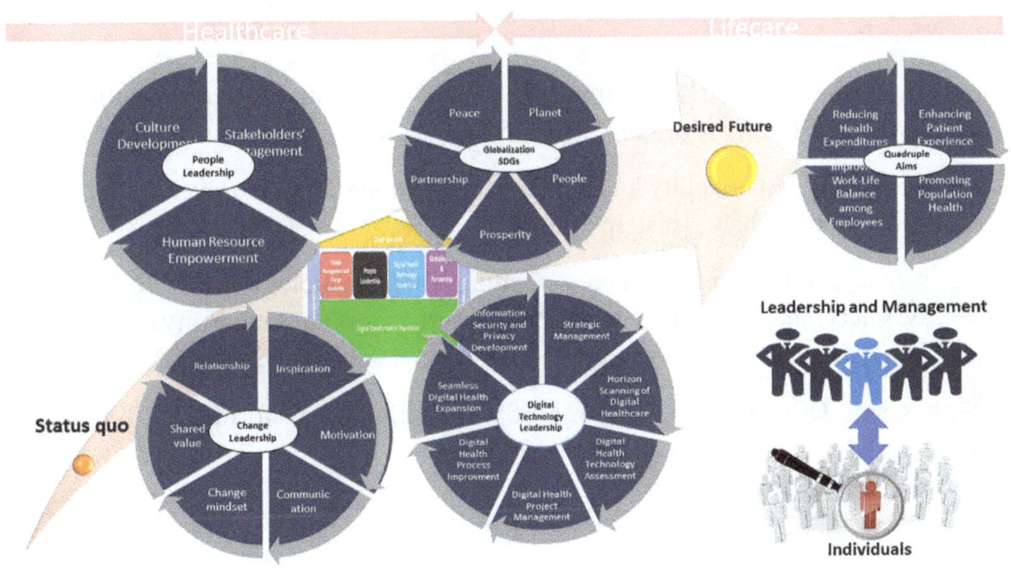

(SDGs) to contribute in five dimensions of SDGs: people, planet, prosperity, peace, and partnership are the essential factors while globalization is our near future.

REFERENCES

Adeyemi, O. A. (2017). *Organizational change and how it effects healthcare employees: A study on employee resistance to change in electronic medical record implementation* (Doctoral dissertation). Colorado Technical University. ProQuest Dissertations & Theses Global database. (10602795 D.M.)

Agarwal, R., DesRoches, C., & Jha, A. K. (2010). The digital transformation of healthcare: Current status and the road ahead. *Information Systems Research, 21*(4), 796–809. doi:10.1287/isre.1100.0327

Allman, S. (2009). Leadership vs. Management. *Successful Meetings, 58*(11), 12.

Anonymous. (2017). Physicians optimistic about digital health. *Physician Practice Perspectives, 36*(1), 6–8.

Arbab Kash, B., Spaulding, A., Johnson, C. E., & Gamm, L. (2014). Success factors for strategic change initiatives: A qualitative study of healthcare administrators' perspectives. *Journal of Healthcare Management, 59*(1), 65–81. doi:10.1097/00115514-201401000-00011 PMID:24611428

Atchison, T. A. (1999). Managing change. *Frontiers of Health Services Management, 16*(1), 3–29. doi:10.1097/01974520-199907000-00002 PMID:10557432

Aziz, L. (2007). *Managing change in healthcare information technology projects: the role of the project manager*. Project Management Institute.

Bauer, J. C. (2002). Rural America and the digital transformation of healthcare: new perspectives on the future...third annual Southern Illinois Healthcare/Southern Illinois University Health Policy Institute, Rural Healthcare: Current Issues and Future Directions, May 31 and June 1, 2001. *Journal of Legal Medicine, 23*(1), 73–83. doi:10.1080/019476402317276678 PMID:11957332

Bennis, W., Sample, S. B., & Asghar, R. (2015). *The art and adventure of leadership*. San Francisco: John Wiley & Sons Inc.

Bodenheimer, T., & Sinsky, C. (2014). From triple to quadruple aim: Care of the patient requires care of the provider. *Annals of Family Medicine, 12*(6), 573–576. doi:10.1370/afm.1713 PMID:25384822

Boone, C. (2018). What is sustainability? *ASU School of Sustainability*. Retrieved from https://schoolof-sustainability.asu.edu/about/what-is-sustainability/)

Bourgeois, R., & Stacy, A. (2007). The impact of information technology on small, medium, and large hospitals: Quality, safety, and financial metrics (PhD dissertation). The University of Texas at Arlington. ProQuest Central; ProQuest Dissertations & Theses Global database. (3288889)

Bowersox, D. J., Closs, D. J., & Drayer, R. W. (2005). The digital transformation: Technology and beyond. *Supply Chain Management Review, 9*(1), 22–29.

Brandrud, A. S., Schreiner, A., Hjortdahl, P., Helljesen, G. S., Nyen, B., & Nelson, E. C. (2011). Three success factors for continual improvement in healthcare: An analysis of the reports of improvement team members. *BMJ Quality &amp. Safety, 20*(3), 251–259. doi:10.1136/bmjqs.2009.038604 PMID:21209149

Brolan, C. E., Forman, L., Dagron, S., Hammonds, R., Waris, A., Latif, L., & Ruano, A. L. (2017). The right to health of non-nationals and displaced persons in the sustainable development goals era: Challenges for equity in universal healthcare. *International Journal for Equity in Health, 16*(1), 14. doi:10.118612939-016-0500-z PMID:28219374

Brown, D. (2007). Horizon scanning and the business environment -- the implications for risk management. *BT Technology Journal, 25*(1), 208–214. doi:10.100710550-007-0022-8

Buvat, J., Crummener, C., Kar, K., Sengupta, A., Solis, B., Aboud, C., & Aoufi, E. H. (2018). *The digital culture challenge: Closing the employee-leadership gap*. Academic Press.

Calvillo, J., Román, I., & Roa, L. M. (2015). How technology is empowering patients? A literature review. *Health Expectations, 18*(5), 643–652. doi:10.1111/hex.12089

Carman, K. L., Dardess, P., Maurer, M., Sofaer, S., Adams, K., Bechtel, C., & Sweeney, J. (2013). Patient and family engagement: A framework for understanding the elements and developing interventions and policies. *Health Affairs, 32*(2), 223–231. doi:10.1377/hlthaff.2012.1133 PMID:23381514

Center for Control Diseases and Prevention. (2016). *Health United States, 2016 with special feature in medical technology*. Retrieved from https://www.cdc.gov/nchs/hus/index.htm

Cohn, D., & Caumont, A. (2016). *10 demographic trends that are shaping the U.S. and the world.* Retrieved from https://www.pewresearch.org/fact-tank/2016/03/31/10-demographic-trends-that-are-shaping-the-u-s-and-the-world/

Cohn, K. H. (2015). Training for physician engagement. *Talent Development, 69*(5), 58–62.

Coile, R. C. Jr. (2000). The digital transformation of healthcare. *Physician Executive, 26*(1), 8. PMID:10788126

Commins, J. (2014). Addressing physician engagement. *HealthLeaders, 17,* 8-10.

Dess, G., McNamara, G., Eisner, A., & Hyun, S. (2019). *Strategic management: Creating competitive advantages* (9th ed.). McGraw-Hill Education.

DowJones. (2016). Press Release: New Study Reveals High Confidence in Digital Transformation Success Despite Major Challenges. *Dow Jones Institutional News.*

Dugani, S. M. D. P., Duke, T. M. D., & Kissoon, N. M. (2016). Transforming health through sustainable development. *Canadian Medical Association. Journal, 188*(10), E213-E214.

Dyrda, L. (2018, February). Hospital Transaction and valuation issue. *Backer's Hospital Review.* Retrieved from https://www.beckershospitalreview.com/hospital-transactions-and-valuation/healthcare-transactions-in-the-era-of-megamergers-and-vertical-integration-q-a-with-jeff-swearingen.html

ECRI. (2011). *AHRQ Healthcare horizon scanning system protocol and operations manual.* Prepared by ECRI Institute under Contract No. HHSA290201000006C. Rockville, MD: Agency for Healthcare Research and Quality.

Faddis, A. (2018). The digital transformation of healthcare technology management. *Biomedical Instrumentation & Technology*, *52*(s2), 34–38. doi:10.2345/0899-8205-52.s2.34 PMID:29775387

Friedman, T. L. (2007). *The world is flat, A brief history of the twenty-first century* (2nd rev ed.). Farrar, Straus, and Giroux Publisher.

Gardenswartz, L., Rowe, A., Digh, P., & Bennett, M. (2003). *The global diversity desk reference: Managing an international workforce.* Pfeiffer.

Gardner, P. J. (2009). Organizational change: All we want is better projects-why so difficult? *AACE International Transactions*, PM.03.01-PM.03.25.

Gill, R. (2003). Change Management or Change Leadership. *Journal of Change Management*, *3*(4), 307–318. doi:10.1080/714023845

Gutiérrez-Ibarluzea, I., Chiumente, M., & Dauben, H.-P. (2017). The life cycle of health technologies. Challenges and ways forward. *Frontiers in Pharmacology*, *8*, 14–14. doi:10.3389/fphar.2017.00014 PMID:28174538

Halvorson, G. C. (2013). The culture to cultivate. *Harvard Business Review*. PMID:24730168

Hartnell, C. (2012). Leadership and organizational culture: An integrative view of leaders as culture creators and culture as social context (PhD dissertation). Arizona State University. ProQuest Dissertations & Theses Global database. (3504099)

Herscovitch, L. (2004). *Resistance to organizational change: Toward a multidimensional conceptualization* (Doctoral dissertation). The University of Western Ontario. ProQuest Dissertations & Theses Global database. (NQ96828)

Hill, C. W., & Hult, T. M. (2018). *Global business today* (10th ed.). McGraw-Hill Education.

Institute for Healthcare Improvement. (2012). *The IHI Triple Aim.* Retrieved from http://www.ihi.org/Engage/Initiatives/TripleAim/Pages/default.aspx

Jiju, A., Snee, R., & Hoerl, R. (2017). Lean Six Sigma: Yesterday, today and tomorrow. *International Journal of Quality & Reliability Management*, *34*(7), 1073–1093. doi:10.1108/IJQRM-03-2016-0035

Kane, G. C. (2015). How digital transformation is making healthcare safer, faster and cheaper. *MIT Sloan Management Review, 57*(1), 0.

Kelly, S. (2016). Creating a culture of continuous improvement and sustainable management systems at Abbott Diagnostics Longford. *Global Business and Organizational Excellence*, *36*(1), 6–24. doi:10.1002/joe.21753

Kluge, E.-H. W. (2008). Ethical aspects of future healthcare: Globalization of markets and differentiation of societies- ethical challenges. *Studies in Health Technology and Informatics*, *134*, 77–87. PMID:18376035

Kotter, J. (1995). Leading change: Why transformation efforts fail. (cover story). *Harvard Business Review*, *73*(2), 59–67.

Kotter, J. (2012). *Leading change. Harvard Business Review.*

Kuza, C. C. (2017). Burnout among critical care nurses and the role of ICU telemedicine (PhD dissertation). University of Pittsburgh. ProQuest Dissertations & Theses Global database. (10831866)

Langlois, E. V., Campbell, K., Prieur-Richard, A., Karesh, W. B., & Daszak, P. (2012). Towards a better integration of global health and biodiversity in the new Sustainable Development Goals beyond rio+20. *EcoHealth*, *9*(4), 381–385. doi:10.100710393-012-0800-8 PMID:23001330

Lawler Iii, E. E. (2014). Sustainable Effectiveness and Organization Development. *OD Practitioner*, *46*(4), 65–67.

Linski, C. M. III. (2013). Process consultation and law enforcement: A practitioner's case study report. *Organization Development Journal*, *31*(4), 63–73.

Lloyd, J., & Ferguson, S. L. (2017). Innovative information technology solutions: Addressing current and emerging nurse shortages and staffing challenges worldwide. *Nursing Economics*, *35*(4), 211–212.

Mace, S. (2015). Mobile patient engagement. *HealthLeaders*, *18*, 62–64.

Manganello, J., Gerstner, G., Pergolino, K., Graham, Y., Falisi, A., & Strogatz, D. (2017). The relationship of health literacy with use of digital technology for health information: Implications for public health practice. *Journal of Public Health Management and Practice*, *23*(4), 380–387. doi:10.1097/PHH.0000000000000366 PMID:26672402

Marshak, R. J., & Grant, D. (2008). Organizational discourse and new organization development practices. *British Journal of Management*, *19*(s1), S7–S19. doi:10.1111/j.1467-8551.2008.00567.x

Mary Norine, W., & Rumsfeld, J. S. (2017). Leading the digital transformation of healthcare. *Journal of the American College of Cardiology*, *70*(21), 2719–2722. doi:10.1016/j.jacc.2017.10.020 PMID:29169479

McCabe, C., & Timmins, F. (2016). Embracing healthcare technology - What is the way forward for nurse education? *Nurse Education in Practice*, *21*, 104–106. doi:10.1016/j.nepr.2016.10.007 PMID:27810650

McCullough, J. S., Casey, M., Moscovice, I., & Prasad, S. (2010). The effect of health information technology on quality in U.S. hospitals. *Health Affairs*, *29*(4), 647–654. doi:10.1377/hlthaff.2010.0155 PMID:20368594

Meskó, B., Drobni, Z., Bényei, É., Gergely, B., & Győrffy, Z. (2017). Digital health is a cultural transformation of traditional healthcare. *mHealth*, *3*, 38–38. doi:10.21037/mhealth.2017.08.07 PMID:29184890

Meskó, B., Radó, N., & Győrffy, Z. (2019). Opinion leader empowered patients about the era of digital health: A qualitative study. *BMJ Open*, *9*(3), e025267. doi:10.1136/bmjopen-2018-025267 PMID:30898816

Mintzberg, H. (2009). *Managing*. Berrett-Koehler Publication, Inc.

Moriarty, J. M. (2014). The modern experience of care: Patient satisfaction as a quality metric after the Affordable Care Act (MA thesis). Boston University. ProQuest Central; ProQuest Dissertations & Theses Global database. (1560379)

Morris, M. (2013). The future of hospitals: Visions of the healthcare landscape in 2035. *Becker's Hospital Review.* Retrieved from https://www.beckershospitalreview.com/hospital-management-administration/the-future-of-hospitals-visions-of-the-healthcare-landscape-in-2035.html

Morse, S. (2018). 82% of clinicians, IT leaders blame burnout on interruptions from tech tools. *Healthcare Finance.* Retrieved from https://www.healthcarefinancenews.com/news/82-clinicians-it-leaders-blame-burnout-interruptions-tech-tools

Nahavandi, A. (2015). *The art and science of leadership* (7th ed.). Pearson Education, Inc.

Nelson, L. P. (2014). Patient engagement solutions. *Health Management Technology, 35*(11), 18–19. PMID:25622456

NewsRx. (2019a). *Artificial Intelligence; Findings from University College London Hospital update knowledge of Artificial Intelligence (Artificial intelligence and computer-aided diagnosis in colonoscopy: current evidence and future directions). Computer Technology Journal.*

NewsRx. (2019b). *Artificial Intelligence; Investigators at Massachusetts General Hospital Detail Findings in Artificial Intelligence (Artificial Intelligence in Surgery: Promises and Perils). Medical Devices & Surgical Technology Week.*

Newswire. (2016). Digital transformation market in healthcare: Global industry analysis and forecast 2015 - 2025. *PR Newswire.*

Office for Civil Rights. (2013). Summary of the HIPAA privacy rule. *U.S. Department of Health & Human Services.* https://www.hhs.gov/hipaa/for-professionals/privacy/laws-regulations/index.html

Olden, P. C. (2003). Hospital and community health: Going from stakeholder management to stakeholder collaboration. *Journal of Health and Human Services Administration, 26*(1/2), 35–57. PMID:15330379

Ommaya, A. K., Cipriano, P. F., Hoyt, D. B., Horvath, K. A., Tang, P., Paz, H. L., . . . Sinsky, C. A. (2018). *Care-centered clinical documentation in the digital environment: Solutions to alleviate burnout.* NAM Perspectives. Discussion Paper, National Academy of Medicine. doi:10.31478/201801c

ONC. (2014). *Connecting health and care for the nation: A shared national wide interoperability roadmap.* Office of the National Coordinator for Health Information Technology (ONC). Retrieved from https://www.healthit.gov/sites/default/files/hie-interoperability/nationwide-interoperability-roadmap-final-version-1.0.pdf

Pinkney, L. M. (2013). *Healthcare reform: Innovative and other proven strategies for successfully managing and implementing organizational change.* University of Maryland University College. ProQuest Central; ProQuest Dissertations & Theses Global database. (3608771)

PMP. (2018). The Project Manager of the Future. *The Project Management Institute.* Retrieved from https://www.pmi.org/-/media/pmi/documents/public/pdf/learning/thought-leadership/pulse/digital-pm-skills.pdf?sc_lang_temp=en

Reifsteck, M. W., & Reese, M. L. (2016). The digital health explosion. A comprehensive strategy is required to remain relevant and responsive. *Healthcare Executive*, *31*(3), 66–67. PMID:27319110

Robbins, S. P., & Judge, T. A. (2017). *Organizational behavior*. Pearson Education, Inc.

Roth, M., & Keller, B. (2019). Modernization through digital transformation. *TD: Talent Development*, *73*(1), 32.

Sarrami, F. P., Travaglia, J., Debono, D., & Braithwaite, J. (2014). Implementing strategies in consumer and community engagement in healthcare: Results of a large-scale, scoping meta-review. *BMC Health Services Research*, *14*(1), 402. doi:10.1186/1472-6963-14-402 PMID:25230846

Scheer, V. (2016). Process Improvement for Implementing and Sustaining Change in Healthcare (Master's thesis). The College of St. Scholastica. ProQuest Dissertations & Theses Global database. (10125146)

Schein, E. H. (2004). Organizational culture and leadership (3rd ed.). The Jossey-Bass Business & Management Series.

Schwarzmüller, T., Brosi, P., Duman, D., & Welpe, I. M. (2018). How does the digital transformation affect organizations? Key themes of change in work design and leadership. *Management Review*, *29*(2), 114–138. doi:10.5771/0935-9915-2018-2-114

Shafran, R. F. (2017). Leading organizational change: A phenomenological study of the nonlinear strategies used by female leaders in global companies (EdD dissertation). Pepperdine University. ProQuest Dissertations & Theses Global database. (10635765 Ed.D.)

Sheri-Lynne, L., & Singh, P. (2007). Leadership development: Learning from best practices. *Leadership and Organization Development Journal*, *28*(5), 444–464. doi:10.1108/01437730710761742

Shuck, B., Twyford, D., Reio, T. G. Jr, & Shuck, A. (2014). Human resource development practices and employee engagement: Examining the connection with employee turnover intentions. *Human Resource Development Quarterly*, *25*(2), 239–270. doi:10.1002/hrdq.21190

Sikka, R., Morath, J. M., & Leape, L. (2015). The Quadruple Aim: Care, health, cost and meaning in work. *BMJ Quality & Safety*, *24*(10), 608–610. doi:10.1136/bmjqs-2015-004160 PMID:26038586

Smith, S., & Saleem, H. (2013). *What has HCI done to institutionalize improvement? A report from 17 countries. USAID Healthcare Improvement Project*. HCI.

Smollan, R. K., & Sayers, J. G. (2009). Organizational culture, change, and emotions: A qualitative study. *Journal of Change Management*, *9*(4), 435–457. doi:10.1080/14697010903360632

Springer, P. J., Clark, C. M., Faan, A., Strohfus, P., & Belcheir, M. (2012). Using transformational change to improve organizational culture and climate in a school of nursing. *The Journal of Nursing Education*, *51*(2), 81–88. doi:10.3928/01484834-20111230-02 PMID:22201273

Stensaker, I., & Meyer, C. (2011). *Change experience and employee reactions: Developing capabilities for change* (Vol. 41). Academic Press.

Tait, I. E. (2013). Comparison of project management software tool use in healthcare and other industries (PhD dissertation). Capella University. ProQuest Central; ProQuest Dissertations & Theses Global database. (3607024)

Thimbleby, H. (2013). Technology and the future of healthcare. *Journal of Public Health Research*, *2*(3), 28. doi:10.4081/jphr.2013.e28 PMID:25170499

Thomas, D. (2014). Leading under pressure, coping practices of executives: A mixed methods study (EdD dissertation). Pepperdine University. ProQuest Central; ProQuest Dissertations & Theses Global database. (3668392)

United Nations. (n.d.). *Communication Materials*. Retrieved from https://www.un.org/sustainabledevelopment/news/communications-material/.

ValueCenter. (n.d.). Change vs. Transformation. *Better Value Center.* Retrieved from https://www.valuescentre.com/

Van Fleet, D. D., & Peterson, T. O. (2016). Improving healthcare practice behaviors. *International Journal of Health Care Quality Assurance*, *29*(2), 141–161. doi:10.1108/IJHCQA-07-2015-0089 PMID:26959895

VerticalNews. (2019). Artificial Intelligence; Researchers at Royal Adelaide Hospital Target Artificial Intelligence (Artificial Intelligence for Sex Determination of Skeletal Remains: Application of a Deep Learning Artificial Neural Network To Human Skulls). *Journal of Robotics & Machine Learning,* 2367.

Vukovic, V., Favaretti, C., Ricciardi, W., & de Waure, C. (2018). Health Technology Assessment evidence on e-health/m-health technologies: Evaluating the transparency and thoroughness. *International Journal of Technology Assessment in Health Care*, *34*(1), 87–96. doi:10.1017/S0266462317004512 PMID:29455685

Wade, V. A., Taylor, A. D., Kidd, M. R., & Carati, C. (2016). Transitioning a home telehealth project into a sustainable, large-scale service: A qualitative study. *BMC Health Services Research*, *16*(1), 1–10. doi:10.118612913-016-1436-0 PMID:27185041

Walsh, M. N., & Rumsfeld, J. S. (2017). Leading the digital transformation of healthcare. *The ACC Innovation Strategy*, *70*(21), 2719–2722. doi:10.1016/j.jacc.2017.10.020 PMID:29169479

Wang, L., & Alexander, C. A. (2013). Automated identification technology and information security in digital hospitals. *International Journal of Information and Network Security*, *2*(5), 348–359. doi:10.11591/ijins.v2i5.3914

Weiner, L. J. (2016). Improving physician engagement. *HealthLeaders, 19,* 8-10.

Weinstein, R. S., Lopez, A. M., Krupinski, E. A., Beinar, S. J., Holcomb, M., McNeely, R. A., ... Barker, G. (2008). Integrating telemedicine and telehealth: Putting it all together. *Studies in Health Technology and Informatics*, *131*, 23–38. PMID:18305320

Weston, S. (2017). The real challenge for digital transformation is not your technology. *CIO*.

World Health Organization. (2011). *m-Health New horizons for health through mobile technologies.* World Health Organziation.

Chapter 6
Professional Practices for Digital Healthcare

Sisira Edirippulige
Centre for Online Health, The University of Queensland, Australia

Buddhika Senanayake
https://orcid.org/0000-0002-2278-2889
Centre for Online Health, The University of Queensland, Australia

ABSTRACT

Digital health is quickly becoming an integral part of healthcare services. Research evidence suggests that digital health can benefit stakeholders involved in healthcare including patients and care providers. As digital health continues to integrate into routine healthcare, practitioners may require new knowledge, skills, and competencies to make the best use of it and to be able to communicate with an increasingly digitally enabled consumer. While much effort has been made to systematic education and training relating to digital health, which is an important aspect in developing the digital health workforce, it is important that governments and health systems consider digital health education and training as an important element in the process of implementing digital health within health services. Digital health education must be given its due recognition and support so that the future heath workforce has an opportunity to develop required knowledge and skills relating to digital health.

INTRODUCTION

Digital health is growing. The intentions of digital health include providing *administrative advantage* (e.g. to improve efficiency, and reduce costs through digitisation); *clinical advantage* (e.g. electronic prescribing to improve patient safety, electronic health records (EHR) to facilitate sharing amongst practitioners); to *overcome impediments* to service delivery (e.g. remote consultation, or remote-access to medical imaging); and to *help patients to self-manage* their health (e.g. apps for monitoring chronic conditions, or sharing information amongst providers using a personally-controlled EHR) (Sandhu, 2020; Greenes & Shortliffe, 1990).

DOI: 10.4018/978-1-7998-3274-4.ch006

There is a strong rationale for seeking alternative methods for delivering healthcare using innovative technologies (Hadeel & Sandhu, 2021; Sandhu, 2020; Venkatesh & Davis, 2000; & Davis, 1989). Traditional business models and infrastructure of healthcare organisations are ill-equipped to sufficiently adapt to, or finance, the global health trends of aging populations, declining birth rates, increasing non-communicable chronic disease, poverty, migration and increasing rates of infectious disease. These factors all impose significant logistical and financial hardships for those striving to provide ubiquitous effective and ethical healthcare. The digital transformation of healthcare with information communication technology provides one avenue to better enable patient centred care. Although digital health is growing rapidly in the healthcare industry the education and training component plays a critical role to uplift the future uptake of digital innovation. This chapter explores the current evidence regarding education and training for digital health and discovers the potentials to strengthen digital health in the field of learning and training.

While digital health is not new, advances in technology, in particular, the availability of mobile devices and ubiquitous connectivity, means that services are no longer physically limited to a health facility, or limited only to clinicians (McConalogue, Davis, & Connolly, 2019). Modern healthcare systems increasingly comprise digital hospitals providing services to digital health-consumers. Many governments and health systems have made attempts to introduce telehealth services, a few of which have become large and well-integrated, such as the Ontario Telemedicine Network in Canada (Edirippulige & Armfield, 2017) and Veteran's Affairs Telehealth in the USA (Kampmeijer, Pavlova, Tambor, Golinowska, & Groot, 2016). The interest in telehealth to improve healthcare services is global. A number of European countries have implemented various telehealth projects; and some countries have conducted large research studies to establish an evidence base (Dattakumar, Gray, Henderson, Maeder, & Chenery, 2012; Marschang, 2014). Global organisations such as the World Health Organisation (WHO) have been promoting telehealth, particularly in low and middle income countries in Asia, Africa, and Latin as a new way to address critical health challenges (Gray, Dattakumar, Maeder, Butler-Henderson, & Chenery, 2014; Smith, 2011).

Some governments have made important policy changes to encourage and incentivise the use of digital health. For example, the Australian federal government introduced reimbursement for certain video-based consultations involving general practitioners, specialists, Aboriginal health workers, nurse practitioners and midwives (Bryant, 2014). In the USA, forty-six states, and Washington DC provide reimbursement for some video-based consultations under their Medicaid programs which supports the healthcare costs of those on low incomes and those living with certain disabilities (Lannan, 2015).

Alongside the increase in the use of telehealth, a flourishing industry of medical, technology and clinical service businesses has grown. The size of the market is difficult to reliably estimate. One group of analysts have suggested that it could be as large as USD $43.4 billion by 2019 (Cope, 2011) while another group were more conservative in their estimate of USD $36.3 billion by 2020 (Gill, 2014).

As digital health continues to integrate into routine healthcare, practitioners may require new knowledge, skills, and competencies to make the best use of it and to be able to communicate with an increasingly digitally-enabled consumer. Almost thirty years ago in 1990, Greenes *et al.* foresaw this need: '*horizontal integration of eHealth into healthcare practices requires the integration of eHealth into medical education*' (Greenes & Shortliffe, 1990). Meanwhile, the lack of education and training (E&T) has been highlighted as an impediment for health professionals to use digital health (Sandhu 2020; Edirippulige & Armfield, 2017; Kampmeijer et al., 2016). While universities may be a logical place to provide digital health E&T, a study involving thirty Australian universities in 2012 (largely by survey, response rate ~25%; supplemented by interviews) concluded that the future health-professional workforce was not being adequately educated to achieve competence to work with digital health (Dattakumar et al., 2012; Gray et al., 2014).

While much effort has been made to establish the evidence base relating to the clinical use of digital health, little has been done to understand the E&T needs for practicing digital health within clinical services. Lack of proper understanding of E&T needs may be a reason for the lack of systematic E&T in this field. The recent national study highlighted that no Australian medical curriculum provides formal E&T to future medical practitioners about digital health (Edirippulige, Brooks, et al., 2018).

However, in recent years, there has been an increased interest in digital health E&T in various sectors. For example, the Australian Digital Health Agency has highlighted the importance of workforce development and E&T has been identified as one of the strategic priorities.

LITERATURE REVIEW

The concept of 'digital health' is broad and complex. There are many different definitions associated with digital health and they may vary depending on the context. However, the common aspects of all these definitions are the delivery of healthcare services and information and communication technologies (ICT). As a result, there are a number of different terms associated with this disciple. Some commonly used terms include telemedicine, mHealth, telehealth, health informatics, medical informatics. (Iyawa, Herselman, & Botha, 2016).

There are many definitions of digital health and e-health. The World Health Organization defines digital health as 'the use of information and communication technologies (ICT) for health including treating patients, conducting research, educating the health workforce, tracking diseases and monitoring public health' (World Health Organisation, 2016). This has evolved from the original World Health Organization (WHO) definition of e-health which is as 'the transfer of health resources and healthcare by electronic means'.

Human resources for health is an essential component of an efficient health system. Policymakers should rethink their health workforce strategies to build up competencies and skill mix to meet changing health needs in the future. Countries are taking many actions in health workforce education, retention and reorientation of work processes and of cadres. Many national stakeholders and international development agencies are involved to incorporate digital health into health workforce enhancement (Nancarrow, 2015).

The development of Internet-based technologies, which have significantly changed the way people engage with the data that surrounds their lives. The Internet was considered to be a place that had the potential to change society in fundamental ways. In the context of healthcare, these expectations were reinforced by views that foresaw the capacity of digital technology to create a more cost-effective way of delivering healthcare. Moreover, the proliferation of digital technologies across all sectors of society would lead to increased utilization of and reliance upon digital solutions within the healthcare sector (Rich & Miah, 2014).

Technology is the main factor in the emergence and the development of e-Health. As we have learned, the following are the major technical aspects that have made an impact:

- Developments in computing, the Internet and information technology;
- Development and expansion of networks and telecommunication infrastructure;

- The rapid adoption of technology by society (Rogers, 1995);
- The technological innovation of medical devices, digital cameras, and physiological sensors.

There are plenty of health benefits of Information, Communication, and Technology (ICT). It improves health service delivery, increasing efficiency, reduces operating costs, reduces administrative costs, and enabled entirely novel ways of going about healthcare management. This definition includes clinical, educational, administrative and research health related activities that are carried out at a distance (Bashshur, Reardon, & Shannon, 2000). Therefore, when we place the word 'clinical' in front of 'telehealth', we are talking about the application of ICTs for medical consultations, diagnosis, treatment, monitoring, patient follow up, case discussion, etc. Digital health consisted of several components to provide health services: i.e. telemedicine/ telehealth, health informatics, mobile health, etc.:

- **Telemedicine:** Telehealth is defined as 'the use of information and communication technology (ICT) to deliver health services, expertise and information over distance.' (5) Many, including the World Health Organisation (WHO), use the terms 'telehealth' and 'telemedicine' interchangeably, while others draw distinctions between the two. A Cochrane review concluded that the terms overlap and that 'telemedicine is considered to be the use of communication and information technologies to deliver clinical care where the individuals involved are not at the same location. They can either be two healthcare professionals or a healthcare professional and a patient. Telehealth includes this definition, and also covers telecommunication to deliver non-clinical services such as research and health education promotion' (Currell, Urquhart, Wainwright, & Lewis, 2000). Telemedicine includes telephone and email contact between patients and health professionals, videoconferencing between patients and health professionals and remote patient monitoring, where devices are used in the patient's home to send information to health professionals. There are two main approaches used in telehealth – the real-time approach and the store-and-forward approach. The real-time ('synchronous') approach means that the parties involved interact at the same time using information and communication technologies (ICTs);
- **Health Informatics:** The history of electronic health information exchange (health informatics) is in part matched by the evolution of telemedicine. Clinicians have sought to exploit technological development and progress to overcome everyday logistical issues they face with delivering their services. The ability to electronically transmit text and image-based anatomical pathology, clinical pathology and radiology diagnostic data greatly enhanced the evolution of telemedicine;
- **Mobile Health:** From the world-wide infiltration of mobile communication devices and innovation offerings by advanced networking technologies, a specific field within e-Health has emerged, i.e. mobile health or m-Health. m-health is the fastest growing segment of ICT-based healthcare; devices include smartphones, tablets, global positioning system (GPS) devices, mobile telehealth, and physiological monitoring devices. The latest statistics from April 2019 reveal that mobile devices and transmitters are now in the hands of more people and communities than any other type of communication device. The number of mobile connections exceeds the total population in the world (7.7 billion) and the average number of mobile connections per unique mobile user is 1.52 (We are social, 2019).

World Health Organization (WHO) defines mHealth as medical and public health practice supported by mobile devices, such as mobile phones, patient monitoring devices, personal digital assistants (PDAs), and other wireless devices. mHealth involves the use of voice, video, images and, short messaging services (SMS), general packet radio service (GPRS), third/ fourth and fifth-generation mobile telecommunications (3G/4G and 5G systems), global positioning system (GPS), and Bluetooth technology (World Health Organization, 2011). Digital technologies are becoming an important resource for health services delivery and public health. Mobile wireless technologies are particularly relevant, due to their ease of use, broad reach, and wide acceptance (Hadeel & Sandhu, 2021; Venkatesh & Davis, 2000; & Davis 1989).

- **SMS:** This is the most accessible technology as all mobile phones are SMS capable. SMS is often used to send reminders and motivational prompts (keeping health related appointments, reminders about set goals); the recipient can then use SMS to send back data relative to the intervention;
- **Cameras:** Photos for dermatology review (lesions, etc), photographic evidence of progress;
- **Native Applications:** Via programming interfaces, developers can build special purpose applications – users can log journals relating to their health and health-related goals and participate in online communities for progress monitoring, peer support and motivation. Chronic disease sufferers have a variety of mobile-application programs available to assist them in managing their diseases, i.e. asthma, diabetes, hypertension, heart failure;
- **Automated Sensing:** Mobile phones act as receivers, storage devices and transmitters of data from medical and wellness devices like measuring scales, blood pressure monitors, heart rate monitors, glucometers, portable ECGs, pedometers, ultrasounds;
- **Interfacing With the Internet:** The capacity of mobile devices to be continuously connected to the internet means that the transfer of data to care providers can be automatic and immediate. This allows for the timely review of data by the remote care provider enabling earlier intervention if warranted (World Health Organization, 2011).

Digital health comprise providing administrative advantage (e.g. to improve efficiency, and reduce costs through digitisation); clinical advantage (e.g. electronic prescribing to improve patient safety, electronic health records (EHRs) to facilitate sharing amongst practitioners); to overcome impediments to service delivery (e.g. remote consultation, or remote access to medical imaging); and to help patients to self-manage their health (e.g. apps for monitoring chronic conditions, or sharing information amongst providers using a personally-controlled EHR).

METHODOLOGY

A thorough literature review was performed to identify facts for the research topic. The electronic databases such as "PubMed", "Google Scholar", Medline, Scopus, Emtree and "HINARI" were used to gather data. Keywords such as education and training, digital health, mHealth, health workforce were entered in order to get comprehensive coverage of relevant literature. Citation information along with notes and abstracts were downloaded to Endnote X6 software. Citation and reference lists were made using Endnote X6 software in Harvard APA style –sixth edition.

The exploratory review was conducted on peer-reviewed publications published between January 2000 and April 2019. The reason for limiting searches to this narrow period was due to change in technology and teaching and learning styles rendering findings of earlier studies unsuitable for current contexts. As the study aimed to collate all evidence regarding education and training for digital health, all the potential studies that strengthen digital health in the field of learning and training were included. The review also considered any type of study (quantitative, or qualitative) if adequate information (to assess successful implementation or utilization) on the service delivered was described. Articles related to healthcare models, technical feasibility studies, case studies, letters, and published comments were excluded (inadequacy of information to reliably assess usefulness). Publications with no abstracts and non-English articles were also excluded. Grey literature was not searched.

SOLUTIONS AND RECOMMENDATIONS

Digital Health and Patient-Centred Healthcare

Patient-centred care is a healthcare model that places the patient at the centre of the care instead of the disease or illness. It considers a patient's cultural tradition, personal preferences, and values, family situations, social circumstances and lifestyles as well as the clinical aspects of diagnosis, potential treatment, rehabilitation or advice on healthy behaviours. 'Patient-centred care is an approach to the planning, delivery, and evaluation of healthcare that is grounded in mutually beneficial partnerships among healthcare providers, patients, and families' (Australian Commission on Safety and Quality in Healthcare, 2011).

In the traditional, disease-centered model, physicians make almost all treatment decisions based largely on clinical experience and data from various medical tests. In a patient-centered model, patients become active participants in their own care and receive services designed to focus on their individual needs and preferences, in addition to advice and counsel from health professionals. This model was first described by the Institute of Medicine (US) in its landmark publication 'Crossing the quality chasm: A new health system for the 21st century' (Institute of Medicine, 2001).

Patient-centred care directly improves quality and safety and empower patients. Empowered healthcare consumers require access to high quality medical information and an up to date personal electronic health record. Having a personal electronic health record is vital for the future vision of timely, effective and up-to-date personalised care.

Just like patients, healthcare teams need access to the best possible and most recent information about their patients' health status (European Commisssion, 2004). A single electronic repository for such information, that all participants in a person's healthcare can contribute to and access, is viewed as critical for the success of many e-health innovations. Consider the efficiencies that can be gained if all relevant information from ongoing disease monitoring (including patient well- being and quality of life indicators), diagnostic and treatment data can be made available to all participants in the multi-disciplinary care team including the patient. A vision for the future e-Health patient is to provide enhanced self-management interventions and individually tailored case management; problems can be quickly identified and clinical information and treatment goals shared between the healthcare team and the patient (Australian Health Minister's Conference, 2008).

Digital health provides equal access to health irrespective of location: Digital health is viewed as an eloquent resolution to the inequity of healthcare access for those that dwell in underserved or geographically disadvantaged communities. This also applies to metropolitan dwellers disadvantaged by age, illness or disability. In particular electronic healthcare records and telemedicine applications are viewed as a tool that will assist in 'closing the gap' of Indigenous Australian life expectancy, mental health, maternity services, paediatric services of ear, nose, and throat and aged care healthcare inequities (Dods, Alem, & Nepal, 2012).

In summary, digital health provides greater patient engagement through health related websites, apps, tools and wearable technology with gamification and incentives. It promotes healthier and safer communities: the Internet of things, smarter policy, regulation, and response. Digital health technology is productive and provides targeted care: Genomic and precision medicine, digital therapeutics. Finally, it secures the systematic high quality and safer care with electronic medical records and digital hospitals, improved decision support systems, information sharing, and interoperability smart systems and integration and automation (Queensland Health, 2017).

The Changing Role of Health Workers in the Digital Era

Nurses play a critical role in almost every sphere of healthcare such as primary, community and tertiary care. Nurses, regardless of specialty or work setting, treat patients, educate patients and the public about various medical conditions, and provide advice and emotional support to patients' family members. Nurses are responsible for recording patients' medical histories and symptoms, help perform diagnostic tests and analyse results, operate medical machinery, administer treatment and medications and help with patient follow-up and rehabilitation. Research has shown that there is a clear relationship between the number of nurses and the quality of care. Shortage and mal-distribution of nurses is a serious problem (Yogesan, Bos, Brett, & Gibbons, 2009). There is a significant disproportional distribution of nurses within and among countries. For example, while the United States have 773 nurses per 100,000 population, the number of nurses in Uganda for the same size population is 6 (International Council of Nurses, 2005). The disparity of nurses in urban and rural communities is a significant problem in both developing and developed countries.

These shortcomings can be addressed through nursing informatics. According to the official definition of the American Nursing Association (ANA), nursing informatics is the 'specialty identifying, collecting, processing, analysing and managing data'. Although this definition solely concentrates on the information, it is believed that nursing informatics should also incorporate the aspects of the delivery of care. It is apparent that the definitions are continuing to evolve. In broader terms, telehealth is a tool for healthcare delivery, diagnosis, consultation, treatment, and transfer of medical data/images and education by using ICT (i.e. interactive audio, visual, and data communications) at a distance. Multi-Sensory Stimulation Environment (MSSE) was designed with the assistance of robotic technology and mobile applications for children with Autism Spectrum Disorder identifying their need for rehabilitation and special educational purposes (Vladimir et al., 2018).

In general terms, telenursing is the use of ICT for delivering healthcare services at distance by nurses. Telenursing can be used in both healthcare setting or a non-institutional setting – that is at home or in an assisted-living facility (Wootton, Kvedar, & Dimmick, 2006). Telenursing applications may include real time techniques, for example videoconferencing or telephony and store and forward techniques, for example, email or web-based applications. Through interactive video systems, patients can contact on-call nurses and arrange for a video consultation. This kind of application is particularly helpful for children and adults with chronic conditions and long-term illnesses. Telenursing can also help patients and families to be active in care, such as self-management of chronic conditions. It is useful to support patients in the home, to support remote nurses, to promote and support self-care, to improve medication management and compliance, and cost-saving method.

Healthcare professionals (doctors, nurses, pharmacists, and other allied healthcare professionals) can utilize digital health for their clinical advantage (e.g. electronic prescribing to improve patient safety, electronic health records (EHRs) to facilitate sharing amongst practitioners and to *overcome impediments* to service delivery (e.g. remote consultation, or remote-access to medical imaging); and to *help patients to self-manage* their health (e.g. apps for monitoring chronic conditions, or sharing information amongst providers using a personally-controlled EHR).

Vision and Strategic Goals for Digital Health

The WHO has prepared a five year global strategy for digital health for from 2020-2024. There are four main goals. First, it is essential to promote global collaboration and advance the transfer of knowledge on digital health. It provides the platform to advance the implementation of national digital health strategies and strengthen governance for digital health at the global and national levels. The final goal is to advocate for people centred health systems that are enabled by digital health (World Health Organisation, 2019).

A Ten-year vision is developed for digital health in Queensland, Australia. The first priority is to build a consistent and sustainable capability. It strengthens the systems, infrastructure, and enabling tools as well as establishing the frameworks, standards, and governance required to support greater sharing and linkage of trusted information *(to be achieved within three years) (Queensland Health, 2017).*

The second priority is to integrate, grow and expand digital health and digital workforce capabilities. Apply the technology required to integrate, optimise, grow and expand digital health and digital workforce capabilities. This focus will shift capabilities to the creation of the next generation of digital health solutions including integrated technologies, devices and workflows and the integration of big data to enhance decision support, health system planning and performance reporting *(to be achieved within 5 years) (Queensland Health, 2017).*

The third priority is to scale digital health that can enable new and alternative models of healthcare, delivering treatment outcomes that are beyond the current realms of possibility. It promotes taking full advantage of technology and building capability to change the way that patients access care, where that care is provided, and the manner in which care is centred on patients.

Evidence for the of Digital Health on Workforce

Understanding the E&T Needs for Different Clinical Populations/Stakeholders

A study conducted to explore the progress of eHealth in the Australian medical curriculum by the University of Queensland showed that there is consensus on the importance of eHealth to current and future clinical practice, but there are other priorities and no strong drivers for change. Systemic problems inhibit the inclusion of eHealth in medical education, in which the curriculum is described as 'crowded' and with competing demands, and because accrediting bodies (such as Australian Medical Council) do not expect eHealth competence in medical graduates. Therefore, there is no external pressure for its inclusion. Unless and until accrediting bodies recognise and expect competence in eHealth, it is unlikely that it will enter the curriculum; consequently, the future workforce will remain unprepared (Edirippulige, Brooks, et al., 2018).

A qualitative study of the careers and professional practices of graduates from an e-health postgraduate programme (e-health study at UQ) declared that the digital health programme helped in their career development and more importantly, the current occupation of the majority of respondents was related to health or medicine, and most had worked in an e-health related job since graduating. The overall, level of satisfaction regarding the learning experience doing e-health study at UQ was also very high (Edirippulige, Armfield, & Smith, 2012).

A literature review was conducted to describe the delivery of education and training in telehealth/telemedicine in 2016, which identified nine studies (out of 388 reviewed studies) for final review. Programs from five countries were represented and articles were spread across telemedicine and clinically oriented journals. Education and training in telehealth has been provided as both university level and vocational courses using conventional classroom based delivery methods and e-learning. Reported curriculum items included terminology, clinical applications, the evidence-base, and technological aspects. Currently most recognized universities, public and private organizations have offered telehealth courses within their formal degree program. In addition, Continuous Professional Development (CPD) courses have incorporated telehealth and digital health as essential topics during their curriculums. These CPD courses targeted a range of professionals including health policy makers; telehealth service coordinators; medical doctors; engineers; clinical psychology trainees; nurses; public health professionals; private sector informatics professionals; and information technology professionals (Edirippulige & Armfield, 2017).

Key Topic Areas Relevant to Professional Practices

A study conducted in the UK developed and define domains of competence and associated learning outcomes needed by healthcare graduates to commence working in a digital healthcare environment. It generally applies to all healthcare professionals including doctors, nurses, and allied health professionals. Six key domains of competence were identified.

The agreed domains were: 1) Digital Health: work as a practitioner in the digital healthcare environment; 2) Accessing Data: access and interpret patient data to inform clinical decision-making; 3) Communication: communicate effectively with healthcare professionals and patients in the digital environment; 4)Generating data: generate data for and about patients within the EPR; 5) Multidisciplinary working: work with healthcare professionals with and alongside EPRs; and 6) Monitoring and audit: monitor and improve the quality and safety of healthcare. These domains can be used by academics to guide the integration of EPRs into undergraduate healthcare programmes (Pontefract & Wilson, 2019).

The Association of Faculties of Medicine of Canada and Infoway (2015) launched physician in–training project with the objective of improving clinical practice and patient care by supporting medical students and doctors in their adoption (Rogers, 1995) and use of digital health technologies. The next generation competency based medical education model identified digital health as an essential component for better patient outcomes. They developed 33 virtual patient cases by incorporating the use of digital health to improve patient safety (Baker, Charlebois, Lopatka, Moineau, & Zelmer, 2016).

Suitable Delivery Modes to Provide Relevant Knowledge, Skills, and Competencies

The clinical informatics curriculum was designed for psychiatric residents to improve their skills and competencies for EMR and tele-psychiatry. The e-curriculum in clinical informatics included electronic diagnostics and treatments, mobile apps and devices, EMR, big data, and data science, etc. The exposure therapy through virtual and augmented reality devices and optimizing technology based learning and self-care are identified as key competencies of education and training (Torous, Chan, Luo, Boland, & Hilty, 2018).

Another study was conducted in Australia to assess students' perceptions of the value of an eHealth practicum. The majority of students agreed that the practicum allowed them to gain necessary skills in eHealth applications and provided students with an opportunity to explore ways of using different eHealth tools for the delivery of healthcare at a distance. The study shows that a practical component in eHealth teaching was well received by students. While online teaching is appropriate for providing knowledge, the opportunity to develop practical skills may encourage students to use eHealth techniques in their future practices (Edirippulige, Smith, Armfield, Bensink, & Wootton, 2012).

Another study evaluating the Education ''Clinical Telemedicine/e-Health'' in the Curriculum of Medical Students at the University of Zurich showed that the overall satisfaction and understanding of telemedicine as a supplement in traditional medical consultations increased among students. Most of the students indicated that they would use telemedicine for chronically ill and elderly patients. The positive assessment of the module indicates the successful introduction of the topics of telemedicine and e-health to medical students at the University of Zurich. It was well evident that the students gained confidence and basic skills throughout the course (Brockes, Grischott, Dutkiewicz, & Schmidt-Weitmann, 2017).

Another study examined self-reported knowledge and perception changes associated with an e-health course offered to university undergraduate students in Australia. Students believed the course helped them to improve their knowledge regarding key aspects of e-health. It is important to design an e-health curriculum targeting competencies to provide the necessary knowledge and skills to help students practice e-health in their professional careers (Edirippulige, Samanta, & Armfield, 2018).

Levels of Qualification and Competencies

e-Health is steadily integrating into modern health services, making significant changes in the way health services are traditionally delivered. To work in this new environment, healthcare workers are required to have new knowledge, skills, and competencies specific to e-Health. New research has found that the main motivating factors for studying e-Health were 'relevance to current practice' and 'e-Health is the future'. The participants highlighted the opportunity to 'acquiring relevant knowledge' and 'having exposure' were key benefits offered by the e-Health education program. Participants believed that the postgraduate e-Health program had an influence on their professional practice and the majority of them had worked in the field of e-Health since their graduation. Their professional roles mainly involved the 'implementation of e-Health in health service settings' and the 'use of e-Health in clinical practice'. While e-Health may be steadily integrating into modern health services, e-Health specific job opportunities are still relatively limited. e-Health workforce development must be given priority (Edirippulige, Smith, Wickramasinghe, & Armfield, 2018).

FUTURE RESEARCH DIRECTIONS

It is quite obvious that Information and communication technologies have not been harnessed systematically to improve the health of populations in developing countries. Although developed countries are using modern technology to empower those who use information by providing them with a choice of information to be accessed in their own time and by allowing them to put their own information on the web. Developing countries are par below the standard level compared to developed countries. The current digital divide is more dramatic than any other inequity in health or income. Therefore, it is essential to encourage policymakers in developing countries to embrace digital health by investing in research related to health informatics and e-health. The way forward for these developing countries is to exploit the full interactivity of the internet, which allows rapid feedback and change to continuously mold information into useful knowledge (Edejer, 2000). Although knowledge based economy with digital health is a novel concept, it tends to neglect human values, the impact of the natural environment, and holism which are essential to nurturing a humanitarian health system (Ženko, Mulej, & Potocan, 2017).

The rapidly rising aging population is a challenge for most of the developed countries as they consume more and more healthcare resources for long periods. The cost of healthcare spending is increasing rapidly and the governments are searching for cost-effective healthcare models to maintain their quality of care. Mental health, substance abuse, and domestic violence are emerging challenges for health systems. More importantly, digital health is a vital tool that can be utilized for most of these new health challenges. Poor communication between health authorities and medical curriculum experts have created a barrier to incorporate digital health in a timely manner, as it is essentially required at health service delivery. Some health managers are not geared enough to rethink and redesign healthcare models and resist innovative approaches to new challenges. Less sustainable funding for digital health research to improve systems and patient outcomes is another challenge (Queensland Health, 2017). Personal data privacy and security are another challenge for digital health limiting its implementation. This should be addressed sensitively to uplift the growth of digital health (Filkins et al., 2016). The future direction of the healthcare industry is determined by the quality of education and training provided for healthcare professionals and to general public on digital health and its practical applicability in day-to-day practice. There should be a uniform agreement between all stakeholders regarding the core education components of digital health and its practical implications similar to fundamental disciplines in medical, para-medical and health science streams.

CONCLUSION

Digital health is experiencing steady growth. Innovators and investors alike see the potential in technologies that can transform the face of healthcare by leveraging data to improve diagnosis, treatment, outcomes and the overall patient experience. The new opportunities offered by digital health are generous, with a variety of uses ranging from disease detection and diagnosis, self-management of chronic conditions, psychological support and clinical decision-making. This novel, patient-centered and technology-driven approach has also created openings for new players to break into the market.

While evidence relating to the benefits and effectiveness of digital health is growing, the workforce development relating to digital health has been paid little or no attention. The utility of digital health in clinical practice requires significant changes in the traditional way of practice. Systematic education and training is needed for delivering essential knowledge and skills for healthcare providers to use digital health in their routine practice. Education research has a major role to play in establishing evidence relating to the needs, content, and methods of delivery of digital health education and training for different groups. The development of digital health curriculum must be evidence-based.

REFERENCES

Australian Commission on Safety and Quality in Healthcare. (2011). *Patient-centred care: Improving quality and safety through partnerships with patients and consumers.* Retrieved from Sydney: https://www.safetyandquality.gov.au/wpcontent/uploads/2012/03/PCC_Paper_August.pdf

Australian Health Minister's Conference. (2008). *National e-Health Strategy Summary.* Melbourne: Australian Government.

Baker, C., Charlebois, M., Lopatka, H., Moineau, G., & Zelmer, J. (2016). Influencing Change: Preparing the Next Generation of Clinicians to Practice in the Digital Age. *Healthcare Quarterly, 18*(4), 5–7. doi:10.12927/hcq.2016.24569 PMID:27009699

Bashshur, R. L., Reardon, T. G., & Shannon, G. W. (2000). Telemedicine: A new healthcare delivery system. *Annual Review of Public Health, 21*(1), 613–637. doi:10.1146/annurev.publhealth.21.1.613 PMID:10884967

Brockes, C., Grischott, T., Dutkiewicz, M., & Schmidt-Weitmann, S. (2017). Evaluation of the Education "Clinical Telemedicine/e-Health" in the Curriculum of Medical Students at the University of Zurich. *Telemedicine Journal and e-Health, 23*(11), 899–904. doi:10.1089/tmj.2017.0011 PMID:28498779

Bryant, A. (2014). *An interpretative phenomenological analysis of student engagement in learning at the middle level* (Education Doctoral Theses Paper). Northeastern University. Retrieved from https://repository.library.northeastern. edu/files/neu:336553

Cope, J. (2011). Entrepreneurial learning from failure: An interpretative phenomenological analysis. *Journal of Business Venturing, 26*(6), 604–623. doi:10.1016/j.jbusvent.2010.06.002

Currell, R., Urquhart, C., Wainwright, P., & Lewis, R. (2000). Telemedicine versus face to face patient care: Effects on professional practice and healthcare outcomes. *Cochrane Database of Systematic Reviews*, (2): Cd002098. doi:10.1002/14651858.Cd002098 PMID:10796678

Dattakumar, A., Gray, K., Henderson, K. B., Maeder, A., & Chenery, H. (2012). *We are not educating the future clinical health professional workforce adequately for e-health.* Academic Press.

Davis, F. D. (1989). Perceived usefulness, perceived ease of use, and user acceptance of information technology. *MIS quarterly*, 319-340. competence: Findings of an Australian study. *Studies in Health Technology and Informatics, 178*, 33–38.

Dods, J., Alem, L., & Nepal, S. (2012). *Caring for the last 3%: Telehealth potential and Broadband implications for remote Australia. CSIRO ICT Centre.*

Edejer, T. T.-T. (2000). Disseminating health information in developing countries: The role of the internet. *BMJ (Clinical Research Ed.), 321*(7264), 797–800. doi:10.1136/bmj.321.7264.797 PMID:11009519

Edirippulige, S., & Armfield, N. R. (2017). Education and training to support the use of clinical telehealth: A review of the literature. *Journal of Telemedicine and Telecare, 23*(2), 273–282. doi:10.1177/1357633X16632968 PMID:26892005

Edirippulige, S., Armfield, N. R., & Smith, A. C. (2012). A qualitative study of the careers and professional practices of graduates from an e-health postgraduate programme. *Journal of Telemedicine and Telecare*, *18*(8), 455–459. doi:10.1258/jtt.2012.gth107 PMID:23209263

Edirippulige, S., Brooks, P., Carati, C., Wade, V. A., Smith, A. C., Wickramasinghe, S., & Armfield, N. R. (2018). It's important, but not important enough: eHealth as a curriculum priority in medical education in Australia. *Journal of Telemedicine and Telecare*, *24*(10), 697–702. doi:10.1177/1357633X18793282 PMID:30343657

Edirippulige, S., Samanta, M., & Armfield, N. R. (2018). Assessment of Self-Perceived Knowledge in e-Health Among Undergraduate Students. *Telemedicine Journal and e-Health*, *24*(2), 139–144. doi:10.1089/tmj.2017.0056 PMID:28708457

Edirippulige, S., Smith, A. C., Armfield, N. R., Bensink, M., & Wootton, R. (2012). Student perceptions of a hands-on practicum to supplement an online eHealth course. *Journal of Medical Internet Research*, *14*(6), e182–e182. doi:10.2196/jmir.2029 PMID:23246840

Edirippulige, S., Smith, A. C., Wickramasinghe, S., & Armfield, N. R. (2018). Examining the Influence of E-Health Education on Professional Practice. *Journal of Medical Systems*, *42*(11), 215. doi:10.100710916-018-1084-5 PMID:30276486

European Commisssion. (2004). *E-Health, Making Healthcare Better for European Citizens: An Action Plan for a European E-health Area*. Retrieved from https://ec.europa.eu/digital-single-market/en/news/e-health-making-healthcare-better-european-citizens-action-plan-european-e-health-area

Filkins, B. L., Kim, J. Y., Roberts, B., Armstrong, W., Miller, M. A., Hultner, M. L., ... Steinhubl, S. R. (2016). Privacy and security in the era of digital health: What should translational researchers know and do about it? *American Journal of Translational Research*, *8*(3), 1560–1580. PMID:27186282

Gill, M. J. (2014). The Possibilities of Phenomenology for Organizational Research. *Organizational Research Methods*, *17*(2), 118–137. doi:10.1177/1094428113518348

Gray, K., Dattakumar, A., Maeder, A., Butler-Henderson, K., & Chenery, H. (2014). *Advancing ehealth education for the clinical health professions: Final report 2014*. Academic Press.

Greenes, R. A., & Shortliffe, E. H. (1990). Medical informatics. An emerging academic discipline and institutional priority. *Journal of the American Medical Association*, *263*(8), 1114–1120. doi:10.1001/jama.263.8.1114

Hadeel, A., & Sandhu, K. (2021). PLS Model Performance for Factors Influencing Students Acceptance of Elearning Analytics Recommender. *International Journal of Virtual and Personal Learning Environments*.

Institute of Medicine. (2001). *Crossing the Quality Chasm: A New Health System for the 21st Century*. Washington, DC: The National Academies Press.

International Council of Nurses. (2005). *Summary- Global shortage of registered nurses*. Author.

Iyawa, G. E., Herselman, M., & Botha, A. (2016). Digital Health Innovation Ecosystems: From Systematic Literature Review to Conceptual Framework. *Procedia Computer Science*, *100*, 244–252. doi:10.1016/j.procs.2016.09.149

Kampmeijer, R., Pavlova, M., Tambor, M., Golinowska, S., & Groot, W. (2016). The use of e-health and m-health tools in health promotion and primary prevention among older adults: A systematic literature review. *BMC Health Services Research*, *16*(S5), 290. doi:10.118612913-016-1522-3 PMID:27608677

Lannan, K. (2015). *Interpretative phenomenological analysis: Exploring the formative experiences of community college students enrolled in remedial courses* (Doctoral dissertation). Colorado State University. Retrieved from https://dspace.library.colostate.edu/handle/10217/170325

Marschang, S. (2014). *Health inqualities and eHealth: 2014 eHealth Forum, Report of the e-Health stakeholder Group*. Retrieved from Athens: http://www.ehealth2014.org/wpcontent/

McConalogue, E., Davis, P., & Connolly, R. (2019). Health Technology Assessment: The Role of Total Cost of Ownership. *Business Systems Research*, *10*(1), 180–187. doi:10.2478/bsrj-2019-0013

Nancarrow, S. A. (2015). Six principles to enhance health workforce flexibility. *Human Resources for Health*, *13*(1), 9. doi:10.1186/1478-4491-13-9 PMID:26264184

Pontefract, S. K., & Wilson, K. (2019). Using electronic patient records: Defining learning outcomes for undergraduate education. *BMC Medical Education*, *19*(1), 30. doi:10.118612909-019-1466-5 PMID:30670000

Queensland Health. (2017). *Digital Health Strategic Vision for Queensland 2026*. Author.

Rich, E., & Miah, A. (2014). Understanding digital health as public pedagogy: A critical framework. *Societies (Basel, Switzerland)*, *4*(2), 296–315. doi:10.3390oc4020296

Sandhu. (2020). Digital Systems Innovation for Health Data Analytics. In *Handbook of Research on Optimizing Healthcare Management Techniques*. IGI Global.

Smith, J. A. (2011). Evaluating the contribution of interpretative phenomenological analysis. *Health Psychology Review*, *5*(1), 9–27. doi:10.1080/17437199.2010.510659

Torous, J., Chan, S., Luo, J., Boland, R., & Hilty, D. (2018). Clinical Informatics in Psychiatric Training: Preparing Today's Trainees for the Already Present Future. *Academic Psychiatry*, *42*(5), 694–697. doi:10.100740596-017-0811-4 PMID:29047074

Venkatesh, V., & Davis, F. D. (2000). A theoretical extension of the technology acceptance model: Four longitudinal field studies. *Management Science*, *46*(2), 186–204. doi:10.1287/mnsc.46.2.186.11926

Vladimir, R.-B., Jorge, G.-M., Martín, L.-N., Yaroslava, R.-B., Javier, C.-R., Diego, Q.-P., ... Verónica Cevallos, L.-W. (2018). A Hybrid System to Support the Psychological Intervention for Children With Autism: A Proposal Based on Knowledge Modeling and Intelligent Technologies. *International Journal of E-Services and Mobile Applications*, *10*(4), 74–100. doi:10.4018/IJESMA.2018100105

We are social. (2019). *Digital 2019, Q2 Global Digital Statshot*. Retrieved from https://wearesocial.com/blog/2019/04/the-state-of-digital-in-april-2019-all-the-numbers-you-need-to-know

Wootton, R., Kvedar, J., & Dimmick, S. L. (2006). *Home Telehealth: Connecting care within community.* London: Royal Society of Medicine Press.

World Health Organisation. (2016). *Global diffusion of eHealth: Making universal health coverage achievable. Report of the third global survey on eHealth.* Retrieved from Geneva, Switzerland: https://apps.who.int/iris/bitstream/10665/252529/1/9789241511780- eng.pdf?ua=1

World Health Organisation. (2019). *Global Strategy on Digital Health 2020-2024.* Author.

World Health Organization. (2011). mHealth: New horizons for health through mobile technologies; Global Observatory for eHealth series. Author.

Yogesan, K., Bos, L., Brett, P., & Gibbons, M. C. (2009). *Handbook of Digital Homecare.* Springer-Verlag Berlin Heidelberg.

Ženko, Z., Mulej, M., & Potocan, V. (2017). Knowledge-cum-values Management belongs to the Way out from Global Crisis. *Business Systems Research, 8*(1), 113–123. doi:10.1515/bsrj-2017-0009

ADDITIONAL READING

Edirippulige, S., Brooks, P., Carati, C., Wade, V. A., Smith, A. C., Wickramasinghe, S., & Armfield, N. R. (2018). It's important, but not important enough: eHealth as a curriculum priority in medical education in Australia. *Journal of Telemedicine and Telecare, 24*(10), 697–702. doi:10.1177/1357633X18793282 PMID:30343657

Nancarrow, S. A. (2015). Six principles to enhance health workforce flexibility. *Human Resources for Health, 13*(1), 9. doi:10.1186/1478-4491-13-9 PMID:26264184

Pontefract, S. K., & Wilson, K. (2019). Using electronic patient records: Defining learning outcomes for undergraduate education. *BMC Medical Education, 19*(1), 30. doi:10.118612909-019-1466-5 PMID:30670000

Wootton, R., Kvedar, J., & Dimmick, S. L. (2006). *Home Telehealth: Connecting care within community.* London: Royal Society of Medicine Press.

KEY TERMS AND DEFINITIONS

eHealth: The use of information and communications technology in support of health and health-related fields.

Electronic Health Record: Is a digital version of a patient's paper chart. It is real-time, patient-centered records that make information available instantly and securely to authorized users.

Health Informatics: The interdisciplinary study of the design, development, adoption, and application of IT-based innovations in healthcare services delivery, management, and planning.

Health System: All activities whose primary purpose is to promote, restore, and maintain health.

mHealth: Medical and public health practice supported by mobile devices, such as mobile phones, patient monitoring devices, personal digital assistants (PDAs), and other wireless devices.

Telehealth: Use of telecommunication techniques for the purpose of providing telemedicine, medical education, and health education over a distance.

Telemedicine: The delivery of healthcare services, where distance is a critical factor, by all healthcare professionals using information and communication technologies for the exchange of valid information for diagnosis, treatment and prevention of disease and injuries, research and evaluation, and for the continuing education of healthcare providers, all in the interests of advancing the health of individuals and their communities.

Chapter 7
Digital Employability Skills and Training Needs for the Indian Healthcare Industry

Esha Jain
The NorthCap University, Gurugram, India

ABSTRACT

The utilization of computerized innovation in wellbeing applications is encountering a huge blast in huge part because of growing human services costs and the impediments of one-on-one treatment to meet the psychological well-being needs of the populace. Specifically, cell phone applications for wellbeing have become popular, which gives chances to grow current consideration past the customary facility setting. The objectives of this study were to identify the employability skills and training needs in the digital healthcare industry. Results showed that all the eight skills are important for the training of line service staff (e.g., communication, ICT, work engagement, teamwork, cognitive). As per the response, handling situations is one of the most critical skills required to perform the job followed by self-management, planning and organizing, and analytical skills. However, the type and requirement of skills vary from person to person.

INTRODUCTION

Handling worldwide wellbeing challenges requests the suitable utilization of accessible advancements. Albeit computerized wellbeing could essentially improve human services get to, use, quality, and results, understanding this plausibility requires faculty prepared in advanced wellbeing. There is developing proof of the advantages of advanced wellbeing for improving the presentation of wellbeing frameworks and results in created nations. Training is an ongoing process for enhancing the skills of the employees to achieve the current and future obligations associated with the job (Colombo & Stanca, 2008). Training not only imparts the requisite skills at all levels of the organization but intends at shifting the behavioral patterns of the employees too in a way that is pleasant to accomplish the administrative objective, efficiency, and expansion (Sharma, 2014). Training pattern differs from one organization to other depend-

DOI: 10.4018/978-1-7998-3274-4.ch007

ing on the needs of high management, a technology available (Colombo & Stanca, 2008), the attitude and readiness of the organizations to get advantage from training which will elevate the performance, experience, enhance the skills and knowledge of employees (Noe & Schmitt, 1986). Training is also important for growth, expansion, innovations (Montesino, 2002); it helps the organizations deal with the external and internal changes, especially the rising competition between the private hospitals of Delhi NCR. It is critical to promote the interest of training in such organizations. This study will focus on line services offered by the health sector; low patient satisfaction is posing a great threat of hospitals, which may compel the top management of these hospitals to prepare the training programs in order to elevate the skills and capabilities of their employees (Halfhill & Nielsen, 2005).

In the current changing economic scenario and increasing competition (Cekada, 2010), it is not enough for organizations to have a solid financial condition, modernized technology, upgraded systems since for the competitive survival an organization requires a highly skilled and quality human resource to subsist in long run (O'Driscoll & Taylor, 1992). The healthcare industry is on the boom with respect to other sectors like IT, Pharmaceutical and others and is becoming the major contributor to the total G.D.P of India. With the increase in competition between private sector hospitals in Delhi / NCR, the importance of training increases so as to provide quality medical services, increase organizational commitment, increase the performance of the workers and reducing turnover intentions (Agut et al., 2003). It is fundamental to accomplish Training Need Analysis to identify each individual aptitude and holes before drafting any training program for them. This tailored training program will be more effective and would yield a high return on investment. The study is meant to endeavor at describing the staff grounded on the Employability Skills Set and making 'Preparing Chart'. Aptitudes will be evaluated at all the authoritative pecking order (line administrations) level to recognize the capability/insufficiency and adequacy dimensions of the abilities.

Here are numerous verticals in the health-care sector, for this investigation medicinal administrations portion which incorporates, line administrations, bolster administrations and assistant administrations has been considered (Figure 1).

Training is used as a tool to develop and amend employees to survive in today's scenario. It is essential for an organization to identify employees and organization training needs accurately through training need analysis before conducting a training program which ultimately contributes to the development of existing realism of the association and gear up for the upcoming requirements. Several mobile applications like Medlife, 1mg, PharmaEasy, Practo, mfine, Netmeds, etc. are playing a significant role in the digitization of the healthcare industry which is really helping the patients 24*7 to get on-time treatment and medicines in the case of emergency.

The main objectives of the chapter are:

- To recognize the training requirements of personnel in the digital healthcare industry.
- To analyze the areas for imparting training for optimum utilization of employment skills.

The secondary objectives are:

- To analyze the requirement of communication skills in a training program module.
- To analyze the requirement of information and communication technology skills in a training program module.
- To analyze the requirement of work engagement skills in a training program module.

Figure 1. Aspect of hospital services

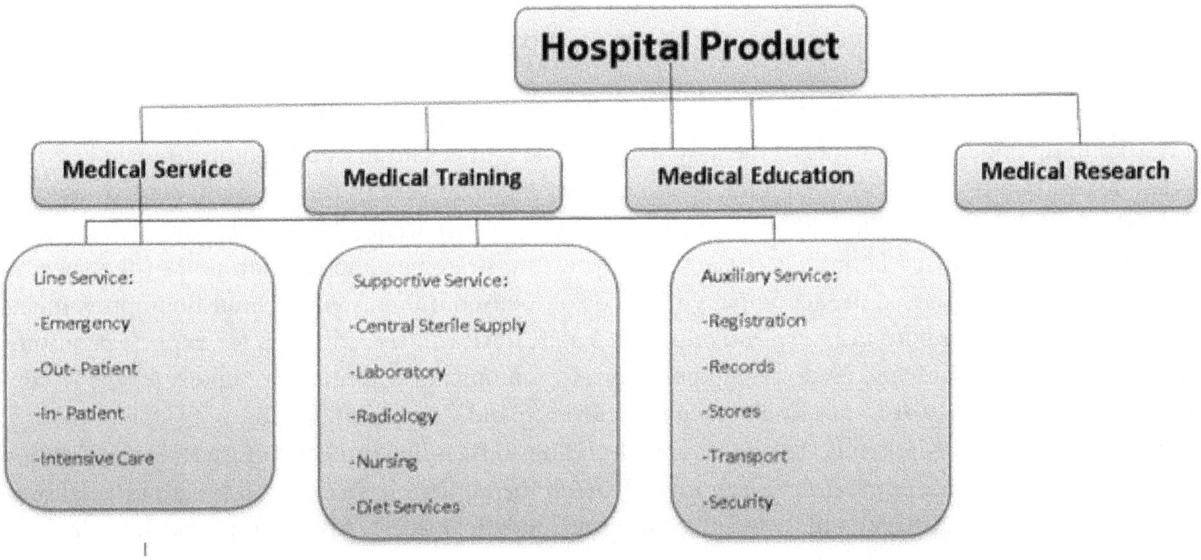

- To analyze the requirement of teamwork skills in a training program module.
- To analyze the requirement of cognitive skills in a training program module.
- To analyze the requirement of self-management skills in a training program module.
- To analyze the requirement of planning and organizing skills in a training program module.
- To analyze the requirement of analytical skills in a training program module.

BACKGROUND

Many researchers have discussed the importance of training need analysis, training effectiveness, on-the-job and off-the-job training methods in various sectors. I have read 40 research papers with the combination of the following keywords "Training Need Analysis", "Healthcare Industry", "Employability Skills", "Training Effectiveness" for searching the research papers. The database of Google Scholar was used for conducting the literature review. Following papers were reviewed and gaps were realized:

Sharma (2014) has done a study to compare the significance and execution of administrative training in India among various mechanical parts in the light of non-concurrent modern development in the most recent two decades which has unevenly contacted different business associations. With the end goal of the investigation, associations were isolated at two dimensions. At the main dimension, they were isolated among worldwide and Indian origin point classification and at the subsequent dimension among administration and assembling class. A 2×2 full factorial plan with inconsistent numbers is utilized to examine fundamental just as collaboration impacts. A sample size of 542 was taken which includes training experts, top/general administrators and trainee representatives. The author at long last inferred that Indian origin associations missed the mark as far as significance is given and execution of training capacity contrasted with global organizations and found that Indian companies and manufacturing companies must devote more time and investment in imparting training in their organization but the biggest limitation of this paper is that, though he emphasize on the importance of training he has not mentioned anywhere about the areas on which training should be imparted. Another main limitation of this study was that it was focussed on large organizations in India and may not be representative of small organizations.

Singh and Singh (2014) have done a research to make a similar investigation of the changing needs of the Training and Developments of the associations when all is said in done and health-care services division specifically in perspective on the post monetary advancement of the nation uncommonly with the coming of MNCs Healthcare Sectors in India. It was an experiential investigation dependent on pilot overviews, organized coordinated meetings, syndicate strategies and opinion poll of the specialists. The outcomes proposed the accompanying kinds of focused training viz. Scholastic improvements and technical upgrades both in-house and outhouse for all staff; Multi - skilling's for explicit positions; Human abilities for senior and predominant positions; Communication aptitudes uniquely for the Receptions, Public Relations, Customer Relations and Grievance and Complaint dealing with staff; Strategic aptitudes for all Sales, Marketing, Publicity, and Branding staff; Behavioral and attitudinal fortification trainings; and Employee commitment trainings. Though the authors have cited all the areas according to their knowledge, they haven't included cognitive and analytical skills. Also, teamwork skills are very much essential which was missed in their research.

Alnidawy (2015) has done a research to recognize the effect of statistic factors (sex, age, instructive capability, the quantity of long periods of experience) on the achievement of the training in the advancement and improvement of the presentation of the Human Resources and Organizational Performance in the Jordanian health sector and to distinguish the troubles looked by the training procedure and approaches to address them. The author utilized the descriptive way to deal with the impact of the autonomous factors on the dependent factors so as to accomplish the targets of the study and to analyze the hypothesis results. It was discovered that the most dynamic elements vital for the accomplishment of the training process from the trainer's perspective were the constancy to train and raise the proficiency of learners through leading instructive and instructional classes. It was discovered that the serious issues looked by the coach during the preparation procedure are the absence of functional use of the aptitudes gained by the trainees.

Heckemann et al. (2015) reviewed and collated ebb and flow research proof on the impact of animosity the executives training for medical attendants and nursing understudies working when all is said in done emergency clinics. Concentrates distributed between January 2000 and September 2011 in English, French or German were mulled over, and it was surveyed with the 'Quality Assessment Tool for Quantitative Studies'. Primary results for example frames of mind, certainty, aptitudes, and knowledge were gathered. Altogether, nine pieces of research were incorporated. Two had a feeble, six a moderate, and one a solid report plan. All examinations detailed expanded certainty, improved demeanor, abilities, and learning about hazard components post-training. There was no noteworthy change in the frequency of patient animosity. It was closed with the view that preparation does not lessen the frequency of forceful acts and hostility should be handled at an authoritative dimension.

Trochimiuk (2015) aimed to exhibit and survey proficient advancement open doors for more established representatives in SME. During the time spent work area look into, the researcher has perceived a few attributes of preparing exercises directed by SMEs. The administration of more seasoned representatives' expert advancement is talked about based on chosen look into discoveries, for example, CATI and CAPI reviews led in the structure of the "Far-reaching system of actuation of individuals matured

50+" venture completed by the Department of Human Resource Management at Kozminski University in 2010–2012. It was viewed that training needs analysis is essential before imparting training. Training provided in public sectors is better than those of the private sector. It was found that older employees are less interested in training than younger employees.

Yang et al. (2015) examined the component composition of the employability aptitudes model for passage level in staff in China. An overview was directed with 25 lodgings inside eight urban communities in China. The proposed estimation model was tried utilizing exploratory factor analysis and corroborative factor analysis. The AMOS programming package was utilized to test 15 estimation scale items, which brought about the distinguishing proof of the four aptitude measurements of employment execution and self-administration, association and time the board, innovativeness, and development, and critical thinking. After exploratory and corroborative factor analysis, both the convergent and discriminant validity were observed to be acceptable. This exploration was the first empirical study to build up a reasonable, worthy, and refreshed model of employability aptitudes for passage level inn workers in Chinese lodgings.

Diab and Ajlouni (2015) tested the impact of training on the employee's performance and the nature of therapeutic administrations on Jordanian private emergency clinics. The information of this examination was gathered through a (380) poll disseminated for a wide range of occupations in the Jordanian private clinics. The outcomes showed that there's a solid connection between the training segment in general and the independent factors (application the phases of training process, training programs decent variety, and utilized present-day innovation in training programs), there is a variety impact of the training segment (consolidated) on the Performance of employees, nature of medicinal administrations, and authoritative responsibility. Also, the most compelling on is the quality of medicinal administrations, the least powerful one is the hierarchical responsibilities, and there's no impact of the utilized current innovation in preparing programs as one of the training areas on the authoritative duties. On the light of the investigation results, the accompanying proposals might be submitted make a fitting administrative atmosphere, yearly training arrangement, for the way toward training and giving suitable motivating forces to the learners, expanded the financial backing assigned for training, in the Jordanian private emergency clinics, gave laborers chance to pick the training programs, and excused regulatory choices in regards to these programs.

Hassan et al. (2016) reviewed three training components specifically the length, approach and region and two individual qualities: instruction level and experience of a learner to evaluate their effect on undertaking and relevant elements of execution. The investigation included employment execution as the dependent variable. Job execution has been additionally separated into task execution and contextual execution so as to evaluate the effect of training on the two elements of a trainee's performance. Task execution has been caught by posing inquiries from the representative in regard to undertaking related dimensions of exertion, duty, and accomplishments while contextual execution has been estimated as far as inquiries concentrating on pro-social behavior and aimed to help collaborators. Separate polls were intended for staff and the chief to evaluate the job execution before as well as after the finishing of the training program. Consequences of the research undertaken upheld a positive effect of time and on the job training approach for subsequent execution of trainees with a better dimension of education. It was additionally discovered that the experience of learners significantly affects contextual execution while no impact on task execution of trainees.

Kitsiou et al. (2016) evaluated the training needs of nurses in all public hospitals in Cyprus and to investigate relations between demographic and occupational characteristics and training needs. A cross-sectional study with 385 nurses was conducted in all public hospitals in Cyprus from October 2014 to

January 2015. Nurses completed the "Training Needs Analysis Questionnaire" that includes 30 skills and five scales: research/audit, communication/teamwork, clinical tasks, managerial tasks, and management/supervision. Nurses stated that all 30 skills were important for the nursing role. Among them 7 skills were considered as very important, 22 as important and only one as less important. Nurses self-estimated their performance as very high in five skills, as high in 23 skills and as moderate in two skills. Moreover, they stated that after the appropriate training, their performance could be improved with a very important degree in 21 skills and to an important degree in nine skills. Nurses without an MSc/Ph.D. degree had greater training needs in research/audit scale than nurses with an MSc/Ph.D. degree and they consider their training as an important issue and that will help them to improve their clinical performance.

van Harten et al. (2016) examined the connection between employers' ventures (through job qualities and administrative help) and representatives' business openings, with employability, conceptualized as apparent state-of-the-art aptitude and eagerness to change, as an intervening variable. The hypothesis was tried utilizing structural equation modeling on survey data gathered from 1,626 representatives of three Dutch emergency clinics. Reliable with the hypothesis, the outcomes showed that job qualities and administrative help were in a roundabout way identified with representatives' convictions on business openings, with the relationship intervened by forward-thinking ability and readiness to change. Further, administrative help is legitimately identified with employees' business openings. This paper demonstrated that businesses, by giving an appealing and testing work in blend with satisfactory supervisory help, can improve their representatives' employability and business openings.

Messum et al. (2017) elicited perspectives on ongoing alumni and senior directors about abilities expected to work in HSM (Health Services Management). For this, senior directors and ongoing alumni working in health services administrations were recognized from a placement database utilized at NSW University and were messaged a typical poll. An aggregate of 38 senior directors and 42 ongoing alumni finished messaged studies, rating significance and abilities watched for 44 employability aptitudes items. Items were apprised by the literature and subject analysis of commercials for alumni health management positions. There was a solid understanding between the two groups on significant employability abilities, and the best seven things on which they concurred were all conventional in nature. It was discovered that for senior health managers, the most significant employability aptitudes were all conventional abilities (integrity and moral conduct, interpersonal skills, cooperation, adaptability and receptiveness, written communication abilities, coordinated effort, mindfulness, need setting, arranging and long-lasting learning). Change management and spending plan/money related administration aptitudes came next pursued by need setting, planning aptitudes, capacity to examine nature, reasonable reasoning, innovativeness and advancement, vital reasoning and autonomous reasoning.

Through investigating the clinicians' scientific research level and weakness ***Huang et al. (2017)*** carried out targeted clinical research training systematically, then strengthened their utilization of clinical resources and data, and finally promoted the transformation of scientific research results. Filling and submitting the online questionnaires through WeChat, a popular chatting tool in China, physicians from 13 affiliated hospitals of a university in Shanghai had joined this research. Results 507 valid questionnaires have been received online. As for the needs for training, the top three topics were how to design a clinical research in a standardized style, how to practice the methodology and how to utilize the statistical skills into clinical trials were included and it was found that standardized design and writing of clinical trial protocols according to the CONSORT (Consolidated Standards of Reporting Trials) and SPIRIT (Standard Protocol Items: Recommendations for Interventional Trials), and the application of epidemiological and statistical methods were still shortboards that most clinicians need to improve urgently, also were what they most concerned about at the same time. So, they found it necessary for physicians to receive systematic clinical research training to enhance their scientific research capacity.

Boyd et al. (2019) viewed that given the fluctuation of ED (Emergency Departments) staffing and individual supplier abilities, current POCUS (Point-of-care ultrasound) utilization and preparing needs among doctors working in EDs was to a great extent obscure. They led a forthcoming observational across the country investigation of all VA facilities utilizing an electronic study in a joint effort with the VA's Healthcare Analysis and Information Group (HAIG). The examination was regarded to be non-look into by the Investigational Review Board of the University of Texas Health Science Center (Protocol Number: HSC20160445N). The electronic review was disseminated to the Chiefs of staff (COS) at all VA Medical Centers across the nation (n = 144) among April and July 2016 and discovered high rates of support (N70%) from ED Service Chiefs to acquire POCUS training for their doctors. For all demonstrative and procedural POCUS applications, the level of POCUS clients craving extra training was reliably higher than POCUS non-clients. Among POCUS clients, extra training in diagnostic applications was most wanted for surveying volume status (92%), profound venous thrombosis (88%), stomach aortic aneurysm (87%), and gallbladder/bile pipes (85%). For all EM POCUS applications, it was discovered that present utilization was related to a craving for extra training in that application.

Ellahham et al. (2019) showed that protected plan, security holds, safe fall flat, and procedural shields are key methodologies, though cost, hazard, and vulnerability ought to be distinguished for all potentially specialized frameworks. It is additionally recommended that reasonable direction and conventions ought to be recognized and imparted to all partners to create and embrace more secure AI applications in the medicinal services setting.

Sarker et al. (2019) explored the extent and spectrum of online pharmaceutical practices along with the unique patterns and challenges in Bangladesh and found 23 online shops fitting the inclusion criteria. Regarding the products, online shops were selling over-the-counter medicine (43.48%), prescription medicine (30.43%), herbal products (52.17%), medical device (69.57%), healthcare products (69.57%) and other general products (39.13%). Regarding medicine, 7(30.43%) online pharmacies were selling prescription medicine and out of these 7 pharmacies, the majority of them (85.71%) had the option to upload prescriptions. Only 2(8.70%) of the online shops were using both Bengali and English as operating language and the rest of them were using only English.

Sisodia and Agrawal (2019) viewed that an association needs an individual with high employability abilities and found that these aptitudes positively affect patient consideration and well-being, treatment adherence, and patient fulfillment. They further proposed that to remain aggressive, medicinal services suppliers need to adjust their current workforce by furnishing them with viable preparation.

Analysis of the Literature Review

After conducting intensive literature review, it was found that number of researches are in existence for healthcare industry emphasizing on employability skills and training needs of employees at different levels of organization, but none of the studies much focused on all employability skills for which training is required and it was agreed in the studies that Indian starting point associations miss the mark as far as significance is given and execution of preparing capacity when contrasted with worldwide organizations and advising Indian organizations to devote more time and investment in imparting training but nowhere it told about the skills on the training is required. Few studies focused on types of specialist training but didn't include cognitive skills, analytical skills, and teamwork skills which is very much required in the healthcare industry. Some researchers found that there was no practical training given to employees, which is a serious threat as you can't tell an employee how to do ultrasound or how to inject without proper hands-on training and experience and few showed all the positive outcomes of a training program to healthcare employees but the type of training, based on which employability skills was not very much defined. Some studies also put emphasis on training needs and their impact on employability skills, but the details of skills were not clearly identified. One or two studies took four different dimensions of skills which were credible i.e., job performance and self-management, organization and time management, creativity and innovation, and problem-solving but they also ignored teamwork and cognitive skills. Some put the whole emphasis on genetic skills only and ignored specialized skills. So, in the present study, all the gaps are identified and taken into consideration like teamwork skills, analytical skills, ICT skills, work engagement skills, cognitive skills, self-management skills, analytical skills and planning, and organizing skills.

SCOPE AND SIGNIFICANCE

Training is pivotal for organizational improvement and achievement. A representative will turn out to be increasingly effective and beneficial on the off chance that he is trained well. Training and advancement are exceptionally indispensable in any firm that goes for advancing. It will help any organization in expanding the profitability of representatives, prompts less supervision which aides in cost-cutting and prevalent can concentrate on greater basic leadership issues, reduction of errors, and mishaps which is extremely critical at any rate for medicinal services industry as a solitary carelessness may prompt patient's life. It can likewise help in pooling the ability together and makes collaboration impacts the work environment. At times, training additionally helps in giving a reactant stage to representatives to impart their plans to the board. It has been shown that a couple of laborers may yearn for a place of power inside the business, however since there is no activity improvement program set up, these individuals don't discover the chance to exhibit their ability or further develop these covered aptitudes. Empowering agents to go to these activities distinguishes the pioneers of tomorrow inside current work power. They believe they have a place with the organization that they work for and the best way to compensate it is by giving the best administrations they can. Something else is Employee turnaround costs time and cash. Training makes a sentiment of trust in the brains of the representatives. It gives them security in the working environment. Subsequently, work turnover and non-attendance rates will be decreased. It will further address employee shortcomings and expanded consistency alongside solidarity and aptitudes improvement. This study will essentially give a chance and broad structure for the advancement of HR's specialized and conduct aptitudes in an organization which at last outcomes in ideal asset usage, in addition, it additionally helps the trainees in achieving self-improvement. The study will be valuable for the employees as well as the employer of the healthcare industry as it helps in understanding the training need at a different level for the skills, required at different levels of the healthcare industry in the digital age.

RESEARCH METHODOLOGY

Research Design

The exploration configuration alludes to the general system that you decide to incorporate the various parts of the investigation in an intelligible and legitimate manner, in this way, guaranteeing you will adequately address the examination issue; it comprises the diagram for the assortment, estimation, and examination of information. This investigation is descriptive in nature.

Sample Size

The sample size measures the number of individual samples measured or observations used in a survey or experiment. In this study, the sample size is 376. The sample size is a very important feature in research. The sample size should not be very low; if the sample size is low it won't provide better and accurate results.

Sampling Design

Sampling is a means of selecting a subset of units from a target population for the purpose of collecting information. Respondent-driven sampling is used to reach the target set. In this sampling technique, first of all, one respondent from the healthcare sector was identified. This respondent act as a "seed" and it has given the reference of three people and further those three people acted as "seed". This sampling method is just like "snowball" sampling, with less data redundancy.

Scaling Technique

Scaling is the strategy of estimating and relegating the items to the numbers as per the predefined rules. At the end of the day, the way toward finding the deliberate items on the continuum, a constant grouping of numbers to which the articles are doled out is called scaling. Likert Scale is used in this study with five parameters from 1-5, where 1 is lowest and 5 is highest.

Data Collection

The questionnaire consists of eight elementary employability skills required in the digital healthcare segment. The following skills are communication skills, IT skills, Work-engagement skills, teamwork skills, cognitive skills, Self-management skills, Planning and Organizing skills and Analytical skills.

First, respondents have contacted either face to face or through phone calls and explained to them the reason for performing this survey. Few respondents replied over the e-mails sent to them. However, few have filled the form in person. Any type of biased-ness was kept away while respondents were filling the questionnaire. In all, 91 questionnaires were filled. However, 15 were rejected as they were partially filled.

Tools Used

Some tools that were used in this research were Pie charts which help in understanding the collected data in a better way.

DATA ANALYSIS AND INTERPRETATION

Through the questionnaire, which consists of 8 questions, the following result was administered. The respondents were asked about the nature of the job. The questionnaire consists of questions on the importance of communication, teamwork, and handling of a critical patient, problem-solving and others. Effective communication is advantageous for each person and association achievement. It was positioned among the highest employability aptitude required in Healthcare Industry. There are a few sorts of correspondence subsist in the HR, which incorporates oral, composed, undivided attention and nonverbal, where undivided attention is a fundamental prerequisite for a triumphant healthcare experience. As per the responses generated (fig 2), this can be analyzed that empathetic listening is more important than active listening or Writing Skills. Line service staff who handles all in and out of patients' needs to be an emotional listener. He should have adequate skills to handle emergency situations and patients. In this era, when everything is computerized, the use of IT skills cannot be neglected. Because of advancement and revolutionizing in the Healthcare sector, it is important to create, spur and train their representatives. Line service Staff should be well equipped in IT skills, as they also handle the front desk and patient-related inquiries. The result shows that people have higher adaptability towards ICT related Skills (fig 3).

Work Psychology comprises of disposition, culture mindfulness, promptness, participation records, peace-making, unwavering ness or uprightness towards the association, responsibility towards seniors and individual appearance. In the healthcare industry, which is pre-dominantly service-oriented, and needs a maximum working hour, it is essential to maintain work engagement skills. These skills vary from being loyal to the profession, maintaining the integrity of work, maintaining work-life balance and keeping oneself aware of the environment. The study shows that most of the respondents think it is important to have work-life balance skills. A healthy balance will protect from stress and getting fatigued (fig 4). The success of any organization depends on the team and the healthy competition that exists. The healthcare industry is the perfect amalgamation of staff from security, nurse, reception, doctors, surgeons, managers and others. However, there is small preparing for collaboration aptitudes is given to the Healthcare staff. In the digital healthcare industry, where patient well-being and results are reliant on solid interdisciplinary cooperation, their group-based preparation achieves a significant position. The study clearly depicts that people feel it is important to be satisfied as a team (fig 5). They feel it is important that everyone is respected individually in a team. The work of every person in the team should be well recognized, this would make an individual more effective. Cognitive skills are those base specialized aptitudes expected to play out a vocation. These abilities go about as an advantage in practically all professions and with the moving scenario the healthcare associations face, increasing strain to construct a relational workplace. The study reveals that for line service staff cognitive skills include handling situations, resolving complaints and feasible planning. As per the response, handling situations is one of the most critical skills required to perform the job (fig 6).

It is important for an employee to be self-managed who includes effective presentation skills, time-management skills, and anger-management. Mindfulness, self-inspiration, self-administration, social-mindfulness, and social-abilities are the center capability for healthcare administrators. As per the result (fig 7), it is important to have effective anger management skills. For line service staff, who handles even the critical patients, should handle people with cool. It is important for line service staff to have effective planning and organizing skills. This skill includes tactic knowledge that includes experience and expertise in the field. Operational knowledge which is everyday work. Motivational skills are essential to keep the patients happy and positive. As per the data 38 percent, people believe that motivational skills are more important in work (fig 8). Individuals having solid scientific abilities can watch and examine circumstances in intelligent and efficient vista. For line service staff analytical skills varies from decision making, logical skills, and visionary skills. Line service staff should have effective logical skills to give hand treatment to patients, to decide how to deal with them and to discuss their things abstractly.

FINDINGS

Digital Healthcare center comprises an expansive range of well-being callings including audiologists, dietitians, restorative researchers, word related advisors, physiotherapists, psychologists, radiation therapists, etc. Training programs will be more effective if attention is given to ensuring that the work-group climate is supportive & encourage change in personal development.

- Both healthcare and hospitality companies know the relevance of quality certification; have the knowledge and understanding of the implementation of quality principal and practices in the organization.
- Training effects on the development of procedural knowledge skills are for technical skills.
- Self-efficacy and training motivation of trainee subsequently affects their learning, reactions and transfer motivation.
- Indian companies and manufacturing companies must devote more time and investment in imparting training in their organization.
- Generic teamwork skills training had a significant and positive impact on both cognitive and skill-based outcomes.

The outcome of the study shows that all eight skills are important for line service staff. However, the type and requirement of skill vary from person to person. Before tailoring any training program for them, it is important to quantify the skill on three parameters proficiency/deficiency and sufficiency.

SOLUTIONS AND RECOMMENDATIONS

- The effect of worker work and vocation dispositions on digital training viability should be increasingly engaged.
- Research ought to be directed to decide whether vocation arranging exercises improve digital preparing adequacy.
- Actual post-training transfer data may improve the validity.
- More training programs should be provided to the employees so that they can help the general public in accessing the digital facilities to save time in case of emergency.

- Facilities for providing emergency treatments or in case of crucial illness should be given more importance.

LIMITATIONS

The sample size taken for the study is limited and confined to a specific region. In this study, only the employees' perspective is discussed. Trainers, as well as patients perspectives, should also be considered. The sample size was small. Future studies will express the simultaneous and dynamic nature of the relationship between training decisions and economic performance. Research should also be conducted to determine if career-planning activities enhance training effectiveness. Research focuses on large organizations only.

FUTURE RESEARCH DIRECTIONS

A large portion of the writing has not contacted a couple of aptitudes like ICT and work brain science; however, the rising interest of innovation-based framework has expanded the utilization of ICT in the working environment. One of the most important skills, teamwork skills, was missed everywhere, which is very necessary for any healthcare organization. So, a further qualitative, as well as quantitative investigation, can be considered keeping in view all the employability skills and its impact can be evaluated by analyzing the efficiency and effectiveness of any employee or team. Empirical analysis can also be done for all the given skillsets to check the real impact value on the skills of an employee. Secondly, the greater part of the exploration effort is bound outside India. For an industry that is blasting so quick and representative's higher number of individuals, it ends up imperative to choose, train or hold them according to the aptitude meter.

CONCLUSION

Well-being examination has progressed in multifaceted nature in late decades with considerable decent variety in substance and viewpoint. The aftereffects of this review recommend that there is considerable specialized and inspirational potential among the healthcare industry to upgrade the examination limit of well-being administration. In view of the aftereffects of the study in the present setting of expanded administration and financial weights, the accomplishment of huge numbers of these outcomes will challenge. It is along these lines basic that examination limit advancement is confined as far as how it can increase the value of administrations, regardless of whether it is improving administration proficiency at the neighborhood level, to creating mediations or projects that advantage benefits over the well-being framework.

Results shown that all the eight skills are important for the training of line service staff viz. communication (empathetic listening training is more important than active listening or Writing Skills), ICT (people have higher adaptability towards ICT related Skills), work engagement (most of the respondents think it is important to have work-life balance skills), teamwork (people feel it is important to be satisfied as a team), cognitive (for line service staff cognitive skills includes handling situations, resolving complaints and feasible planning. As per the response handling situation is one of the most critical skill required to perform the job), self-management (employees prefer effective presentation skills over anger management skills), planning and organizing (38% people believe that motivational skills are more important in work followed by operational knowledge and tactic knowledge by 37% and 25% respectively), and analytical skills (preference of logical skills over decision making followed by visioning skills). However, the type and requirement of skill vary from person to person. For line service staff the parameter of skill varies with the kind of work they are involved in. Few of them must be great empathetic listeners, while few need to be best with a compilation of reports and emails. Therefore, it becomes important to tailor the training programs as per the nature of the job and its demand. It is also suggested that there is considerable specialized and persuasive potential among the healthcare industry to improve the exploration limit of health administration.

REFERENCES

Aguilera, A. (2015). Digital Technology and Mental Health Interventions: Opportunities and Challenges. *Arbor, 191*(771), a210. doi:10.3989/arbor.2015.771n1012

Agut, S., Grau, R., & Peiró, J. M. (2003). Competency needs among managers from Spanish hotels and restaurants and their training demands. *International Journal of Hospitality Management, 22*(3), 281–295. doi:10.1016/S0278-4319(03)00045-8

Alnidawy, A. A. B. (2015). The Effect of Identifying Training Needs on the Effectiveness of the Training Process and Improving the Individual and Organizational Performance: Applied Study in the Jordanian Health Sector. *International Journal of Business Administration, 6*(4), 48.

Boyd, J. S., LoPresti, C. M., Core, M., Schott, C., Mader, M. J., Lucas, B. P., ... Colon-Molero, A. (2019). Current use and training needs of point-of-care ultrasound in emergency departments: A national survey of VA hospitals. *The American Journal of Emergency Medicine, 37*(9), 1794–1797. doi:10.1016/j.ajem.2019.02.043 PMID:30878406

Cheng, E. W., & Ho, D. C. (2001). The influence of job and career attitudes on learning motivation and transfer. *Career Development International, 6*(1), 20–28. doi:10.1108/13620430110381007

Curioso, W. H. (2019). Building Capacity and Training for Digital Health: Challenges and Opportunities in Latin America. *Journal of Medical Internet Research, 21*(12), e16513. doi:10.2196/16513 PMID:31850849

Diab, S. M., & Ajlouni, M. T. (2015). The influence of training on employee's performance, organizational commitment, and quality of medical services at Jordanian private hospitals. *International Journal of Business and Management, 10*(2), 117. doi:10.5539/ijbm.v10n2p117

Ellahham, S., Ellahham, N., & Simsekler, M. C. E. (2019). Application of Artificial Intelligence in the Healthcare Safety Context: Opportunities and Challenges. *American Journal of Medical Quality, §§§*, 1062860619878515. PMID:31581790

Fassaert, T., van Dulmen, S., Schellevis, F., & Bensing, J. (2007). Active listening in medical consultations: Development of the Active Listening Observation Scale (ALOS-global). *Patient Education and Counseling*, *68*(3), 258–264. doi:10.1016/j.pec.2007.06.011 PMID:17689042

Freshman, B., & Rubino, L. (2002). Emotional intelligence: A core competency for healthcare administrators. *The Health Care Manager*, *20*(4), 1–9. doi:10.1097/00126450-200206000-00002 PMID:12083173

Hall, D. (2011). Debate: Innovative teaching to enhance critical thinking and communication skills in healthcare professionals. *The Internet Journal of Allied Health Sciences and Practice*, *9*(3), 7.

Hassan, H., Asad, S., & Hoshino, Y. (2016). Connecting the Post-Training Task and Contextual Performance with the Essentials of Training Program and Characteristics of Trainees. *International Journal of Business and Management*, *11*(4), 11. doi:10.5539/ijbm.v11n4p48

Heckemann, B., Zeller, A., Hahn, S., Dassen, T., Schols, J. M. G. A., & Halfens, R. J. G. (2015). The effect of aggression management training programmes for nursing staff and students working in an acute hospital setting. A narrative review of current literature. *Nurse Education Today*, *35*(1), 212–219. doi:10.1016/j.nedt.2014.08.003 PMID:25200511

Huang, H., Zhang, S., Feng, T., Zhu, J., Zheng, Z., Tao, Y., & Qian, B. (2017). Questionnaire analysis of clinical research capacity and training needs for physicians at university hospitals. *Chinese Journal of Medical Science Research Management*, *30*(4), 293–299.

Husain, M. Y., Mokhtar, S. B., Ahmad, A. A., & Mustapha, R. (2010). Importance of employability skills from employers' perspective. *Procedia: Social and Behavioral Sciences*, *7*, 430–438. doi:10.1016/j.sbspro.2010.10.059

Iliashenko, O., Bikkulova, Z., & Dubgorn, A. (2019). Opportunities and challenges of artificial intelligence in healthcare. In *E3S Web of Conferences* (Vol. 110, p. 02028). EDP Sciences. doi:10.1051/e3sconf/201911002028

Jain, E., & Yadav, A. (2017). Marketing and Technology: Role of Technology in Modern Marketing. *IOSR Journal of Business and Management*, *19*(5), 49–53. doi:10.9790/487X-1905064953

Kitsiou, A., Galanis, P., Bilali, A., Vraka, I., & Theodorou, M. (2016). Training needs of nurses in public hospitals in Cyprus. *Nursing Care & Research/Nosileia kai Ereuna*, (46).

Leggat, S. G. (2007). Effective healthcare teams require effective team members: Defining teamwork competencies. *BMC Health Services Research*, *7*(1), 17. doi:10.1186/1472-6963-7-17 PMID:17284324

Mackey, T. K., Kuo, T. T., Gummadi, B., Clauson, K. A., Church, G., Grishin, D., ... Palombini, M. (2019). 'Fit-for-purpose?'–challenges and opportunities for applications of blockchain technology in the future of healthcare. *BMC Medicine*, *17*(1), 68. doi:10.118612916-019-1296-7 PMID:30914045

Madan, M., & Jain, E. (2017). Impact of organizational culture & climate on managerial effectiveness: An empirical study. *Delhi Business Review*, *16*(2), 47–57.

Menvielle, L., Audrain-Pontevia, A. F., & Menvielle, W. (Eds.). (2017). *The digitization of healthcare: New challenges and opportunities*. Springer. doi:10.1057/978-1-349-95173-4

Messum, D., Wilkes, L., Peters, C., & Jackson, D. (2017). Senior Managers' and Recent Graduates' Perceptions of Employability Skills for Health Services Management. *Asia Pacific Journal of Cooperative Education, 18*(2), 115–128.

O'Driscoll, M. P. P. J. T., & Taylor, P. J. (1992). Congruence between theory and practice in management training needs analysis. *International Journal of Human Resource Management, 3*(3), 593–603. doi:10.1080/09585199200000167

Sarker, S. K., Bhas, G., Paul, R., Pal, H., Yusuf, M. A., & Eva, E. O. (2019). E-Pharmacy Utilization on the Spectrum of Digital Pharmaceutical Practices, Patterns and Challenges in Bangladesh. *Journal of Shaheed Suhrawardy Medical College, 11*(1), 43–47. doi:10.3329/jssmc.v11i1.43178

Sharma, H. (2014). Importance and performance of managerial training in Indian companies–an empirical study. *Journal of Management Development, 33*(2), 75–89. doi:10.1108/JMD-11-2013-0144

Sheldon, L. K. (2005). Communication in oncology care: The effectiveness of skills training workshops for healthcare providers. *Clinical Journal of Oncology Nursing, 9*(3), 305–312. doi:10.1188/05.CJON.305-312 PMID:15973840

Simoni, J. M., Kutner, B. A., & Horvath, K. J. (2015). Opportunities and challenges of digital technology for HIV treatment and prevention. *Current HIV/AIDS Reports, 12*(4), 437–440. doi:10.100711904-015-0289-1 PMID:26412082

Singh, G. K. G., & Singh, S. K. G. (2008). Malaysian graduates' employability skills. *UNITAR e-Journal, 4*(1), 15-45.

Singh, N., & Singh, B. N. (2014). Recent Trends in Training and Developments in Indian Health-Care Sectors in the Changed Economic Scenario. International Journal of Scientific and Research Publications, 20.

Trochimiuk, R. (2015). Professional Development of Older Employees in Small and Medium Enterprises. *Journal of Management and Business Administration. Central Europe, 23*(1), 80–95.

van Harten, J., Knies, E., & Leisink, P. (2016). Employer's investments in hospital workers' employability and employment opportunities. *Personnel Review, 45*(1), 84–102. doi:10.1108/PR-05-2014-0115

Yang, H., Cheung, C., & Fang, C. C. (2015). An empirical study of hospitality employability skills: Perceptions of entry-level hotel staff in china. *Journal of Hospitality & Tourism Education, 27*(4), 161–170. doi:10.1080/10963758.2015.1089510

APPENDIX

Figure 2. Showing responses for communication skills

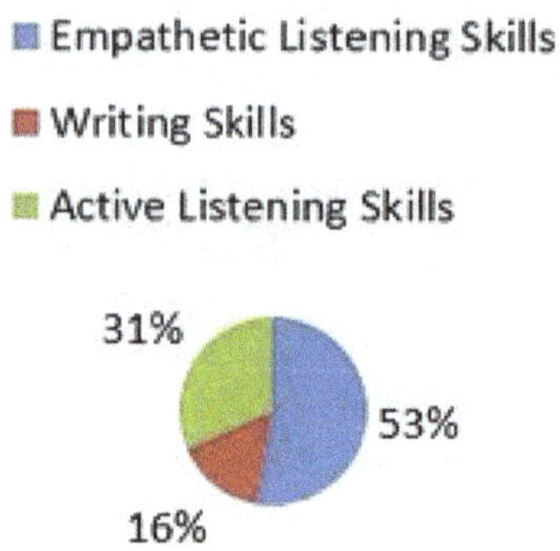

Figure 3. Showing responses for ICT skills

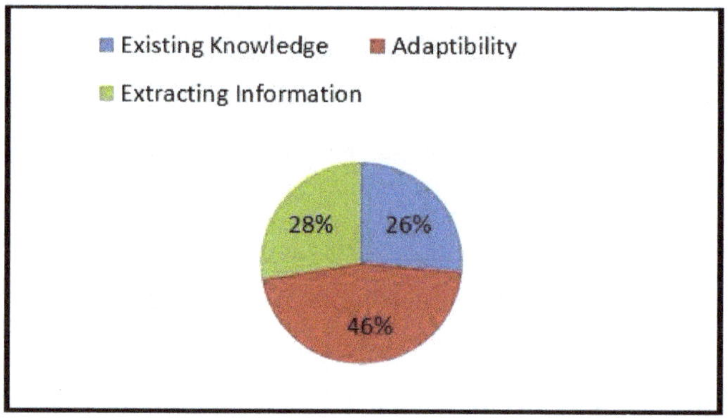

Figure 4. Showing responses for work-engagement skills

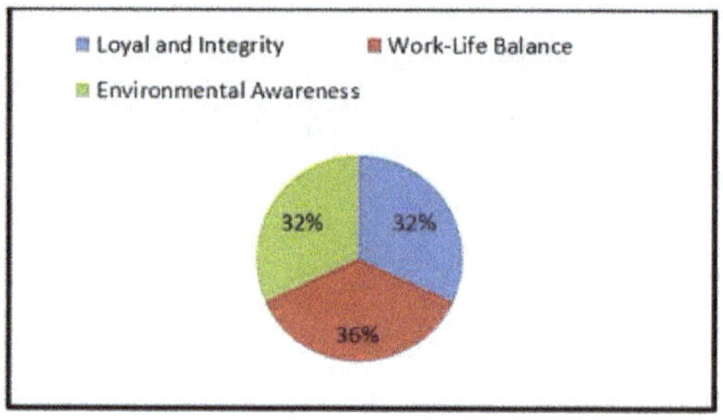

Figure 5. Showing responses for team-work skills

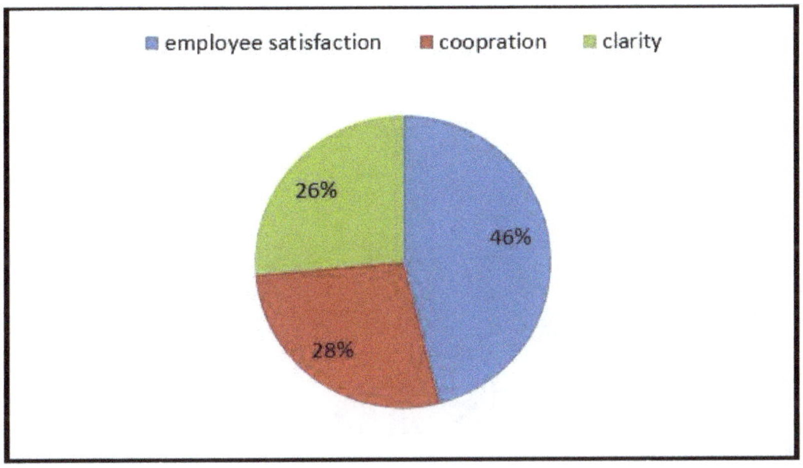

Figure 6. Showing responses for cognitive skills

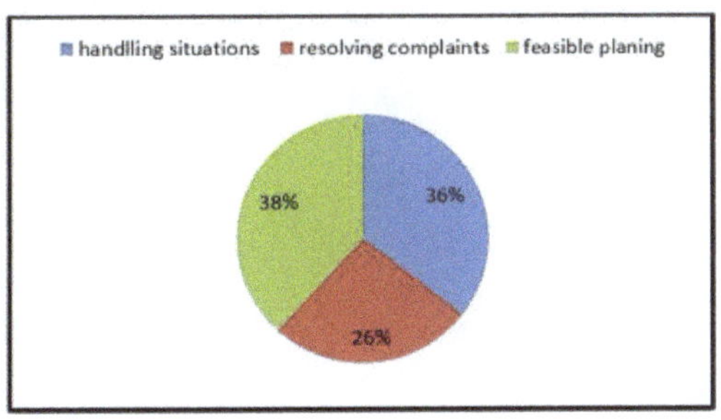

Figure 7. Showing responses for self-management skills

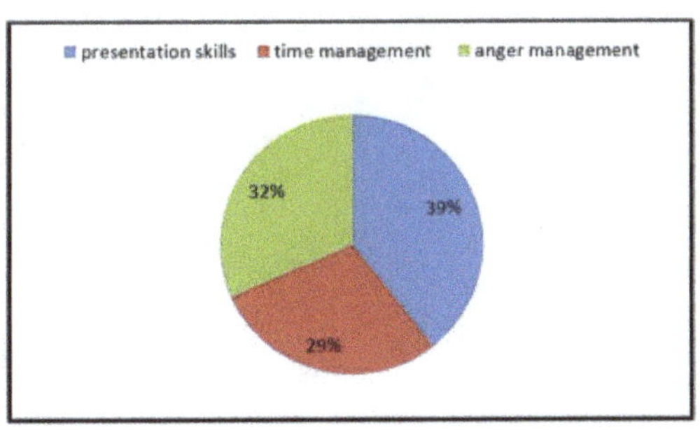

Figure 8. Showing responses for planning & organizing skills

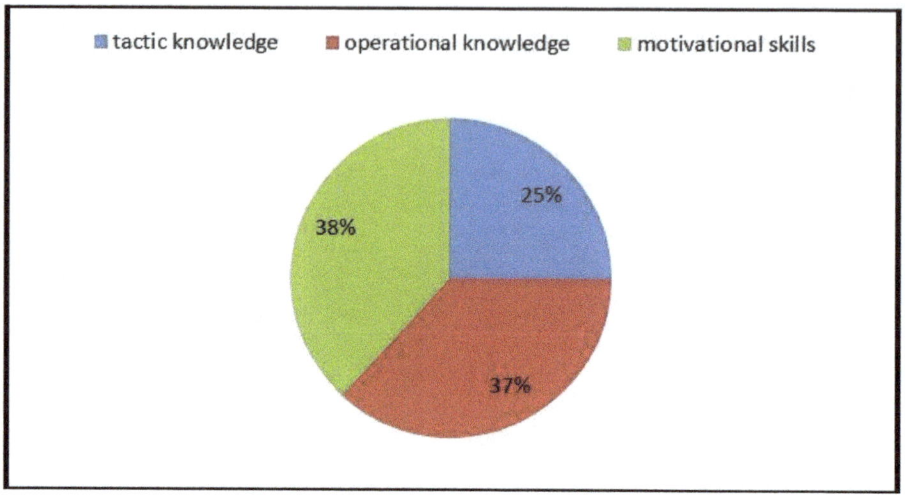

Chapter 8
My Digital Healthcare Record:
Innovation, Challenge, and Patient Empowerment

Anita Medhekar
https://orcid.org/0000-0002-6791-4056
Central Queensland University, Australia

Julie Nguyen
https://orcid.org/0000-0003-1018-0079
Central Queensland University, Australia

ABSTRACT

In the 21st century, the digital revolution is disrupting every sector of the economy. Australia has adopted the digital healthcare technological revolution such as My Health Record (MyHRC) to improve healthcare practice for clinicians/medical professionals and empower consumers to provide positive health management experience with a patient-centred approach to digital health revolution and digital literacy. My Health Record has its benefits, but it has been a challenge for the healthcare practitioners, hospital staff, as well as patients as consumers to accept, embrace, and uptake digital technologies and manage their healthcare records amidst concerns of slow adoption by the patient, data privacy, and implications of the secondary use of their personal data by non-government entities.

INTRODUCTION

In the 21st century, developed countries, have adopted digital health technological revolution to improve healthcare practices for clinicians/medical professionals, and provide positive experience to the consumers and the community at large. It has been a challenge for the healthcare practitioners, hospital administrative staff as well as patients to accept, embrace and uptake digital technologies and manage their healthcare records amidst concerns of slow adoption by the patient/consumers because of personal data privacy and security issues (Walsh et al., 2018). The main aim of embracing digital or e-Health technologies in healthcare, is to transform and provide world class healthcare system and hospital facilities and em-

DOI: 10.4018/978-1-7998-3274-4.ch008

power the patients to participate online, access their health information, communicate and control their personal health records and choose the right healthcare provider and treatment to improve their health and well-being (Archer et al., 2011; Baldwin, Singh, Sittig & Giardina, 2017; Kim & Johnston, 2002; Queensland Health, 2017; Sittig, 2002; Wood et al., 2013).

Medical technological innovation includes a wide range of products and services to treat medical conditions and diseases, for example, innovative healthcare services, medical devices such as e-Health, digital health record tools, healthcare transportation, 3D printing of medical products, tele-medicine, information technology, tele-health, mobile health technologies, artificial intelligence, health informatics and 'My Health Record' ['MyHRC'] (Guo, Chen & Mehta, 2017).

Digital revolution is disrupting every sector of the economy including healthcare in Australia. Digital revolution is driven by innovators of healthcare technologies, investors/entrepreneurs, medical professionals, healthcare providers and government policy makers to bring about a change in healthcare ecosystems. Any innovation, such as technological e-Health innovation needs to be diffused to be widely adopted and used effectively for its perceived advantage derived from its use and application (Lee, Hsieh & Hsu 2011; Roger, 2003).

Usually government policies and regulation drive or squash any type of innovation. It is essential that digital e-Health innovation is healthcare provider-friendly as well as patient-friendly (Hemsley, et al., 2016; Hemsley et al., 2017). A human and a patient-centred approach to digital health revolution, such as ''MyHRC'' will help to change the patient experience and empower them to embrace digital technologies and engage with digital technologies to access and manage their own health records with positive healthcare experience (Australian Government, 2016a & 2016b). Greenhalgh et al. (2010) describe it as a shift from 'specialists-driven' to 'patient-driven' self-managed care as we move from 'information-age' to' industrial-age', which empowers the patients/consumers.

There are many benefits of adopting e-health to the clinicians as well as to patients, who are empowered to engage with their 'MyHRC' to manage their health effectively. However, there are also many challenges in terms of English language literacy, internet literacy, health literacy, and key stakeholders' such as government and healthcare providers responsibility in ensuring privacy and safety of patient's data online (Russo, Sittig, Murphy & Singh, 2016; Sittig, Belmont & Singh, 2018; von Wagner, Steptoe, Wolf & Wardle, 2009). Literature review indicates publications on digital healthcare innovation, such as 'MyHRC' and mobile health adoption and patient empowerment is relatively an emerging new area of research.

This exploratory research examines the benefits and challenges of adopting digital MyHRC in Australia. The objective of this chapter is as follows. The first introductory section of the chapter introduces the growing importance and significance of digital health innovation and adoption in developed countries. Section two, provides the literature review on digital health innovation and patient literacy regarding digital health. Section three, discusses the case study example of Australia in adopting digital health strategies such as 'MyHRC'. Section four, lists the benefits and challenges from healthcare providers and patients/consumer perspective in adopting digital health platforms. Section five, presents discussions and recommendations for healthcare policy implications and proposes a model for diffusion of innovation of 'MyHRC', which can be tested in the future. Section six, provides conclusion and future research directions to advance the knowledge in the field of digital healthcare innovation and patient empowerment.

LITERATURE REVIEW

Digital Health Innovation: Electronic Health Records

Queensland Health has identified four key roles for digital health system: **(i)** *Promoting wellbeing* by thorough healthy behaviour to improving health of people in Queensland. **(ii)** *Delivering healthcare* by emphasising access, equity and quality in healthcare delivery for all. **(iii)** *Connecting healthcare* by tackling funding, policy and delivery barriers, in order to make the health system work better for consumers and communities. **(iv)** *Pursuing innovation* by developing evidence-based models that work, promoting research and translating it into better healthcare practice (Queensland Health, 2017).

This chapter considers online 'MyHRC' as a subset of digital health technological application. Rogers (2003) model of diffusion of innovation theory has been used by researchers to predict technology usage or adoption of internet technology. Diffusion of Innovation Theory identifies four characteristics of innovation: **(i)** advantage, **(ii)** compatibility, **(iii)** complexity, and **(iv)** observability (Rogers, 2003). These diffusion of innovation characteristics can be applied to e-Health such as the use of 'MyHRC' and Mobile Health applications, discussed in section five.

A scoping literature review by Archer et al. (2011) consisting of qualitative and quantitative journal articles about patient-centred personal health records system was looking at its architecture/design, functionality, cost/financing issues, implementation, application, privacy/security, benefits, barriers to acceptance, adoption, and use, satisfaction, health self-management, health education and lifestyle, and clinical outcomes in Canada and the USA. They conclude that patients, primary care provider/ general partitioner has access to patient's electronic medical records. According to their scoping review findings electronic health records functionality is more 'physician-oriented' rather than 'patient-oriented', as physicians use these records for "advising and supporting patients in education and health self-management" (Archer et al., 2011, p.515).

On the other hand, 'MyHRC' share most confidential personal information with patients, physician/ clinicians, administrative staff, and health insurance providers, which also engages patients in managing their healthcare issues and records related to sickness, diagnostic results, x-rays, and prescribed medications. Protecting the security, privacy and confidentiality of the online electronic health/clinical records is critical, as the data can be infected with viruses and lost, hacked, stolen and misused without patients consent for example by the health insurance, agencies, employers and hospital administrators. Andrews, Gajanayake and Sahama (2014) quantitative survey in Queensland, 750 Australian people up to the age of 65, who had not used 'MyHRC' because of lack of trust, perceived risks involved in using and sharing the online health record system, and privacy and confidentiality breach related to their personal health records. Further, a study conducted in Denmark and New Zealand found that respondents were very concerned about the security risk and privacy of the integrated private e-Health records/data stored online (Chhanabhai & Holt, 2007; Zurita & Nøhr, 2004). Trust in e-Health technology and usage are also researched by Atienza et al. (2015) and Georgiou and Prgomet, (2018). The key themes identified from the selected 14 papers was about trust related to privacy and confidentiality, quality of e-Health and effectiveness and its sustainability (Georgiou & Prgomet, 2018).

Atienza et al. (2015) mixed-methods study about the U.S consumers attitudes and perceptions about privacy and security of health summary records with 24 focus group interviews with 256 participants from diverse geographical locations and demographic characteristics. Consumers as patients are not only concerned about privacy of their health information as to who is accessing, seeing, and using their personal health records, and security regarding unauthorised access, use and sharing their records; but also with the knowledge and user-friendly applications of online technologies such as tablet note books and smart-phone mobile health devices on which health information can be accessed (Lin & Bautista, 2017). Furthermore, Atienza et al. (2015) findings generated three themes concluding that, **(i)** consumers consider the trade-offs of privacy and security of health information exchanged that is costs of privacy and security versus the potential benefits of using mobile-Health devises for accessing their health information. **(ii)** Control over health information used, shared and exchanged, and **(iii)** Trust in mobile technology use of health applications to share information and trust in the healthcare provider/general practitioner influencing people behaviour to use mobile devices for sharing health information.

Further, Greenlalgh et al. (2010) mixed methods study in England found that patients perceived HealthSpace neither useful or easy to use to self-manage their health records. Policy makers according to their study hoped that adopting HealthSpace will empower patients, lower National Health Service costs, provide better quality of data, personalise healthcare, and improve patient health literacy. Zulman et al. (2011) survey regarding use of personal health record system by veteran affairs found that 79% of respondents were interested in sharing their personal health information with someone outside of their health system and 25% with non-veteran healthcare provider.

Australian study found that, protection of private data, ease of use of e-Health records, lack of interest and lack of integration of health records with the existing health systems, privacy and security of personal information of the patent is critical for the health consumer and healthcare professionals (Andrews et al., 2014; Lehnbom, McLachlan & Brien, 2012). Therefore, Haas, Wohlgemuth, Echizen, Sonehara and Müller (2011) consider confidentiality, availability and integrity as the three essential goals for ensuring that personal online health records of the patients are confidentially secured, and available and accessed by those who have the authority to use it with integrity and accountability in order to maintain patient's safety and privacy for effective and efficient delivery of healthcare to the patient over their lifetime. A comparative study also found that security and privacy requirements are essential for developing online integrated health records of the patient's data (Farzandipour, Sadoughi, Ahmadi & Karimi, 2010).

Various other international studies identified lack of awareness of benefits lack of interest, concerns about data privacy, safety and security, internet and communication technology related issues, inadequate skills of the user, to understand and use the information, technology and health the benefits derived from information access, sharing and use of 'MyHRC' (Ludwick & Doucette, 2009; Nambisan, Kreps & Polit, 2013; Stevenson & Nilsson, 2012; Yoo et al., 2013).

A systematic literature review of 49 articles by Fernández-Alemán, Carrión Señor, Lozoya and Toval (2013) found that, security and privacy of patient's electronic health records and regulation around security and privacy policy is a concern given that countries are moving away from paper-based to online integrated electronic health records. The study of literature identified five main characteristics related to patient's electronic health records safety and security: **(i)** compliance related to ensuring privacy, safety standards and regulation of electronic health records, **(ii)** information systems acquisition, development and maintenance of encrypted user's data on the server for confidentiality reasons, **(iii)** access and control to authenticate origin of data source and user of the data by user name and password identity, **(iv)** communications and operations management of the type of information exchanged through audit trials, and **(v)** human resources education and training of medical and non-medical professional staff is essential to ensure information security and privacy issues of e-Health records of the patient's sensitive data.

Farzandipour et al. (2010) comparative study on e-Health records security in Australia, Canada and the USA conclude that, not just medical professionals and patients but all computer users should be aware of their online information security through relevant training. Therefore, continuous education and training of the human resources during service is essential for reducing the potential risk to patient safety, data security and privacy in a healthcare service delivery environment. Further, Fernando and Dawson (2009) Australian study with 26 clinicians in three large hospitals found that hospital clinicians were not trained to use and understand the information regarding privacy and security implementation effectively and identify confidential and sensitive private information of the patients, resulting in suboptimal patient safety and healthcare outcomes. Furthermore, the Health Information Management Association of Australia Limited (HIMAA) is registered with Australian Skills Quality Authority (ASQA) to ensure training of health information professional employees of certificate IV in clinical classification and a clinical coding unit for understanding and implementing anonymity, privacy and security coding rules for patient private health records and data usage (HIMAA, 2019).

Another Australian study by Hanna et al. (2017) where they interviewed 12 patients over the phone to explore their own experience of using personally controlled electronic health records identified two key advantages of using 'MyHRC's. (i) Improved quality of healthcare delivery due to information sharing, and (ii) enhanced capacity of the patient for self -management of their health issues. Further, Kerai, Wood and Martin (2014) study, where they interviewed 80 senior citizens in Australia to get their perspective on electronic health record usage found that 84% of the participants were not ready to take on the responsibility of using the system due to lack of knowledge of online usage and preferred their general practitioner's medical practice to manage their health records.

For the online health record system to be fully beneficial, effective to provide patient-centred care, it should be widely accepted, simple, easy to use and accessible to both the patients and the healthcare providers to share and communicate health information in a timely manner to empower the patients. A qualitative pilot study of patient experience in using 'My HealtheVet' in the USA found that, their health records positively influenced to improve communication with the healthcare provider, enhanced the knowledge of their health and improved self-care, increased greater participation, as when to seek care for follow-up action and also it was a challenge to have so much health information, which empowered them to improve their quality of care. There is thus an association between internet and health literacy and health empowerment that is patient's use of e-Health record portals (Coughlin et al., 2018).

Therefore, it is essential that patients also have English language literacy, as well as knowledgeable in the use of internet and health literacy to adopt, engage and manage their online health records to improve self-management of healthcare and have a choice what to keep or delete from online summaries of health reports (Baldwin et al., 2017; Bratan, Stramer & Greenhalgh, 2010; Hemsley et al., 2016; Hemsley, Rollo, Georgiou, Balandin & Hill, 2018; von Wagner, 2009).

Patient Digital Health Literacy

World Health Organization (2019) has defined health literacy as "the cognitive and social skills which determine the motivation and ability of individuals to gain access to, understand, and use information in ways which promote and maintain good health. Health literacy means more than being able to read health information pamphlets and successfully take doctors' appointments. By improving people's access to health information and their capacity to use it effectively, health literacy is critical to empowerment" (WHO, 2019). Nations with multicultural migrant population in Australia, Canada, New Zealand, United Kingdom and USA, digital e-Health health literacy is essential. Health literacy is defined as an individual's ability and skills to read, understand and use medical and healthcare information from western socio-cultural context (Williams & Cooper 2006).

There is an association between general health literacy, digital-literacy, empowerment and to learn about online health information with the use of digital health technologies, in order to make decisions to achieve positive healthcare outcomes. Usually, in developed or developing countries, low income and education levels of the people, is associated with people with low socio-economic, Aboriginals and Torres Strait Islanders, or culturally and linguistic diverse background with low levels of health literacy (Birru et al., 2004; Paasche-Orlow, Parker, Gazmararian, Nielsen-Bohlman & Rudd, 2005; Mitchell & Begoray, 2010; Walsh et al., 2018; von Wagner et al., 2009). Therefore, developing adequate levels of health literacy depends on numerous internal and external factors such as family environment, education, self-learning, cognitive ability, and prior knowledge (von Wagner et al., 2009).

Walsh et al. (2018) Australian study applied content analysis method to analyse online 'MyHRC's information quality on government and non-government organisations website to identify key themes. Further, they examined the use of e-Health resources, knowledge, registration and barriers to use faced by the consumers. Their research findings identified key themes to determine health information quality which were from Government Department of Health and created for the Australian public when developing these health record information sites. Other information resources related to 'MyHRC' registration, privacy issues and benefits of use were mentioned in the resources, which was meant for the people with high literacy rate and excluded population with low health literacy, to engage online with healthcare professionals and health service providers to manage their summary of health records (Walsh et al., 2018). Therefore, people with low literacy levels regarding the use of internet computers and e-Health records hesitate to use and click only a couple of times on electronic health information (Birru et al., 2004).

Access to and use of internet based digital technologies, along with health information quality is the most important step in health literacy and understanding how to engage online and manage 'MyHRC' (Walsh et al., 2019). In case of Australia, an online content analysis study by Walsh et al. (2019) found that since 2016, there was some improvement on assessing health information quality and usability of 'MyHRC'. Their study also found that there was an increase in 'My-HRC' related information resources specially from non-government organisations for users from non-English speaking backgrounds, video resources, and information regarding security of data, patient/user privacy and post-registration use of information by patients and the doctors. However, usability of health information resources, information quality and 'MyHRC' system still needed to be improved and enhanced, because people with low digital/computer usage literacy and health literacy found it difficult to access and use 'MyHRC's and will be hesitant to register and use 'MyHRC' or e-Health platforms due to low literacy levels.

Clark et al. (1998) and Clark, Starr-Schneidkraut and Windsor (1994) proposed a framework for self-management of diseases by the patient, by determining what is the effective way of controlling the disease to achieve one's personal goal of improving health and wellbeing. Clark et al. (1988) self-regulation model was based on three assumptions: **(i)** Several internal and external factors predispose a person to manage a disease. **(ii)** Disease management by patients is the conscious use of various strategies. **(iii)** The patients' perception of outcome/s is related to their health and wellbeing.

Further, according to Clark, Gong and Kaciroti (2001), disease management by a person depends on the internal factors like the knowledge about their own health problems and word-of-mouth information from friends and relatives regarding the disease and external factors like financial means, literacy levels and recommendations by the doctor/clinicians. Clark et al. (2001) emphasise that self-regulation model for disease management is a continuous and a reciprocal process. Furthermore, access and literacy regarding use of mobile wireless health technologies such as smart-phones, mobile-Health, internet, telemedicine and tablets are widely used for self-management of health, health information literacy, health communication, in developed and developing countries rural remote areas for "providing low costs and effective communication" (Gleason, 2015, p.114) of information sharing between the patient's general practitioner and local healthcare worker.

In case of 'MyHRC' use ethical, regulatory and equal access questions are raised. The patient is empowered to make choices and decide what personal records should be in 'MyHRC' online to be accessed by the doctor or hospital's administrative staff (Australian Government, 2016a). Various studies about Australia mention about ethical, legal, regulatory and equal access rights issues related to adopting and use of 'MyHRC' by people in general, and mainly those with intellectual and communication disability to be able to make a choice to use e-Health record system and empower themselves (Fry, Spriggs, Arnold & Pearce, 2014; Hemsley et al., 2017; Spriggs, Arnold, Pearce & Fry, 2012; van Dooren, Lennox & Stewart, 2015).

RESEARCH METHODOLOGY

The research methodology undertaken was qualitative exploratory approach, examining the origin and implementation of the MyHRC by the Australian Government. The source of qualitative data collection was the government MyHRC websites and the related literature. The social science exploratory research, which is considered primary method for theory advancement was used along with case study-based research as the preferred method of choice by researchers for developing and proposing new theoretical models (Creswell, 2014; Yin, 2017). Authors explored and examined various Australian government documents, related to digital 'MyHRC' regulatory acts, 'MyHRC' privacy and confidentiality acts, available online, regulatory requirements and current relevant literature and proposed a conceptual model for digital MyHRC: *Innovation, Adoption, Literacy and Empowerment,* which can be tested in the future.

DIGITAL HEALTH INNOVATION: CASE OF AUSTRALIA – MY HEALTH RECORD

In the Australian context, the relatively new electronic health record is called 'My Health Record'. Online 'MyHRC' is a digital collection of patient's meetings with the doctor, results of x-ray, allergies, diagnostic reports, such as blood tests, prescription medicine records at one central place, which can be accessed by the medical practitioner and the patients with access to internet, rather than with every doctor that the patient visits. Therefore, it provides a secure online summary of an individual's health information from various clinical settings entered by healthcare providers (e.g. specialists, doctors, and allied health professionals) and the individual. This may include information regarding the individual's medical appointment dates and times, health professional's details, past medical conditions, allergies, pathology and radiology results (e.g. blood tests and x-rays), medication prescription and treatment plan (Australian Digital Health Agency {ADHA}, 2019).

The Australian Government initially launched nationwide the personally controlled electronic health record (PCEHR), an opt-in model provided by National E-Health Transition Authority in July 2012 and nearly 2.6 million (11%) had registered, and since March 2016, it was relaunched as 'MyHRC' an opt-out model operated by Digital Health Agency (Department of Health, 2016). For administration related to use, privacy and regulation, MyHRC is underpinned by, various regulatory acts introduced by the Australian Commonwealth Government **(i)** *Healthcare Identifier Act 2010,* **(ii)** *My Health Record Act 2012',* **(iii)** *My Health Record Regulations 2012, and* **(iv)** *My Health Record Rule 2016, and Privacy Act 1988* to provide access, identify the user, privacy and confidentiality of patient records and the rules governing the electronic health records (Australian Government, 2016a; Commonwealth of Australia, 2012 & 2015).

My Health Record allows for healthcare providers to share patient health information to improve effectiveness of healthcare and reduce healthcare costs. It may also aid in improving health outcomes and patient satisfaction by engaging individuals in decision-making, encouraging active patient participation in their health management plan, enabling effective communication between individuals and their healthcare provider, and enabling a strong patient-clinician relationship (Otte-Trojel, de Bont, Rundall & van de Klundert, 2014). Torrens and Walker (2017) study found that females were more likely to register and use 'MyHRC' online than males. Moreover, middle-aged males, older females and adolescents of both sexes had lowest registration on My Health Record.

The Australian Government (2019c) reports a 90.1% national participation rate for My Health Record as at 28th of July 2019. This is the rate of people who chose not to opt-out as a percentage of those who meet the eligibility criteria for Medicare (Australian Government, 2019c). State wise participation rate is Australian Capital Territory (86.7%), New South Wales (90.2%), Northern Territory (93.6%), Queensland (91.2%), SA (89.3%), Tasmania (90.3), Victoria (89.3), and Western Australia (90.4%). Further, an approximate of 16,400 healthcare provider organisations have registered with My Health Record (Australian Government, 2019c). The number and types of healthcare providers organisation registered are as follows: General Practice Organisations (7,240), Public Hospitals and Health Services (832), Private Hospitals and Clinics (190), Pharmacies (4770), Aged Care Residential Services (239), Pathology and Diagnostic Imaging Services (119) and, Other categories of healthcare providers Including Allied Health (2960).

The Health Portfolio Budget Statements 2018-19 released by the Australian Government confirms the continuing investment of $200 million to continue the operation of the 'MyHRC' system (Australian Government, 2019a). This is in additional to the existing national investment of more than $1 billion (Tomlinson, 2019). This will further improve health outcomes by enhancing patient self-management and continuity of care across all healthcare services in Australia. (Australian Government, 2019a).

Concerns around reliability, privacy and security of 'MyHRC' has also been raised in Australia by the public. Further, there are increasing concerns around secondary use of personal information by the Australian Government, such as for the use of information to assess social welfare eligibility and research for the public good. Furthermore, the fear of My Health Record database breach by cyber attackers were rapidly heightened by untimely reports in July 2018, by various international media organisations that 1.5 million Singaporean citizens' health records had been breached (BBC, 2018). It was reported that the Singapore Prime Minister Lee Hsien Loong's personal information was targeted after a similar incident in the previous year targeting the military service (BBC, 2018).

The Australian Government's implementation of 'MyHRC' has generated widespread controversy and debate in Australia. This mainly stemmed from the transition between the original opt-in model of the Personally Controlled Electronic Health Record to the opt-out model of the My Health Record. Australians who wished to not have a 'MyHRC' were informed to opt-out via the 'MyHRC' website and/ or the help line by the 15th of October 2018. This opt-out period was soon extended to 31st of January 2019 following increasing reports of problems with opting out of My Health Record (ADHA, 2018a).

All Australians who did not to elect to opt-out will have a 'MyHRC' created for them automatically. However, individuals who may eventually decide to have a My Health Record do have the option to register at any time to create a record (ADHA, 2018).

Australian Commission on Safety and Quality in Healthcare {ACSQHC}, commissioned report by Shaw, Hines, and Kielly-Carroll (2017) findings identified five key areas of digital health interventions: **(i)** electronic patient portals, **(ii)** Electronic patient reminders on mobile phone technologies, **(iii)** information-sharing by electronic discharge summaries, **(iv)** computerises provider order entry and electronic prescription, and **(v)** clinical decision support systems. Shaw et al., (2017) concluded following extensive research, a synthesis of systematic reviews; and interviews with informants from Australia, the US and the UK that:

Introducing digital health initiatives into healthcare organisations can produce significant benefits to patients and healthcare providers. Improvements to quality, safety and efficiency of patient care are achievable via digital interventions. The literature indicates that a combination of digital interventions may yield greater benefit (Shaw et al., 2018, p.6).

The Chief Executive of e-Health Queensland, rightly comments, "Digital healthcare is one of the most important revolutions in healthcare. Our digital hospitals and other digital healthcare capabilities not only relieve some of the pressures of public hospital infrastructure but are also providing highly connected and interactive models of care that support personalised, precise and well-informed treatment of patients across care settings and care teams. This means improved safety, quality of care and faster treatment for patients" (Queensland Health, 2017).

Health information on 'MyHRC', is viewed online with an access to internet on any device, anytime, anywhere in the world. It helps to keep check on our health over our life time. Healthcare providers and doctors can access patient's important healthcare information if they cannot talk under anaesthetic, to know about patient's prescription medicine, allergies, family history of diseases, pathology and radiology tests results and medical condition of diagnostic results (ADHA, 2019). Australian Commission {ACSQHC} report mentions various benefits generated from digital initiative in health for healthcare providers and patients, such as improved outcomes, improved patient centeredness, improved appropriateness of healthcare, reduction in preventable harm to the patient, and reduction in unwarranted variation (Shaw et al., 2017).

The following section lists the benefits and challenges from digital health innovation.

BENEFITS AND CHALLENGES OF DIGITAL HEALTH INNOVATION

Benefits: Adoption and Use of Digital 'MyHRC'

Introduction of online 'MyHRC' has numerous benefits to healthcare providers and patients/consumers to make the healthcare management and delivery integrated, efficient and effective.

- Adopting 'MyHRC' system which is a subset of e-Health, can provide improved capabilities to the providers and the patient for data reporting, recording data using software offline, analysis and feedback for improving healthcare delivery and optimal patient outcome.

- Availability of patient information in an integrated manner to the healthcare providers for effective delivery of quality treatment.
- Increased patient empowerment and participation, provides foundation for patient-centred healthcare management, giving a sense of ownership and satisfaction of the patient by empowering them to manage and use online 'MyHRC' to improve their health and wellbeing.
- Increased empowerment and satisfaction of the key stakeholders/ medical professionals to manage and use online e-Health records in an integrated manner for the benefit of the patient.
- Economic benefit in the use of scarce resources and cost-effectiveness in using e-Health records and 'MyHRC' from the demand side and the supply side, including eliminating paper and logistic of storing and transport costs of posting medical reports to the healthcare stakeholders.

Challenges: Adoption and Use of Digital 'MyHRC'

Introduction of online e-Health or 'MyHRC' by the national healthcare system of countries faces numerous challenges by healthcare providers and patients as listed below.

- Access to affordable and sustainable internet connections.
- Access and affordability of internet communication and electronic devices such as laptop, tablets, smart-phone, and e-Health mobile apps by consumers.
- Availability of financial resources and funding to establish e-Health system and 'MyHRC'.
- Support from the government and hospital / healthcare senior management.
- Affordability and access to electricity, internet connectivity and personal computers by the people/patients to use 'MyHRC'.
- Patient safety related to poor documentation about medication and clinical errors, feedback and treatment.
- Patient health summary data privacy, safety and security.
- Patient health literacy, English language, computer and Internet literacy.
- Education and training regarding patient data privacy, safety and security.
- Professionals, doctors and clinician's (medical and non-medical staff) education and training regarding ethical and medical issues about understanding, use and application of online health information, engagement and communication with the consumers/patient.
- Quality of healthcare data and avoiding human errors in data entry and other technological challenges.
- Linguistic or English language challenges faced by non-English speaking migrants in Australia, to participate on mobile health devises and register for using 'MyHRC'.
- Besides people with low literacy rates, poverty, with mental and physical disabilities, retirees with health problems and those who cannot afford internet and computers, are not able to use 'MyHRC' and thus may be disadvantaged due to being excluded from the system.
- Low confidence and lack of motivation and knowledge to use information technology for access and use of e-Health record or 'MyHRC' by the healthcare providers and the patients, will reduce the percentage of adoption and uptake by the healthcare practitioners and consumers.
- Shortage of human resources trained capabilities in information technology and health informatics to assist the healthcare practitioners and consumers in adopting the technology.

SOLUTIONS AND RECOMMENDATIONS

MyHRC are managed by the patients to restrict access to some or all documents stored. However, in an emergency the doctor can override the safeguard to access information in order to provide the best care. It is particularly important that women, Aboriginal First Nation people and non-English speaking background migrants from culturally and linguistically diverse (CALD) communities in Australia adopt digital health technology such as 'MyHRC' and empower to self-manage their health. This also requires everyone to have access to smart phones, laptop and internet connections. On the other hand, it is essential for the doctors and clinicians to also embrace, access and manage the privacy of their patient 's health records to enhance their clinical practice and provide positive healthcare outcome to the patients.

The challenge is to strike a balance between the quality of healthcare delivery and managing the online digital healthcare records by the clinicians is very important in partnership with the patient. Patient literacy or education that incorporates self-management of digital records, empowers the patient in achieving the goal of improving health in a cost-effective manner. Following steps can be taken to promote digital literacy as well as e-Health literacy so that people can use 'MyHRC' to empower them for their own health benefit.

- Promoting digital health literacy by the healthcare providers is essential, as it facilitates and motivates patients to self-manage and empower themselves and have control over factors that determine their own health with a positive healthcare outcome.
- Improved partnerships and collaboration between healthcare service providers and the patients as consumers to enhance their self-management capabilities, can result in better use and self-management of digital 'MyHRC' to improve health and wellbeing.
- Further, non-government community and multicultural organisations can be funded to provide information sessions and workshops to non-English speaking migrants which are coming from CALD backgrounds including Aboriginal and Torres Strait Islander people with low literacy rates to train them how to register, use and engage with 'MyHRC', to make informed decisions about their ehealth and empower them for their own benefit.
- It is essential for people to not just to have access, know how to use their digital MyHRC, but foremost how to use the computer technology. Technical and Advancing Further Education (TAFE) can be funded to run one semester digital/computer literacy units to teach how to use the computer and internet search engine skills to people with low-literacy and non-English speaking background migrates from CALD backgrounds.
- All key stakeholders such as government at the commonwealth and state levels, department of health, hospitals (public and private), allied healthcare service providers and patients as consumers must work together for the adoption, safety, security, privacy of shared health summaries, for beneficial usage of electronic healthcare system to empower the patient to manage their health and wellbeing in cooperation with the general practitioner.
- Roger's (2003) four characteristics of innovation diffusion theory such as relative advantage, compatibility, complexity, and observability is adapted to the MyHRC Innovation, Adoption, Literacy and Empowerment Model proposed by this paper.

The perceived four characteristics of innovation diffusion and adoption theory as identified by Roger (2003) can be applied to 'MyHRC' as shown in the proposed developed Figure -1- *'My Digital Health-*

care Record: Innovation, Adoption, Literacy and Empowerment Model'. can be empirically tested in the future. This paper contributes a 5th characteristics of Universal Adoptability to e-Health innovation of 'MyHRC'. The five perceived characteristics as independent variables of My Digital Healthcare Record- 'MyHRC' as an e-Health Innovation which can improve healthcare communication and sharing health summaries between the patient and the healthcare provider and provides relative advantage to both, in achieving positive health outcomes.

Figure 1. My digital healthcare record: innovation, adoption, literacy and empowerment model
Source: Proposed Conceptual Model

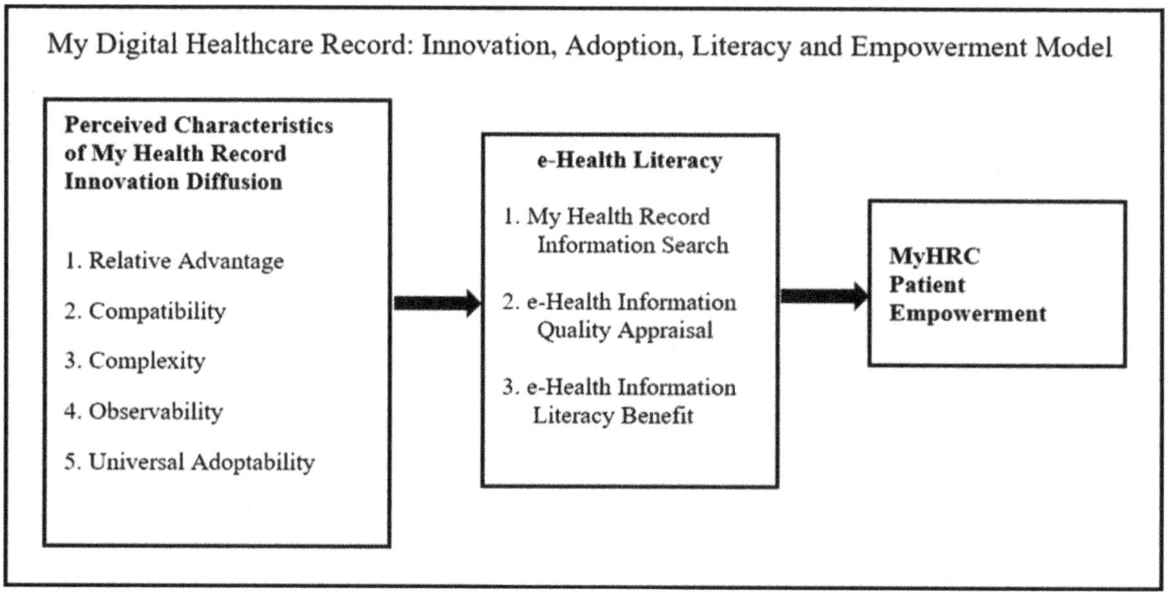

First, '*Relative Advantage*' is defined as "the degree to which an innovation is perceived as being better than the idea it supersedes" (Rogers, 2003, p. 229) and an innovation is considered cost-effective and economical to adopt and use by the society. Second, '*Compatibility*' with electronic information and communication technologies is defined as "the degree to which an innovation is perceived as consistent with the existing values, past experiences, and needs of potential adopters" (Rogers, 2003, p. 240). Third, '*Complexity*' is defined as, "the degree to which an innovation is perceived as relatively difficult to understand and use" (Rogers, 2003, p. 257). Fourth, '*Observability*' refers to "the degree to which the results of an innovation are visible to others" (Rogers, 2003, p. 258), in terms of positive benefits of usage such as patient empowerment and self-management and empowerment of health. Fifth, *Universal Adoptability*, is defined by authors as an ability of everyone or population at large willing to learn new skills and to adopt and engage in new ways of doing things. For example, new ways of using and managing e-Health related online 'MyHRC' summaries by using internet communication technologies.

These five independent variables of innovation diffusion are influenced by three dependent variables of e-Health Literacy: **(i)** the information search about 'MyHRC' registration and usage; **(ii)** health information appraisal of quality of information search and processing information; **(iii)** benefits derived from e-Health information literacy and internet technology literacy to the consumer in context of managing health summaries on line. Therefore, e-Health information literacy in return results in patient empowerment to manage and control their personal health summaries as to who sees and uses it to achieve patient's good health and wellbeing.

FUTURE RESEARCH DIRECTIONS

Future research could collect interview data with the doctors/physicians and the patients/consumers to test the validity of the qualitative findings, followed by quantitative survey with the patients/consumers. Studies can also survey consumer/patient satisfaction with the use of 'MyHRC' by purposeful sampling of diverse population belonging to different demographic groups, education, gender characteristics and rural urban setting, due to digital divide. Such as youth, middle age, retired population, Aboriginal and Torres Strait Islanders, migrants from CALD population sample and people with low and high literacy rate including those who are physical and mentally challenged. The hypothesised relationship between digital health literacy, improves communication and enhances self-care health management can be explored and empirically tested with different groups of people for example youth, retired Australians, Aboriginal and Torres Strait Islanders and CALD migrant population in regional Australia.

CONCLUSION

This chapter concludes that there are many benefits and challenges in adoption and use of digital 'MyHRC' in Australia. It concludes that the use of digital technologies like 'MyHRC' requires health literacy as well as digital literacy which will empower patients to manage their health and wellbeing. The authors identified benefits and challenges and proposed a conceptual model for future data collection and research by qualitative interviews and quantitative survey of the healthcare providers and the users of digital 'MyHRC'. It will lead to better communication between the physician and the patient with the objective of healthcare self-management and empowerment. However, adults and senior citizens still fear privacy and security of patient healthcare data, and therefore show lack of interest in registering and learning to use the health information. People thus do not recognise the potential benefits of use of digital 'MyHRC' in context of improved communication with their general practitioner to manage their health information, resulting in positive healthcare outcomes. Patients therefore need basic health as well as information technology literacy, to be able to communicate and use the online digital health record for their health benefit. Further, income inequality, illiteracy, linguistically diverse ethnic population with poor health and lack of information technology literacy, are few of the major reasons for low up-take of digital 'MyHRC' in Australia.

REFERENCES

Andrews, L., Gajanayake, R., & Sahama, T. (2014). The Australian general public's perceptions of having a personally controlled electronic health record. *International Journal of Medical Informatics, 83*(12), 889–900. doi:10.1016/j.ijmedinf.2014.08.002 PMID:25200198

Archer, N., Fevrier-Thomas, U., Lokker, C., McKibbon, K. A., & Straus, S. E. (2011). Personal Health records: A scoping review. *Journal of the American Medical Informatics Association, 18*(4), 515–522. doi:10.1136/amiajnl-2011-000105 PMID:21672914

Atienza, A. A., Zarcadoolas, C., Vaughon, W., Hughes, P., Patel, V., Chou, W.-Y., & Pritts, J. (2015). Consumer Attitudes and Perceptions on mHealth Privacy and Security: Findings from a Mixed-Methods Study. *Journal of Health Communication, 20*(6), 673–679. doi:10.1080/10810730.2015.1018560 PMID:25868685

Australian Digital Health Agency. (2018a). *My health record opt-out period extended to 31 January 2019.* Available from https://www.myhealthrecord.gov.au/news-and-media/my-health-record-stories/opt-out-period-extended-january-2019

Australian Digital Health Agency. (2018b). *Annual Report 2017-2018.* Available from https://www.digitalhealth.gov.au/about-the-gency/publications/reports/annual-report/Annual_Report_Australian_Digital_Health_Agency_2017-2018_Online.pdf

Australian Digital Health Agency (ADHA). (2019). *MyHRC.* Available from https://www.myhealthrecord.gov.au/for-you-your-family/what-is-'MyHRC'

Australian Government. (2016a). *Welcome to 'MyHRC'.* Available from https://myhealthrecord.gov.au/internet/mhr/publishing.nsf/content/home

Australian Government. (2016b). *'MyHRC's Rule 2016.* Available from https://www.legislation.gov.au/Details/F2016C00607

Australian Government. (2019a). *Health Portfolio Additional Estimates Statements 2018-19.* Department of Health. Available from https://www.health.gov.au/resources/publications/health-portfolio-budget-statements-2018-19

Australian Government. (2019b). *Impact of digital health on the safety and quality of healthcare.* Available from https://www.oaic.gov.au/privacy/other-legislation/my-health-record/

Australian Government. (2019c). *My Health Record Statistics.* Available from https://www.myhealthrecord.gov.au/sites/default/files/my_health_record_dashboard_-_28_july_2019.pdf?v=1565831963

Baldwin, J. L., Singh, H., Sittig, D. F., & Giardina, T. D. (2017). Patient portals and health apps: Pitfalls, promises, and what one might learn from the other. *Health Care, 5*(3), 81–85. PMID:27720139

BBC. (2018, July 20). *Singapore personal data hack hits 1.5m, health authority says.* Available from https://www.bbc.com/news/world-asia-44900507

Birru, M. S., Monaco, V. M., Charles, L., Drew, H., Njie, V., Bierria, T., ... Steinman, R. A. (2004). Internet usage by low-literacy adults seeking health information: An observational analysis. *Journal of Medical Internet Research*, *6*(3), e25. doi:10.2196/jmir.6.3.e25 PMID:15471751

Bratan, T., Stramer, K., & Greenhalgh, T. (2010). 'Never heard of it'– Understanding the public's lack of awareness of a new electronic patient record. *Health Expectations*, *13*(4), 379–391. doi:10.1111/j.1369-7625.2010.00608.x PMID:20579117

Chhanabhai, P., & Holt, A. (2007). Consumers are ready to accept the transition to online and electronic records if they can be assured of the security measures. *General Medicine (Los Angeles, Calif.)*, *9*(1), 8. PMID:17435617

Clark, N. M., Gong, M., & Kaciroti, N. (2001). A model of self-regulation for control of chronic disease. *Health Education & Behavior*, *28*(6), 769–782. doi:10.1177/109019810102800608 PMID:11720277

Clark, N. M., Rosenstock, I., Hassan, H., Wasilewski, Y., Evans, D., Feldman, C., & Mellins, R. (1998). The effect of health beliefs and feelings of self-efficacy on self-management behavior of children with a chronic disease. *Patient Counseling and Education*, *11*(2), 131–139. doi:10.1016/0738-3991(88)90045-6

Clark, N. M., Starr-Schneidkraut, N. J., & Windsor, R. A. (1994). Management of asthma by patients and families. *American Journal of Respiratory and Critical Care Medicine*, *149*(2), 554–556. doi:10.1164/ajrccm/149.2_Pt_2.S54 PMID:8298769

Commonwealth of Australia. (2012). *'MyHRC's Act 2012 (Australia)*. Available from https://www.legislation.gov.au/Series/C2012A00063

Commonwealth of Australia. (2015). *'MyHRC's Regulation 2012 (Australia)*. Available from https://www.legislation.gov.au/Details/F2016C00093

Coughlin, S. S., Stewart, J. L., Young, L., Heboyan, V., & DeLeo, G. (2018). Health Literacy and Patient Web Portals. *International Journal of Medical Informatics*, *113*(1), 43–48. doi:10.1016/j.ijmedinf.2018.02.009 PMID:29602432

Creswell, J. W. (2014). *Research Design: Qualitative, Quantitative, and Mixed Methods Approaches* (4th ed.). Thousand Oaks, CA: SAGE Publications.

Department of Health. (2016, March). MyHRC. Canberra: Australian Government. Available from https://myhealthrecord.gov.au/internet/mhr/publishing.nsf/

Farzandipour, M., Sadoughi, F., Ahmadi, M., & Karimi, I. (2010). Security requirements and solutions in electronic health records: Lessons learned from a comparative study. *Journal of Medical Systems*, *34*(4), 629–642. doi:10.100710916-009-9276-7 PMID:20703917

Fernández-Alemán, J. L., Carrión Señor, I., Lozoya, P. L. O., & Toval, A. (2013). Security and privacy in electronic health records: A systematic literature review. *Journal of Biomedical Informatics*, *46*(3), 541–562. doi:10.1016/j.jbi.2012.12.003 PMID:23305810

Fernando, J., & Dawson, L. (2009). The health information system security threat lifecycle: An informatics theory. *International Journal of Medical Informatics*, *78*(12), 815–826. doi:10.1016/j.ijmedinf.2009.08.006 PMID:19783203

Fry, C. L., Spriggs, M., Arnold, M., & Pearce, C. (2014). Unresolved ethical challenges for the Australian Personally Controlled Electronic Health Record (PCEHR) system: Key informant interview findings. *AJOB Empirical Bioethics*, *5*(4), 30–36. doi:10.1080/23294515.2014.919972

Georgiou, A., & Prgomet, M. (2018). E-Health: Developing trust, confidence, quality and sustainability. *The HIM Journal*, *4*(2), 59–61. doi:10.1177/1833358318808064 PMID:30392402

Gleason, A. W. (2015). mHealth-Opportunities for Transforming Global Healthcare and Barriers to Adoption. *Journal of Electronic Resources in Medical Libraries*, *12*(2), 114–125. doi:10.1080/15424065.2015.1035565

Greenlalgh, T., Hinder, S., Stramere, K., Bratan, T., & Russell, J. (2010). Adoption, non-adoption, and abandonment of a personal electronic health record: Case study of HealthSpace. *Biomedical Journal*, *341*, c5814. PMID:21081595

Guo, U., Chen, L., & Mehta, P. H. (2017). Electronic health record innovations: Helping physicians – One less click at a time. *The HIM Journal*, *43*(3), 140–144. doi:10.1177/1833358316689481 PMID:28671038

Haas, S., Wohlgemuth, S., Echizen, I., Sonehara, N., & Müller, N. (2011). Aspects of privacy for electronic health records. *International Journal of Medical Informatics*, *80*(2), 26–31. doi:10.1016/j.ijmedinf.2010.10.001 PMID:21041113

Hanna, L., Gill, S. D., Newstead, L., Hawkins, M., & Osborne, R. H. (2017). Patient perspectives on a personally controlled electronic health record used in regional Australia: 'I can be like my own doctor'. *The HIM Journal*, *46*(1), 42–48. doi:10.1177/1833358316661063 PMID:27486184

Health Information Management Association of Australia Limited (HIMAA). (2019). *Educational Services for Health Information Professionals*. Available from http://himaa2.org.au/education/?q=node/2

Hemsley, B., Georgiou, A., Carter, R., Hill, S., Higgins, I., van Vlient, P., & Balandin, S. (2016). Use of the 'MyHRC' by people with communication disability in Australia: A review to inform the design and direction of future research. *The HIM Journal*, *45*(3), 107–115. doi:10.1177/1833358316652060 PMID:27269277

Hemsley, B., McCarthy, S., Adams, S., Georgiou, A., Hill, S., & Balandin, S. (2017). Legal, ethical, and rights issues in the adoption and use of the "MyHRC' by people with communication disability in Australia. *Journal of Intellectual & Developmental Disability*, *43*(4), 506–514. doi:10.3109/13668250.2017.1294249

Hemsley, B., Rollo, M., Georgiou, A., Balandin, S., & Hill, S. (2018). The health literacy demands of electronic personal health records (e-PHRs): An integrative review to inform future inclusive research. *Patient Education and Counseling*, *101*(1), 2–15. doi:10.1016/j.pec.2017.07.010 PMID:28864052

Kerai, P., Wood, P., & Martin, M. (2014). A pilot study on the views of elderly regional Australians of personally controlled electronic health records. *International Journal of Medical Informatics*, *83*(3), 201–209. doi:10.1016/j.ijmedinf.2013.12.001 PMID:24382474

Kim, M. I., & Johnston, K. B. (2002). Personal Health Records: Evaluation of Functionality and Utility. *Journal of the American Medical Informatics Association*, *9*(2), 171–180. doi:10.1197/jamia.M0978 PMID:11861632

Lee, Y. H., Hsieh, Y. C., & Hsu, C. N. (2011). Adding innovation diffusion theory to the technology acceptance model: Supporting employees' intentions to use E-Learning systems. *Journal of Educational Technology & Society*, *14*(4), 124–137.

Lehnbom, E. C., McLachlan, A., & Brien, J. A. (2012). A qualitative study of Australians' opinions about personally controlled electronic health records. *Studies in Health Technology and Informatics*, *178*, 105–110. PMID:22797027

Lin, T. C., & Bautista, J. R. (2017). Understanding the Relationships between mHealth Apps' Characteristics, Trialability, and mHealth Literacy. *Journal of Health Communication*, *22*(4), 346–354. doi:10.1080/10810730.2017.1296508 PMID:28323546

Ludwick, D. A., & Doucette, J. (2009). Adopting electronic medical records in primary care: Lessons learned from health information systems implementation experience in seven countries. *International Journal of Medical Informatics*, *78*(1), 22–31. doi:10.1016/j.ijmedinf.2008.06.005 PMID:18644745

Mitchell, B., & Begoray, D. (2010). Electronic Personal Health Records That Promote Self-Management in Chronic Illness. *OJIN: The Online Journal of Issues in Nursing*, *15*(3). doi:10.3912/OJIN.Vol15No03PPT01

Nambisan, P., Kreps, G. L., & Polit, S. (2013). Understanding electronic medical record adoption in the United States: Communication and sociocultural perspectives. *Interactive Journal of Medical Research*, *2*(1), e5. doi:10.2196/ijmr.2437 PMID:23612390

Otte-Trojel, T., de Bont, A., Rundall, T. G., & van de Klundert, J. (2014). How outcomes are achieved through patient portals: A realist review. *Journal of the American Medical Informatics Association*, *21*(4), 751–757. doi:10.1136/amiajnl-2013-002501 PMID:24503882

Paasche-Orlow, M., Parker, R., Gazmararian, J., Nielsen-Bohlman, L., & Rudd, R. (2005). The prevalence of limited health literacy. *Journal of General Internal Medicine*, *20*(2), 175–184. doi:10.1111/j.1525-1497.2005.40245.x PMID:15836552

Queensland Health. (2017). *Digital Health Strategic Vision for Queensland 2026*. State of Queensland: Queensland Health. Available from https://www.health.qld.gov.au/__data/assets/pdf_file/0016/645010/digital-health-strat-vision.pdf

Rogers, E. M. (2003). *Diffusion of innovations*. New York, NY: Simon and Schuster.

Russo, E., Sittig, D. F., Murphy, D. R., & Singh, H. (2018). Challenges in patient safety improvement research in the era of electronic health records. *Health Care*, *4*(4), 285–290. PMID:27473472

Shaw, T., Hines, M., & Kielly-Carroll, C. (2017). *Impact of Digital Health on the Safety and Quality of Healthcare*. Sydney: ACSQHC Available from https://www.safetyandquality.gov.au/

Sittig, D. F. (2002). Personal health records on the internet: A snapshot of the pioneers at the end of the 20th Century. *International Journal of Medical Informatics*, *65*(1), 1–6. doi:10.1016/S1386-5056(01)00215-5 PMID:11904243

Sittig, D. F., Belmont, E., & Singh, H. (2018). Improving the safety of health information technology requires shared responsibility: It is time we all step up. *Health Care, 6*(1), 7–12. PMID:28716376

Spriggs, M., Arnold, M. V., Pearce, C. M., & Fry, C. (2012). Ethical questions must be considered for electronic health records. *Journal of Medical Ethics, 38*(9), 535–539. doi:10.1136/medethics-2011-100413 PMID:22573881

Stevenson, J. E., & Nilsson, G. (2012). Nurses' perceptions of an electronic patient record from a patient safety perspective: A qualitative study. *Journal of Advanced Nursing, 68*(3), 667–676. doi:10.1111/j.1365-2648.2011.05786.x PMID:21781148

Tomlinson, J. (2019). My Health Record implementation in private specialist practice. *The Medical Journal of Australia, 210*(6), S32–S34. doi:10.5694/mja2.50030 PMID:30927474

Torrens, E., & Walker, S. M. (2017). Demographic characteristics of Australian health consumers who were early registrants for opt-in personally controlled electronic health records. *The HIM Journal, 46*(3), 127–133. doi:10.1177/1833358317699341 PMID:28537210

van Dooren, K., Lennox, N., & Stewart, M. (2013). Improving access to electronic health records for people with intellectual disability: A qualitative study. *Australian Journal of Primary Health, 19*(4), 336–342. doi:10.1071/PY13042 PMID:23962451

von Wagner, C., Steptoe, A., Wolf, M. S., & Wardle, J. (2009). Health literacy and health actions: A review and a framework from health psychology. *Health Education & Behavior, 36*(5), 860–877. doi:10.1177/1090198108322819 PMID:18728119

Walsh, L., Hemsley, B., Allan, M., Dahm, M., Balandin, S., Georgiou, A., ... Hill, S. (2019). Assessing the quality and usability of 'MyHRC' within a health literacy framework: What's changed since 2016? *The HIM Journal*, 1–13. doi:10.1177/1833358319864734 PMID:31370712

Walsh, L., Hill, S., Allan, M., Balandin, S., Georgiou, A., Higgins, I., ... Hemsley, B. (2018). A content analysis of the consumer-facing online information about 'MyHRC': Implications for increasing knowledge and awareness to facilitate uptake and use. *The HIM Journal, 4*(6), 106–116. doi:10.1177/1833358317712200 PMID:28589741

Williams, S., & Cooper (2006). Culture-based Literacy and Aboriginal Health. *Canadian Journal of Public Health, 97*(S21).

Wood, S., Schwartz, E., Tuepker, A., Pres, N. A., Nazi, K. M., Turvery, C., & Nichol, W. P. (2013). Patient Experiences with Full Electronic Access to Health Records and Clinical Notes Through the My HealtheVet Personal Health Record Pilot: Qualitative Study. *Journal of Medical Internet Research, 15*(3), e65. doi:10.2196/jmir.2356 PMID:23535584

World Health Organisation (WHO). (2019). *Defining Health Literacy*. Available from https://www.who.int/healthpromotion/conferences/7gchp/track2/en/

Yin, R. K. (2017). *Case study research and applications: Design and Methods*. Thousand Oaks, CA: SAGE Publications.

Yoo, S., Kim, S., & Lee, K. H. (2013). A study of user requests regarding the fully electronic health record system at Seoul National University Bundang Hospital. *Studies in Health Technology and Informatics, 192*, 1015. PMID:23920789

Zulman, D., Nazi, K. M., Turvey, C. L., Wagner, T. H., Woods, S., & An, L. C. (2011). Patient, interest in sharing personal health record information: A web-based survey. *Annals of Internal Medicine, 155*(12), 805–810. doi:10.7326/0003-4819-155-12-201112200-00002 PMID:22184687

Zurita, L., & Nøhr, C. (2004). Patient opinion–EHR assessment from the user's perspective. *Studies in Health Technology and Informatics, 107*(2), 1333–1336. PMID:15361031

ADDITIONAL READING

Australian Commission on Safety and Quality in Healthcare. (n.d.). Publications and Resources. Available from https://www.safetyandquality.gov.au/publications-and-resources

Cillers, L., Viljoen, K. L.-A., & Chinyamurindi, W. T. (2018). A study on students' acceptance of mobile phone use to seek health information in South Africa. *The HIM Journal, 47*(2), 59–69. doi:10.1177/1833358317706185 PMID:28537211

Dehnavieh, R., Haghdoost, A., Khosravi, A., Hoseinnabadi, F., & .... (2019). The District Health Information System (DHIS2): A literature review and meta-synthesis of its strengths and operational challenges based on the experiences of 11 countries. *The HIM Journal, 48*(2), 62–75. doi:10.1177/1833358318777713 PMID:29898604

Hay, P., Wilton, K., Barker, J., Mortley, J., & Cumerlato, M. (2019). The importance of clinical documentation improvement for Australian hospitals. *The HIM Journal, 1-5*. doi:10.1177/1833358319854185 PMID:31303061

Otte-Trojel, T., De Bont, A., Rundall, T. G., & van de Klundert, J. (2016). What do we know about developing patient portals? a systematic literature review. *Journal of the American Medical Informatics Association, 23*(e1), e162–e168. doi:10.1093/jamia/ocv114 PMID:26335985

Sher, M.-L., Talley, P. C., Cheng, Y.-J., & Kuo, K.-M. (2017). How can hospitals better protect the privacy of electronic medical records? Perspectives from staff members of health information management departments. *The HIM Journal, 46*(2), 87–95. doi:10.1177/1833358316671264 PMID:27702792

Yazdanpanah, A., Parsaei, A., & Jeihooni, A. K. (2018). The role of digital marketing in medical tourism industry in point of view of medical tourism policy makers of Shiraz in 2017. *Universal Journal of Pharmaceutical Research, 3*(1), 1–6. doi:10.22270/ujpr.v3i2.128

KEY TERMS AND DEFINITIONS

Digital Health: Digital health also known as e-Health is a system where computer technologies and tele-medicine is used to connect, communicate and manage healthcare information, manage health risk, promote health and wellbeing by the providers/ clinicians and the people/patients. Use of information and communication technologies help to enhance efficient delivery of health information and communication between the physician and the patient and empowers the patient to manage their health and health records.

E-Health Literacy: With the diffusions of internet technology, e-Health literacy means peoples knowledge and skills to use innovative internet and communication technologies and devices such as laptop, tablet, and mobile phone apps to search for health information which is appropriate for health decision making process and communicate effectively with the doctor.

Health Innovation: Disruptive technologies like the use of digital 'MyHRC', e-Health Record is a technological innovation in healthcare used by the healthcare providers, clinicians, nurses, administrators, insurance agencies and the patients. These healthcare innovations empower the people/patients to keep health records, manage and improve our health. For example, digital devices and technologies are used for keeping records of steps taken during the day, daily diet, medicine, sports, and overall wellbeing to improve overall health, wellbeing and knowledge.

Health Literacy: Health literacy is the ability of the people to acquire, read and understand basic healthcare information such as prescription, x-ray and blood tests results, in order to make health related informed decisions for managing and improving one's health and wellbeing.

Mobile Health: Mobile health devices is considered a subset of e-Health. It is the use of internet, tablets and mainly smart-phone devices and mobile phone Apps to adopt, access, communicate and share my health information and records between the patient and the medical doctor in real time to improve health outcomes.

My Health Record: 'MyHRC' is a password and user name protected online information about an individual's health reports. These reports are managed by the patient, who provides permission to allow hospitals, doctors, and other healthcare providers to access these records.

Chapter 9
Digital Recognition of Breast Cancer Using TakhisisNet:
An Innovative Multi-Head Convolutional Neural Network for Classifying Breast Ultrasonic Images

Loris Nanni
Università di Padova, Italy

Alessandra Lumini
https://orcid.org/0000-0003-0290-7354
University of Bologna, Italy

Gianluca Maguolo
University of Padova, Italy

ABSTRACT

In this chapter, the authors evaluate several basic image processing and advanced image pattern recognition techniques for automatically analyzing bioimages, with the aim of designing different ensembles of canonical and deep classifiers for breast lesion classification in ultrasound images. The analysis starts from convolutional neural networks (CNNs) in a square matrix that is used to feed other CNNs. The novel ensemble, named TakhisisNet, is the combination by sum rule of the whole set of the modified CNNs and the original one. Moreover, the performance of the system is further improved by combining it with some handcrafted features. Experimental results obtained on the well-known OASBUD breast cancer dataset (i.e., the open access series of breast ultrasonic data) and on a large set of bioimage classification problems show that TakhisisNet obtains very valuable results and outperforms other approaches previously tested in the same datasets.

DOI: 10.4018/978-1-7998-3274-4.ch009

INTRODUCTION

Breast cancer is one of the main causes of death for women living in western countries (Wild & Stewart, 2014). The diagnosis and the detection of a breast lesion relies upon ultrasound images. This technique is safe, low cost and let radiologists discriminate between benignant and malignant lesions with a very high accuracy. However, the need of an expert doctor to read ultrasound images increases the cost of screening and makes the diagnosis process operator-dependent (Byra, 2018).

In order to support radiologists, the recent innovation in the analysis of digital images led researchers to propose automatic classifiers with the purpose of discriminating between benignant and malignant tumors. E.g. automatic systems based on manually engineered features extracted from ultrasound images and fed into machine learning classifiers like Support Vector Machines (SVMs) are proposed in (Cheng, Shan, Ju, Guo, & Zhang, 2010). However, the recent rise of deep learning lead to the first attempts to use convolutional neural networks to recognize and classify malignant lesions in medical images (Saikia, Bora, Mahanta, & Das, 2019).

Convolutional neural networks (CNNs) are a class of neural networks designed to perform image classification, image segmentation and object recognition (Krizhevsky, Sutskever, & Hinton, 2012). One of the first successful attempt to use CNNs for image classification can be found in (Krizhevsky et al., 2012), where the authors designed a CNN able to outperform any previous classifier on the ImageNet challenge 2012. Since then, every winner of the ImageNet challenge was a CNN. Nowadays, modern CNNs obtain superhuman accuracies on ImageNet (He, Zhang, Ren, & Sun, 2015).

CNNs have already been used on several medical datasets reaching very high performance. In (Pereira, Pinto, Alves, & Silva, 2016) authors used deep CNNs with very small kernels to perform brain tumor segmentation from MRI images; in (Esteva et al., 2017) it is shown that a single CNN could detect keratinocyte carcinomas and malignant melanomas with the same accuracy as expert dermatologists; in (Chi et al., 2017) a fine-tuned version of GoogleNet (Szegedy et al., 2015) is proposed trained to classify thyroid nodules from ultrasound images; the work in (Lakhani & Sundaram, 2017) presented a system to detect pulmonary tuberculosis from radiographies using AlexNet (Krizhevsky et al., 2012) and GoogleNet (Szegedy et al., 2015). In (Byra, 2018) authors proposed a deep learning based method to classify breast cancer from ultrasound images. They used the OASBUD (Open Access Series of Breast Ultrasonic Dataset), a publicly available dataset containing 52 benignant lesions a 48 malignant lesions (Piotrzkowska-Wróblewska, Dobruch-Sobczak, & Byra Michałand Nowicki, 2017). Their approach consisted in combining Fisher Linear Discriminant Analysis (Welling, 2005) and neural style transfer (Gatys, Ecker, & Bethge, 2016).

In this chapter we propose a novel method for the digital classification of breast cancer based on CNNs. The architecture of CNN consists of several convolutional and pooling layers stacked at the beginning of the network. These layers are usually followed by one or more fully connected layers. While the first layers of a CNN can be interpreted as trained feature extractors, the fully connected layers can be thought as a classifier. In particular, the last fully connected layer, after a softmax normalization, returns a probability distribution of the predicted label over the set of the possible classes. Our idea consists in replacing a pooling layer with other CNNs architectures. To be more precise, we add a reshape layer that takes the output of a pooling layer and randomly puts its entries in a square matrix. If the number of features is not a perfect square, the matrix can be padded with some zeros. After this reshape layer, we feed other CNNs with the new matrix. The CNNs on top are trained end-to-end with the first CNN and each of them return its own set of probability distributions. The final ensemble, resulting from the sum rule of such probability distribution is named TakhisisNet, since it is a multi-head convolutional neural network.

Finally, to improve the performance of the system we have experimented the combination by sum rule of TakhisisNet with a set of Support Vector Machine (SVM) trained on handcrafted features.

The chapter is organized as follows. The background describes the prior art for CNNs and the architecture of the two models used in this work: Vgg16 and GoogleNet, After that, the authors describes the proposed method, including the architecture of the TakhisisNet. In the Materials section the authors describe the Breast Ultrasound dataset and other medical datasets used during experimentation, and explain the details of the experimental setup. After that, the authors present the classification results along with a discussion of the findings. Finally, the conclusions for the study are presented.

BACKGROUND

The topology of CNN is divided into multiple learning stages composed of a combination of several types of layers: i.e. convolutional layers, non-linear processing units, subsampling layers, fully connected layers (Liu et al., 2017).

A convolutional layer takes a multi-channel image as an input and outputs a new multi-channel image, which is the discrete convolution between the input and a bank of convolutional kernels (filters). This kind of layers mimics the visual systems of a human eye. Depending on the weights of the kernel, convolutional layers can highlight specific geometric features of the input image like corners and boundaries. Besides, they can interpret the color of a pixel depending on the surrounding context. For example, a little square containing alternated red and yellow pixels will look orange: that is the founding principle of many painting techniques like pointillism. This means that the human eye cannot see the difference between images that might be far from each other in terms of matrix distance. Convolutional layers with suitable weights can compute an approximation of the average of the pixel colors in a small square and mimic this property of human vision, in particular when the input image is noisy. Output of the convolutional kernels is given to non-linear processing units, which helps in learning abstraction and embeds non-linearity in the feature space. This non-linearity produces different patterns of activations for dissimilar responses and thus facilitates in learning of semantic differences in images. Convolutional layers do not decrease the dimension of their input, as a neural network layer is often supposed to do. Hence, they are often followed by a pooling layer. A standard pooling layer is a subsampling unit that divides every channel of the input image in little squares with potential overlap and outputs a new image that has only one pixel for every square of the original image. Since a square has a larger dimension than a single pixel, these layers perform dimensionality reduction. The aim of subsampling is not only to summarize the results but also to make the input invariant to geometrical distortions. The last layers of a convolutional network are usually one or more fully connected layers, which are trained to perform a classification task. Unlike pooling and convolution, a fully connected layer performs a global operation: it takes input from the previous layer and makes a non-linear combination of selected features, which are used for the classification of data. The general architecture of a standard CNN can be found in Figure 1.

We performed our experiments using two different CNN architecture: VGG16 and GoogleNet.

VGGnet (Simonyan & Zisserman, 2015) is a very heavy network that was runner-up in the ImageNet Challenge in 2014. VGGnet (figure 2) is one of the most used architectures for feature extraction from images, due to the simplicity of its uniform architecture. VGGNet is a linear combination of convolu-

Figure 1. Standard CNN architecture

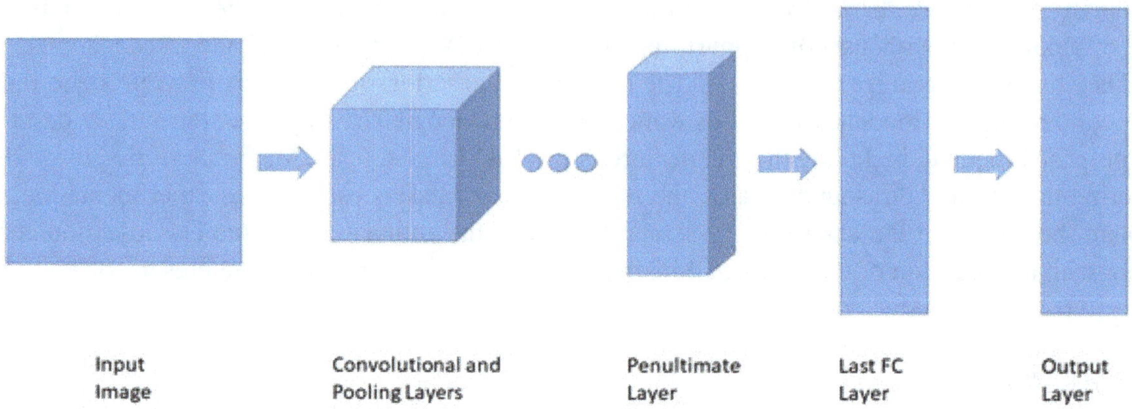

tional layers and pooling layers followed by 3 fully connected layers. Each Convolutional layer has the same configuration including a different number of small size filters (3×3 kernel). Each Max Pooling is designed to half the size of the image. The main limitation of VGG is its high computational cost: despite of the use of size filters, VGG require about 140 million parameters, most of which are given by fully connected layers. VGG16 is a 16 layers deep VGGNet.

Figure 2. VGGNet architecture

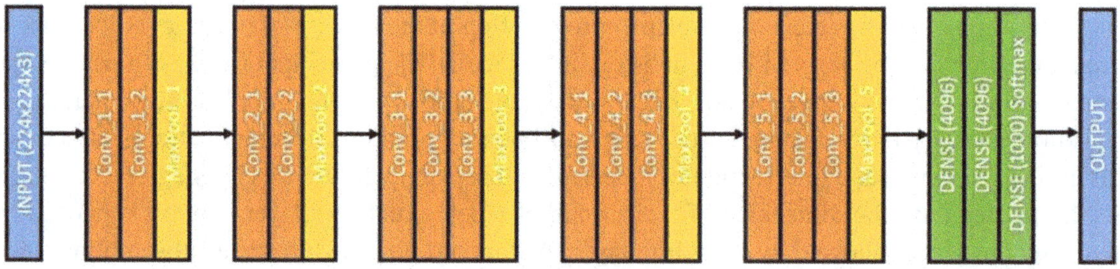

GoogleNet (Szegedy et al., 2015) is a light network that won the ImageNet Challenge in 2014. GoogleNet implements a novel element, named inception module (figure 3), which is a subnetwork consisting of parallel convolutional filters whose outputs are concatenated. GoogleNet uses batch normalization, image distortions and RMSprop optimizer. The use of inception modules that strongly reduce the number of parameters, therefore GoogleNet architecture consists of 22 layers but requires only 4 million parameters.

Figure 3. GoogleNet architecture

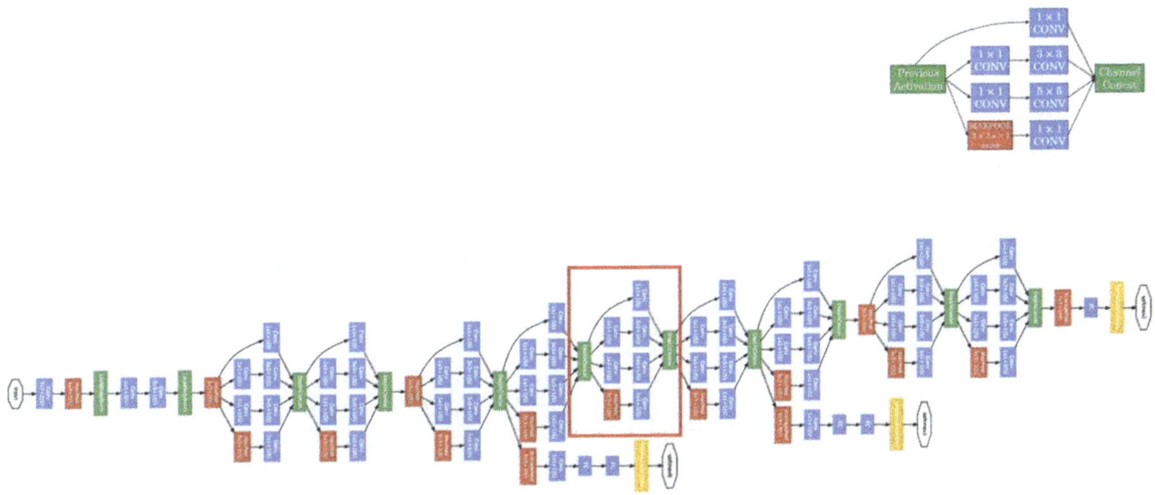

RESEARCH METHODOLOGY: TAKHISISNET ARCHITECTURE

In this chapter we propose a novel CNN architecture based on the fusion of several network: TakhisisNet is a multi head CNN which owes its name to the fictional character of Takhisis, a five-headed dragon. The architecture of the proposed ensemble is shown in figure 4. The "body" of the network is a standard CNN architecture (VGG16 or GoogleNet in this work), from which we extract the output of the Global Average Pooling layer for GoogleNet and the output of the last max pooling for Vgg16.

To be more precise, we add a set of reshape layers that take input from Global Average Pooling layer for GoogleNet and from last max pooling for Vgg16, and randomly reshape it into a square matrix (if the number of features is not a perfect square, the matrix is padded with some zeros). After the reshape layers, we feed other "head"-CNNs with the new matrices. The "head"-CNNs are trained end-to-end with the "body" CNN and each of them returns its own set of probability distributions. Then, we make our predictions by averaging the probability distributions of all the "head"-CNNs and summing it to the probability distribution of the body-CNN.

Besides, it creates an ensemble of neural networks trained end-to-end. In the experiments we used architectures with ten "heads", each head is a different CNN whose input is the output of a reshape layer. Besides, we used the same architecture for the "body" CNN and for the "heads". In the tests reported in this chapter we used 10 "heads" which are finally fused, by weighted sum rule, to the "body" to give the response of TakhisisNet. Before the fusion the scores of both "body" and "heads" are normalized to mean 0 and standard deviation 1 (before the normalization the scores of the heads are combined by sum rule); moreover, the weight of "body" is 2 and the weight of "heads" is 1.

In our experiments we evaluated two different implementations of the reshape layers: the first one is based on a simple randomization of the position of the features inside the output matrix, the second is based on pre-processing the output vector according to a continuous wavelet transform before reshaping.

Figure 4. Proposed TakhisisNet architecture

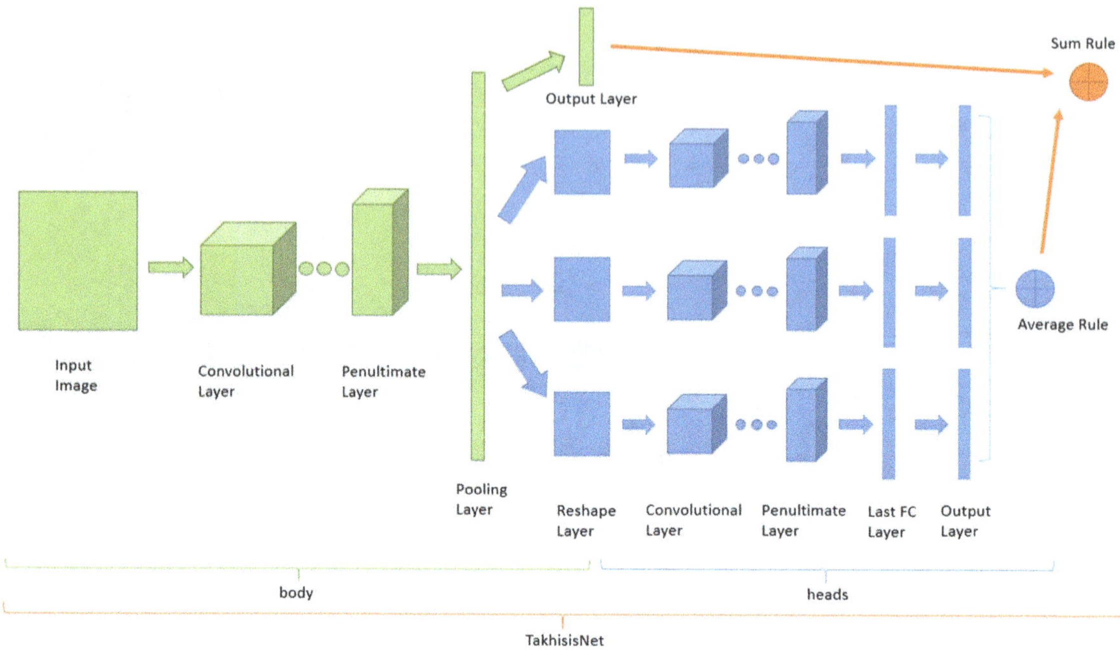

The Wavelet Transform is signal decomposition onto a set of basis function, which is derived from a single prototype wavelet by scaling (dilatations and contractions) as well as translations (shifts).

In this work we use the Meyer mother wavelet (Daubechies, 1992), an orthogonal wavelet that is indefinitely differentiable with infinite support. The number of scales has been set to the length of the feature vector and in the case of feature vector larger than 5000, we reduce it to 5000 to avoid huge computational time. Then the output of the wavelet is resized to the size required by the CNN.

Materials

In order to validate our architecture, we performed experiments on several well-known medical datasets and we test our TakhisisNet on a Breast Ultrasound dataset.

The medical datasets used for preliminary validation, see Table 1, include: the Chinese hamster ovary cells (a proteomic profiling dataset), the 2D HELA, a dataset of cell images from fluorescence microscope acquisition, Locate Endogenous and Locate Transfected, two database of pattern for subcellular location and 6 biological dataset from the IICBU Biological Image Repository (FlyCel, Terminal bulb aging, Lymphoma, Muscle aging, Liver gender, Liver aging) https://ome.grc.nia.nih.gov/iicbu2008/, and three cancer datasets: the Human colorectal cancer dataset, the breast grading carcinoma and the Laryngeal dataset (Moccia et al., 2017). The 13 datasets are summarized in table 1, where the number of classes and samples for each dataset are reported.

The protocol used in our experiments is five-fold cross-validation for 12 of 13 datasets. Since the Laryngeal dataset (Moccia et al., 2017) came already divided in training and testing, we used the suggested testing protocol in that dataset.

Table 1. Descriptive Summary of the Medical Datasets: ShortName, Name, the number of classes (#C), number of samples (#S), URL for downloading, Reference.

Dataset	Name	#C	#S	URL for Download
CH	Chinese hamster ovary cells	5	327	http://ome.grc.nia.nih.gov/iicbu2008/hela/index.html#cho
HE	2D HELA	10	862	http://ome.grc.nia.nih.gov/iicbu2008/hela/index.html
LO	Locate Endogenous	10	502	http://locate.imb.uq.edu.au/downloads.shtml
TR	Locate Transfected	11	553	http://locate.imb.uq.edu.au/downloads.shtml
RN	Fly Cell	10	200	http://ome.grc.nia.nih.gov/iicbu2008/rnai/index.html
TB	Terminal bulb aging	7	970	https://ome.grc.nia.nih.gov/iicbu2008
LY	Lymphoma	3	375	https://ome.grc.nia.nih.gov/iicbu2008
MA	Muscle aging	4	237	https://ome.grc.nia.nih.gov/iicbu2008
LG	Liver gender	2	265	https://ome.grc.nia.nih.gov/iicbu2008
LA	Liver aging	4	529	https://ome.grc.nia.nih.gov/iicbu2008
CO	Human colorectal cancer	8	5000	https://zenodo.org/record/53169#.WaXjW8hJaUm
BGR	breast grading carcinoma	3	300	https://zenodo.org/record/834910#.Wp1bQ-jOWUl
LAR	Laryngeal dataset	3	1320	https://zenodo.org/record/1003200#.WdeQcnBx0nQ

As to breast cancer classification is concerned, we used the OASBUD (Open Access Series of Breast Ultrasonic Data) (Piotrzkowska-Wróblewska, Dobruch-Sobczak, & Byra Michałand Nowicki, 2017), a freely available breast lesion dataset[1]. The dataset includes raw ultrasound data recorded from breast focal lesions corresponding to 52 and 48 scans from malignant and benign lesions of different people, respectively. Two orthogonal scans are available for each lesion, therefore in our system the final score of each lesion is obtained as the sum of the scores of the two orthogonal scans.

In figure 5 some samples from the OASBUD dataset are shown. Since the dataset is quite small, we used the leave-one-out cross validation as testing protocol: the test set consisted of 2 images from the same lesion and the training set consisted of all remaining images.

SOLUTIONS AND RECOMMENDATIONS

In order to validate the TakhisisNet architecture we perform experiments in several medical image classification tasks. In all the experiments the class distribution has not been maintained when splitting the datasets between training and testing (according to the k-fold cross validation testing protocol), and all the input images has been evaluated without ad hoc preprocessing. Since CNNs need input images of a fixed size, we have used the following approach: first the input image is padded to square size to maintain the aspect ratio, then it is resized using bilinear interpolation.

The evaluation of the proposed approaches and the comparison with the literature is performed according to two of the most used performance indicators in image classification: accuracy and AUC. Accuracy is the ratio between the number of true predictions and the total number of samples, while

Figure 5. Samples form the OASBUD dataset

AUC, i.e. the Area Under the ROC-curve, is a performance indicator mainly used for 2-class problems which can be interpreted as the probability that the classifier will assign a higher score to a randomly picked positive sample than to a randomly picked negative one (Huang & Ling, 2005). To validate the experiments the Wilcoxon signed rank test (Demšar, 2006) has been used.

In the first experiment we evaluate the proposed architecture on several well-known medical datasets, comparing the performance of TakhisisNet with its "body"-CNN (i.e. GoogleNet or VGG16) and the ensemble of its "heads"-CNNs. For fine-tuning the networks on each image classification problem we have used the following parameter configuration: learning rate 0.0001, miniBatch size 30, twenty-five epochs to train the "body" CNN, and 100 epochs for training each "head" of the TakhisisNet after the reshape layers. During the training phase a simple data augmentation has been performed (only for "body", not for the "heads") including reflection and scaling on both x and y axes.

In table 2 the performance, in terms of accuracy, of TakhisisNet and its components is reported: the "body" is the standard CNN model (VGG16 or GoogleNet) fine-tuned on the specific dataset, the "heads"

Table 2. Performance (accuracy) obtained by TakhisisNet vs. Body vs. Heads varying the base model (GoogleNet and VGG16) and using the standard random method for the reshape layer.

MODEL	METHOD	DATASET												Avg
		CH	HE	LO	TR	RN	TB	LY	MA	LG	LA	BG	LAR	
GoogleNet	Heads	88.62	83.60	92.00	86.55	44.50	59.18	72.00	60.83	97.33	93.14	80.67	85.76	78.68
	Body	95.08	86.74	93.00	92.73	45.00	57.84	73.33	82.08	91.67	83.43	86.00	85.08	81.00
	TakhisisNet	95.38	87.79	93.80	92.73	49.50	60.10	74.40	83.33	94.00	88.00	87.67	85.83	82.71
VGG16	Heads	94.15	89.88	91.00	85.45	55.50	63.71	78.67	71.67	99.00	96.19	84.00	88.03	83.10
	Body	99.69	93.60	98.20	93.27	69.50	61.44	80.80	85.00	85.33	88.57	93.00	91.44	86.65
	TakhisisNet	99.69	93.72	98.00	93.64	72.50	64.12	83.47	86.25	87.67	91.62	93.00	91.89	87.96

is the fusion by average rule of the 10 heads of the network. From the results in table 2 it is clear that TakhisisNet outperforms both its components in almost all the datasets.

In table 3 the performance obtained varying the reshape method (random or wavelet) is reported. Even if the results in table 2 suggests that VGG16 performs better than GoogleNet in almost all the tested problems, we selected GoogleNet as base model for next experiments since its requirements in terms of memory occupancy and GPU time for training are much lower than for VGG16. Moreover, for a sake of time only a subset of datasets have been evaluated in table 3. For a better comparison some results of table 2 are replicated in table 3. In the last two lines of table 3 we also report the performance of other two ensemble: ENS_HEADS, is the fusion between Heads based on Random and Heads based on Wavelet; ENS_TAK, is the fusion between the two TakhisisNet, the one based on Random and the other based on Wavelet.

Table 3. Performance (accuracy) obtained by TakhisisNet vs. Body vs. Heads varying the reshape method (random and wavelet) and using GoogleNet as base model. The last two rows report the performance of two ensembles.

MODEL (reshape method)	METHOD	DATASET								Avg
		CH	HE	LO	TR	RN	LG	LA	BG	
GoogleNet (random)	Heads	88.62	83.60	92.00	86.55	44.50	97.33	93.14	80.67	83.30
	Body	95.08	86.74	93.00	92.73	45.00	91.67	83.43	86.00	84.20
	TakhisisNet	95.38	87.79	93.80	92.73	49.50	94.00	88.00	87.67	86.10
GoogleNet (wavelet)	Heads	88.92	84.19	92.40	84.18	34.00	94.00	94.10	72.33	80.51
	Body	95.08	86.74	93.00	92.73	45.00	91.67	83.43	86.00	84.20
	TakhisisNet	95.69	87.67	93.40	93.09	47.50	92.67	88.00	87.33	85.66
ENS_heads		90.77	86.28	94.20	89.27	44.00	97.00	93.71	79.67	84.36
ENS_Tak		95.69	87.91	93.60	93.09	49.50	93.67	88.19	87.00	86.08

From the accuracies reported in Tables 2 and 3 and considering the results of the Wilcoxon signed rank test, the following conclusions can be drawn:

- TakhisisNet outperforms the base CNN architecture ("body") with a p-value of 0.005 for both GoogleNet and Vgg16 models;
- ENS-heads outperforms with a p-value of 0.1 both heads-Random and heads-Wavelet;
- Unfortunately, there is not a static performance difference between ENS-Tak and TakhisisNet-Random or between ENS-Tak and TakhisisNet-Wavelet.

The second experiment is focused to the main aim of this work, breast ultrasound image classification. For computational reasons, due to the onerous testing protocol used in the breast ultrasound dataset (i.e. leave-one-out) we have run tests using only GoogleNet. In table 4 the performance of TakhisisNet (based on GoogleNet) are compared with other ensembles designed for a sake of comparison.

The first ensemble, named ENS_HAND is the combination of several SVM (Chang & Lin, 2011) classifiers trained with different handcrafted descriptors (L. Nanni, Brahnam, Ghidoni, & Lumini, 2018):

1. Multithreshold LPQ (MLPQ) (L. Nanni, Brahnam, Lumini, & Barrier, 2014) is a multi-threshold approach applied the LPQ descriptor. The MLPQ features used in our experiments are extracted and combined according to the method proposed in (L. Nanni et al., 2014).
2. Gaussian Of Local Descriptors (GOLD) (Serra, Grana, Manfredi, & Cucchiara, 2015) is a descriptor that models the local features distribution with a multivariate Gaussian, without any quantization.
3. Full BSIF (Loris Nanni, Paci, Caetano dos Santos, Brahnam, & Hyttinen, 2016) is an extension of the Binarized Statistical Image Feature (Kannala & Rahtu, 2012) that assigns each pixel of the input image a n-bit label obtained by means of a set of n linear filters. Full BSIF is a multi-threshold extension of BSIFT used to create an ensemble of classifiers.
4. Full RIC, is a multiscale Rotation Invariant Co-occurrence of Adjacent LBP (RIC) (Nosaka & Fukui, 2014). This variant extracts RIC features using different parameter settings, i.e. varying the LBP radius and displacement among the LBPs. The values used in our experiments are: (1, 2), (2, 4) and (4, 8).
5. LETRIST, the descriptor proposed in (Song, Li, Meng, Wu, & Cai, 2017): a descriptor that explicitly encodes the joint information within an image across feature and scale spaces.

A detailed description of each of these descriptors along with information about the parameter sets used for each descriptor can be found in APPENDIX 1.

The second ensemble, named ENS_DEEP is the combination of several GoogleNets trained with different parameters or data augmentation methods (all the combination have been considered) for a total of 24 CNNs:

1. Batch Size $\in$ {10, 30, 50, 70}
2. Learning rate $\in$ {0.0001, 0.001}
3. Data Augmentation $\in$ {left-right reflection; 4 side reflection + scaling; 4 side reflection + scaling + roto-translation}

The third ensemble, named ENS_TH is the fusion by the sum rule between TakhisisNet[2] and ENS_HAND; notice that before the fusion the scores of both TakhisisNet and ENS_HAND have been normalized to mean 0 and standard deviation 1.

The first line of table 4 is the most performing stand-alone GoogleNet belonging to the ensemble ENS_DEEP chosen considering the performance directly on the test set. Even if in many papers the tuning of parameters is performed selecting the best configuration on the test set, this practice can generate overfitting and it useful only to find an over bound to the performance. Therefore, the resulting network is named GoogleNet_OF. The second line is the most performing GoogleNet selected on the base of the performance in the training set. The third line is a VGG16 network fine-tuned on in the OASBUD dataset. The last two lines of table 4 report the best results published in the literature on this dataset.

Table 4. Comparisons in the OASBUD dataset in terms of AUC

Method	AUC
GoogleNet_OF	0.855
GoogleNet	0.822
VGG16	0.849
ENS_DEEP	0.874
TakhisisNet	0.877
ENS_HAND	0.887
ENS_TH	0.891
(Byra, 2018)	0.847
(Antropova, Huynh, & Giger, 2017)	0.826

From the analysis of table 4 it is clear that the proposed system TakhisisNet obtains performance higher that that reported in the literature (Byra, 2018)(Antropova et al., 2017). Another clear result is the usefulness of the ensemble: GoogleNet obtains an AUC of 0.822, drastically lower than the 0.877 obtained by TakhisisNet. The highest AUC value is equal to 0.887 and has been obtained by the ensemble ENS_TH designed by the fusion of both deep learning and handcrafted features: this fact highlights the diversity among the two methods that can be exploited to improve the overall performance in an ensemble. The ROC curves calculated for the worst and the best performing classifiers (the stand-alone GoogleNet (yellow curve), TakhisisNet (blue curve) and ENS_TH (green curve)) are shown in figure 6. The difference between AUC values was statistically significant according to the Wilcoxon signed rank test (p-value < 0.1).

It is interesting to stress the high performance obtained by ensemble of texture descriptors; it outperforms the method based on CNN. As already show in other works, handcrafted descriptors can outperform deep learning approaches if a large training set is not available, as in the problem faced in this work.

Another interesting result is that we apply the same CNN ensemble validated on several medical datasets and we use a set of handcrafted descriptors that we have already proposed in the literature (L. Nanni, Brahnam, Ghidoni, & Lumini, 2018); we have not optimized our ensemble for the breast ultrasound cancer dataset. That dataset is quite small, so it is risky to optimize a given approach on that

Figure 6. ROC curves of the proposed methods: GoogleNet (yellow curve), TakhisisNet (blue curve) and ENS_TH (green curve)

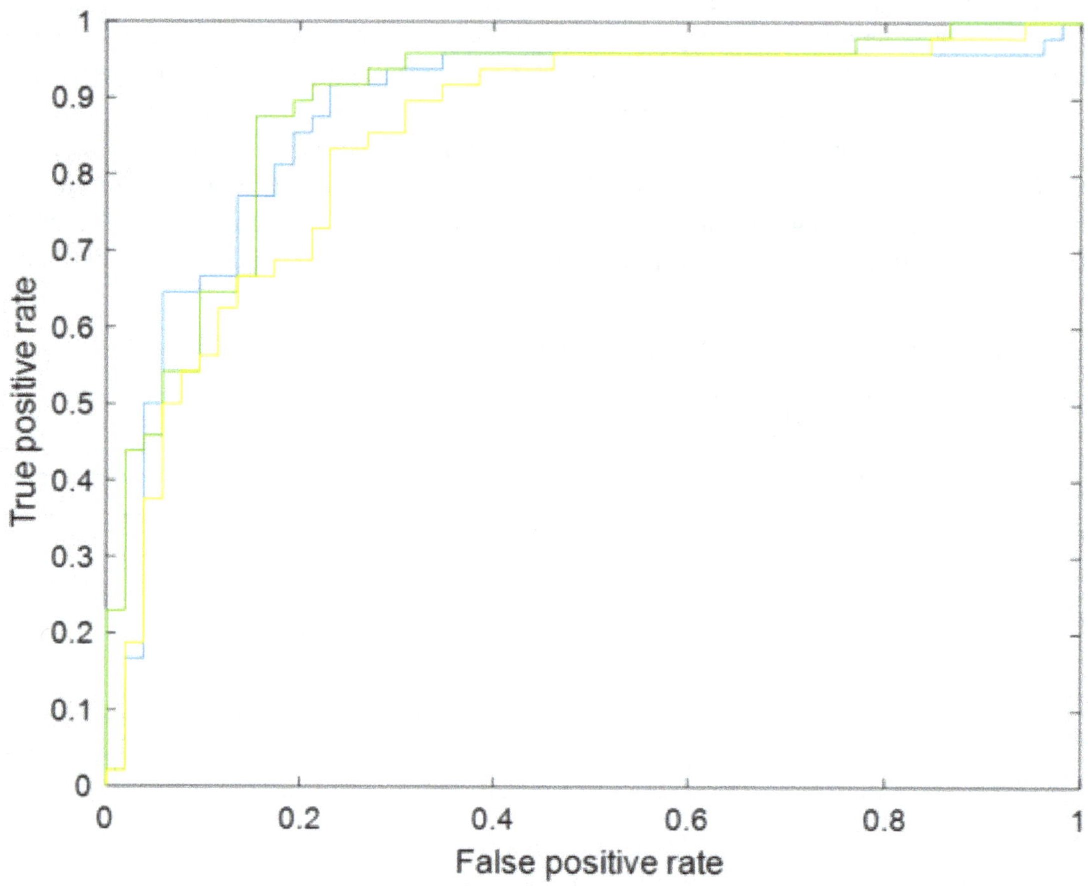

dataset, e.g. in (Byra, 2018), see Figure 7, the performance of their approach is not very stable, to choose which layer to feed their classifier considering the performance on the test set could overfit the system.

As already stressed, the main problem with CNNs is that they need a large training set for the training/ tuning step; we expect to obtain better performance when more patients will be available. For example, the method proposed in (Antropova, Huynh, & Giger, 2017) obtains an AUC of 0.826 in the breast dataset tested in this paper, instead in a larger dataset of 1125 breast lesions an higher performance is obtained: AUC of 0.872.

As shown in Figure 6 our system does not obtain a 100% true positive rate (TPR) with an acceptable false positive rate (FPR), the same problem occurs with (Byra, 2018); anyway also considering those performance indicators we obtain state of the art performance:

With a TPR of ~0.65 our approach obtains an FPR of 0.1, instead (Byra, 2018) obtains a TPR ~0.55 with an FPR of 0.1.

Figure 7. Performance reported in (Byra, 2018) using different layers of VGG19 for the classification; "image" means that the raw imaged are used for feeding their classifier

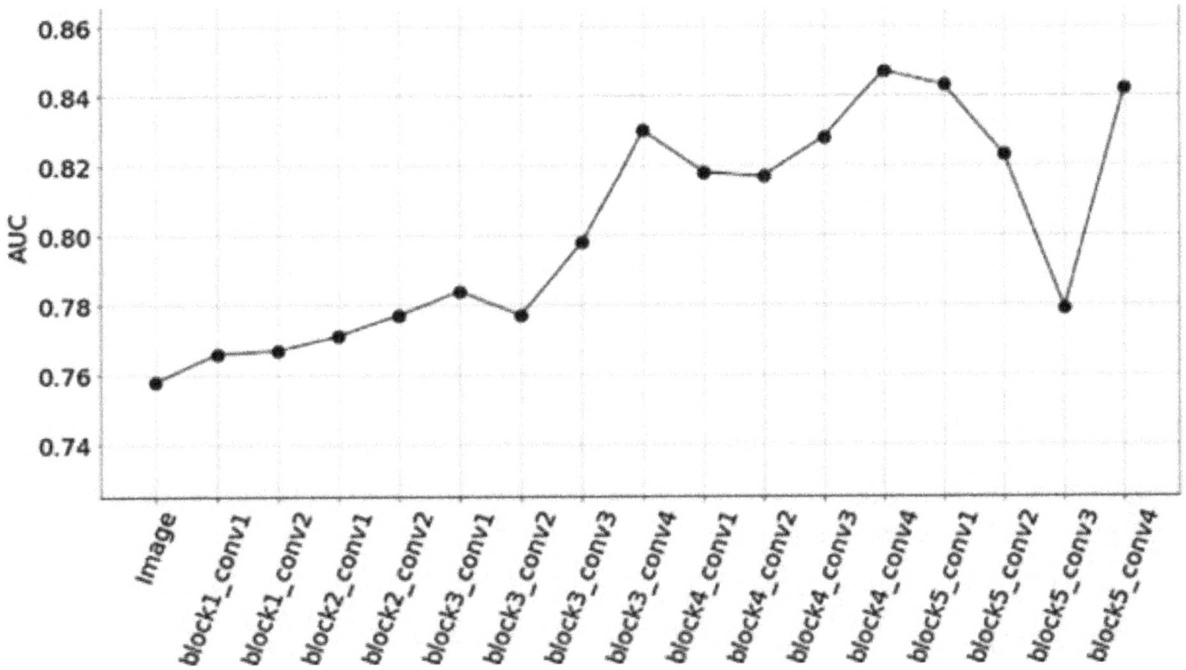

FUTURE RESEARCH DIRECTIONS

Usually, neural networks require large amounts of training data in the order of millions of images, especially when the resolution is low. Nonetheless, our experiments based on fine-tuning pre-trained networks and the fusion of several CNNs shows that very high performance can already be achieved with few training images resulting in performance comparable or even higher than handcrafted descriptors. Although this work used a supervised training approach, i.e. the training images were manually labeled as malignant or benign lesion, there are several attempts in the literature aimed at unsupervised or semi-supervised training of neural networks (Rasmus, Valpola, Honkala, Berglund, & Raiko, 2015)(Erhan, Courville, Bengio, & Vincent, 2010) with some works the medical field (Kallenberg et al., 2016). Therefore, we expect that in the future the size of the training set would not be a problem, given the availability of large datasets of medical images that could be used for training neural networks in an unsupervised, or semi-supervised mode. Finally, we try to couple our idea also to other CNN architectures.

CONCLUSION

The purpose of the present chapter was to propose a novel CNN architecture named TakhisisNet, based on the fusion of a "body"-CNN of a set of "heads"-CNN trained end-to-end with the body. We have tuned and evaluated TakhisisNet on the digital classification of bio-images, and encouraged by the good accuracy achieved, we applied this promising network to breast ultrasound image. The experimental results demonstrate the promising performance of our classification system with a higher AUC than stand-alone approaches. It was unexpected that in this dataset our ensemble of handcrafted descriptors (ENS_HAND) performs better than other famous deep learning approaches: this fact is probably due to the small dimension of the training set; this fact is exploited to maximize the classification performance in this dataset by fusing the proposed TakhisisNet with the handcrafted ensemble. Our approach outperforms state of the art methods of the same dataset.

Even if the proposed system has shown to be robust also with a small training set, we hope that a further improvement can be obtained using large amounts of unlabeled data made available from the very high number of screening participants. Further study for semi-supervised training of TakhisisNet will be explored.

Finally, we share the MATLAB code of TakhisisNet for research purposes at https://github.com/LorisNanni.

ACKNOWLEDGMENT

We gratefully acknowledge the support of NVIDIA Corporation for the "NVIDIA Hardware Donation Grant" of a Titan X used in this research.

REFERENCES

Antropova, N., Huynh, B. Q., & Giger, M. L. (2017). A deep feature fusion methodology for breast cancer diagnosis demonstrated on three imaging modality datasets. *Medical Physics*, *44*(10), 5162–5171. doi:10.1002/mp.12453 PMID:28681390

Byra, M. (2018). Discriminant analysis of neural style representations for breast lesion classification in ultrasound. *Biocybernetics and Biomedical Engineering*, *38*(3), 684–690. doi:10.1016/j.bbe.2018.05.003

Chang, C., & Lin, C. (2011). LIBSVM : A Library for Support Vector Machines. *ACM Transactions on Intelligent Systems and Technology*, *2*(3), 1–39. doi:10.1145/1961189.1961199

Cox, D., & Pinto, N. (2011). Beyond simple features: A large-scale feature search approach to unconstrained face recognition. In *2011 IEEE International Conference on Automatic Face and Gesture Recognition and Workshops, FG 2011* (pp. 8–15). 10.1109/FG.2011.5771385

Csurka, G., Dance, C. R., Fan, L., Willamowski, J., & Bray, C. (2004). Visual categorization with bags of keypoints. In *Proceedings of the ECCV International Workshop on Statistical Learning in Computer Vision* (pp. 59–74). 10.1234/12345678

Daubechies, I. (1992). *Ten Lectures on Wavelets*. Ten Lectures on Wavelets; doi:10.1137/1.9781611970104

Demšar, J. (2006). Statistical Comparisons of Classifiers over Multiple Data Sets. *Journal of Machine Learning Research*, *7*, 1–30. doi:10.1016/j.jecp.2010.03.005

Erhan, D., Courville, A., Bengio, Y., & Vincent, P. (2010). Why does unsupervised pre-training help deep learning? Journal of Machine Learning Research. doi:10.1145/1756006.1756025

Huang, J., & Ling, C. X. (2005). Using AUC and accuracy in evaluating learning algorithms. *IEEE Transactions on Knowledge and Data Engineering*. doi:10.1109/TKDE.2005.50

Kallenberg, M., Petersen, K., Nielsen, M., Ng, A. Y., Diao, P., & Igel, C. … Lillholm, M. (2016). Unsupervised Deep Learning Applied to Breast Density Segmentation and Mammographic Risk Scoring. *IEEE Transactions on Medical Imaging*. doi:10.1109/TMI.2016.2532122 PMID:26915120

Kannala, J., & Rahtu, E. (2012). BSIF: Binarized statistical image features. In *21st International Conference on Pattern Recognition (ICPR)* (pp. 1363–1366). Academic Press.

Liu, W., Wang, Z., Liu, X., Zeng, N., Liu, Y., & Alsaadi, F. E. (2017). A survey of deep neural network architectures and their applications. *Neurocomputing*, *234*, 11–26. doi:10.1016/j.neucom.2016.12.038

Moccia, S., De Momi, E., Guarnaschelli, M., Savazzi, M., Laborai, A., Guastini, L., ... Mattos, L. S. (2017). Confident texture-based laryngeal tissue classification for early stage diagnosis support. *Journal of Medical Imaging (Bellingham, Wash.)*, *4*(3), 34502. doi:10.1117/1.JMI.4.3.034502 PMID:28983494

Nanni, L., Brahnam, S., Ghidoni, S., & Lumini, A. (2018). Bioimage Classification with Handcrafted and Learned Features. *IEEE/ACM Transactions on Computational Biology and Bioinformatics*. doi:10.1109/TCBB.2018.2821127 PMID:29994096

Nanni, L., Brahnam, S., Lumini, A., & Barrier, T. (2014). *Ensemble of local phase quantization variants with ternary encoding* (Vol. 506). Studies in Computational Intelligence; doi:10.1007/978-3-642-39289-4_8

Nanni, L., Paci, M., Caetano dos Santos, F. L., Brahnam, S., & Hyttinen, J. (2016). Review on Texture Descriptors for Image Classiðcation. In *Computer Vision and Simulation: Methods, Applications and Technology*. Nova Science Publisher.

Nosaka, R., & Fukui, K. (2014). HEp-2 cell classification using rotation invariant co-occurrence among local binary patterns. *Pattern Recognition*, *47*(7), 2428–2436. doi:10.1016/j.patcog.2013.09.018

Nosaka, R., Ohkawa, Y., & Fukui, K. (2011). Feature extraction based on co-occurrence of adjacent local binary patterns. In Lecture Notes in Computer Science (including subseries Lecture Notes in Artificial Intelligence and Lecture Notes in Bioinformatics). doi:10.1007/978-3-642-25346-1_8

Ojala, T., Pietikainen, M., & Maenpaa, T. (2002). Multiresolution gray-scale and rotation invariant texture classification with local binary patterns. *IEEE Transactions on Pattern Analysis and Machine Intelligence*, *24*(7), 971–987. doi:10.1109/TPAMI.2002.1017623

Ojansivu, V., & Heikkilä, J. (2008). Blur insensitive texture classification using local phase quantization. In Lecture Notes in Computer Science (including subseries Lecture Notes in Artificial Intelligence and Lecture Notes in Bioinformatics) (Vol. 5099 LNCS, pp. 236–243). doi:10.1007/978-3-540-69905-7_27

Piotrzkowska-Wróblewska, H., Dobruch-Sobczak, K., & Byra Michałand Nowicki, A. (2017). Open access database of raw ultrasonic signals acquired from malignant and benign breast lesions. *Medical Physics*, *44*(11), 6105–6109. doi:10.1002/mp.12538 PMID:28859252

Rasmus, A., Valpola, H., Honkala, M., Berglund, M., & Raiko, T. (2015). Semi-supervised learning with Ladder networks. Advances in Neural Information Processing Systems.

Serra, G., Grana, C., Manfredi, M., & Cucchiara, R. (2015). Gold: Gaussians of local descriptors for image representation. *Computer Vision and Image Understanding*, *134*, 22–32. doi:10.1016/j.cviu.2015.01.005

Simonyan, K., & Zisserman, A. (2015). *Very Deep Convolutional Networks for Large-Scale Image Recognition.* CoRR, abs/1409.1

Song, T., Li, H., Meng, F., Wu, Q., & Cai, J. (2017). LETRIST: Locally Encoded Transform Feature Histogram for Rotation-Invariant Texture Classification. *IEEE Transactions on Circuits and Systems for Video Technology*. doi:10.1109/TCSVT.2017.2671899

Szegedy, C., Liu, W., Jia, Y., Sermanet, P., Reed, S., Anguelov, D., … Rabinovich, A. (2015). Going deeper with convolutions. In *Proceedings of the IEEE conference on computer vision and pattern recognition* (pp. 1–9). IEEE.

ADDITIONAL READING

Arevalo, J., González, F. A., Ramos-Pollán, R., Oliveira, J. L., & Lopez, M. A. G. (2016). Representation learning for mammography mass lesion classification with convolutional neural networks. *Computer Methods and Programs in Biomedicine*, *127*, 248–257. doi:10.1016/j.cmpb.2015.12.014 PMID:26826901

Ciompi, F., Chung, K., Van Riel, S. J., Setio, A. A. A., Gerke, P. K., Jacobs, C., ... van Ginneken, B. (2017). Towards automatic pulmonary nodule management in lung cancer screening with deep learning. *Scientific Reports*, *7*(1), 46479. doi:10.1038rep46479 PMID:28422152

Huynh, B. Q., Li, H., & Giger, M. L. (2016). Digital mammographic tumor classification using transfer learning from deep convolutional neural networks. *Journal of Medical Imaging (Bellingham, Wash.)*, *3*(3), 34501. doi:10.1117/1.JMI.3.3.034501 PMID:27610399

Li, H., Giger, M. L., Huynh, B. Q., & Antropova, N. O. (2017). Deep learning in breast cancer risk assessment: Evaluation of convolutional neural networks on a clinical dataset of full-field digital mammograms. *Journal of Medical Imaging (Bellingham, Wash.)*, *4*(4), 41304. doi:10.1117/1.JMI.4.4.041304 PMID:28924576

Samala, R. K., Chan, H.-P., Hadjiiski, L., Helvie, M. A., Richter, C., & Cha, K. (2018a). Cross-domain and multi-task transfer learning of deep convolutional neural network for breast cancer diagnosis in digital breast tomosynthesis. In *Medical Imaging 2018* (Vol. 10575, p. 105750Q). Computer-Aided Diagnosis. doi:10.1117/12.2293412

Samala, R. K., Chan, H.-P., Hadjiiski, L. M., Helvie, M. A., Richter, C., & Cha, K. (2018b). Evolutionary pruning of transfer learned deep convolutional neural network for breast cancer diagnosis in digital breast tomosynthesis. *Physics in Medicine and Biology*, *63*(9), 95005. doi:10.1088/1361-6560/aabb5b PMID:29616660

KEY TERMS AND DEFINITIONS

AUC: The "Area Under the ROC Curve" (AUC) measures the entire two-dimensional area underneath the entire ROC curve. One way of interpreting AUC is as the probability that the model ranks a random positive sample more highly than a random negative sample.

Convolutional Neural Networks: A convolutional neural network (CNN) is a type of artificial neural network used in image recognition and processing that is specifically designed to process pixel data by means of learnable filters.

Deep Learning: Deep learning is a subset of machine learning that models high-level abstractions in data by means of network architectures, which are composed of multiple nonlinear transformations.

Ensembles of Classifiers: An ensemble of classifiers is a set of classifiers whose individual decisions are combined in some way (typically by weighted or unweighted voting) to classify new samples.

k-Fold-Cross Validation: Cross-validation is a statistical method used to estimate the skill of machine learning models. This approach involves randomly dividing the set of observations into k groups, or folds, of approximately equal size. At each round one different fold is treated at turn as a validation set, and the method is trained on the remaining k-1. Finally, the performance are combined (e.g. averaged) over the rounds.

Leave-One-Out Testing Protocol: Leave-one-out cross-validation (LOOCV) is a particular case of k-fold-cross validation where k is the dimension of the set of observations, therefore each test set includes only one sample.

Machine Learning: Machine learning is an application of artificial intelligence that provides systems the ability to automatically learn and improve from experience without being explicitly programmed. Machine learning focuses on the development of computer programs that can access data and use it learn for themselves.

ROC Curve: A receiver operating characteristic (ROC) curve is a graph showing the performance of a classification model at all classification thresholds. This curve plots two parameters: True Positive Rate vs. False Positive Rate.

ENDNOTES

1 Available at https://doi.org/10.5281/zenodo.545928

2 In this test, each CNN that built TakhisisNet is coupled with different learning rate and batch size (the same values of ENS_DEEP), moreover to boost performance we have used 20 heads instead 10

APPENDIX

In this appendix each of the descriptors used to build the ensemble ENS_HAND is briefly described.
Multithreshold LPQ: MLPQ (L. Nanni et al., 2014) is a multi-threshold approach applied the LPQ descriptor. LPQ (Ojansivu & Heikkilä, 2008) is a texture descriptor that uses the local phase information extracted from the 2-D short-term Fourier transform computed over a rectangular neighborhood of radius R at each pixel position in an image. In (L. Nanni et al., 2014) a multi-threshold version of the simple binary quantizer of LPQ is proposed where the different pixels are encoded with 3 values using a set of thresholds τ around zero:

$$q(x) = \begin{cases} 1, x \geq \\ 0, - \leq x < \\ -1 \mathit{otherwise.} \end{cases}$$

According to (L. Nanni et al., 2014) the quantization is performed using to the following thresholds τ Î {0.2, 0.4, 0.6, 0.8, 1} and concatenating the resulting descriptors. In this study we combine sets of MLPQ extracted by varying the following parameters: the neighborhood size (R Î {1, 3, 5}), the scalar frequency, (*a* Î {0.8, 1, 1.2, 1.4, 1.6}), the correlation coefficient between adjacent pixel values PÎ{0.75, 0.95, 1.15, 1.35, 1.55, 1.75, 1.95}. Each descriptor is used to train a different SVM classifier which are fused by sum rule.
Gaussian Of Local Descriptors: GOLD (Serra et al., 2015) is an improvement of the Bag of Word (BoW) approach (Csurka, Dance, Fan, Willamowski, & Bray, 2004). The original BoW method extracts local features to generate a codebook, which is used to encode the local features into codes that form a global image representation. The codebook generation step is performed through clustering methods on the training set. GOLD is a four-step process that generates the codebook via a flexible local feature representation that is obtained by a parametric probability density estimation. Differently from BoW, GOLD does not requires neither quantization nor a training set. The steps for extracting GOLD features are:

1. Feature extraction: dense SIFT descriptors (Cox & Pinto, 2011) are extracted on a regular grid of the image.
2. Spatial Pyramid Decomposition: the image is decomposed by a multilevel recursive method, and features are softly assigned to regions according to a local weighting.
3. Parametric probability density estimation: for each region local mean and covariance of extracted local descriptors are inferred, according to as a multivariate Gaussian distribution.
4. Projection on the tangent Euclidean space: the final description is the mean concatenated to the projection the covariance matrix on the tangent Euclidean space.

The resulting GOLD descriptor is fed into an SVM classifier with a histogram kernel.
Full BSIF: (Loris Nanni et al., 2016) is an extension of the Binarized Statistical Image Feature (BSIF) (Kannala & Rahtu, 2012) that assigns each pixel of the input image a n-bit label obtained by means of a set of n linear filters. The original BSIF is a local image descriptor constructed by binarizing the responses to *n* linear filters which, differently to previous binary descriptors, are learnt from natural im-

ages using independent component analysis (ICA). BSIF assigns an n-bit label to each pixel of an image using a set of n linear filters. The BSIF descriptor has two parameters: the filter size d (filters are $d \times d$) and the number n of features extracted. In the original BSIF the binarization of a digit d_i (the result of the application of a filter on a pixel) is performed according to a fixed threshold $\tau=0$:

$$b_i = \begin{cases} 1, if\, d_i > 0 \\ 0, if\, d_i \leq 0 \end{cases}$$

Full BSIF is a multi-descriptor version of BSIF obtained by varying the parameters of filter size (d Î {3, 5, 7, 9, 11}) and a threshold τ for binarizing (τ Î {-9, -6, -3, 0, 3, 6, 9}). The resulting 35 combinations of descriptors are used each to train a different SVM that are combined by sum rule.

Full RIC: this is a multiscale Rotation Invariant Co-occurrence of Adjacent LBP (RIC-LBP) (Nosaka & Fukui, 2014). The RIC-LBP features are variants of the standard LBP designed to simultaneously have characteristics of rotation invariance and a high descriptive ability. LBP (Ojala, Pietikainen, & Maenpaa, 2002) is an operator that describes a local region as a binary pattern obtained by thresholding the difference between a center pixel and its neighboring pixels. LBP represents the magnitude relation of intensities, therefore it is robust against changes in illumination among image patterns, but it does not preserve structural information among binary patterns. The CoALBP (Nosaka, Ohkawa, & Fukui, 2011) uses LBP pairs to keep such structural information: the histogram feature generated from CoALBP contains information on the structure of the image, since it describes the frequency of LBP pairs that are located near each other. Rotation invariant is reached in RIC-LBP by using a map table that maps together all the LBP pairs which have rotation equivalence according to a rotation angle θ. Finally, an RIC-LBP histogram is generated from for the entire image. He multi-scale variant of RIC-LBP extracts RIC-LBP features using different parameter settings, i.e. varying the LBP parameters radius and displacement (P,R). The values used in our experiments are: (1, 2), (2, 4) and (4, 8). }). Each resulting descriptor is used to train a different SVM which are combined by sum rule.

LETRIST: (Song et al., 2017) the Locally Encoded TRansform feature hISTogram descriptor is a histogram representation that explicitly encodes the joint information within an image across feature and scale spaces. It consists of the following three major steps: first local texture structures are characterized by a set of transform features their correlation is calculated by applying linear and non-linear operators on the extremum responses of directional Gaussian derivative filters in scale space. Second, these transform features are binarized into by scalar quantization. Third, the discrete texture codes are aggregated into a compact histogram representation using cross-scale joint coding. In this work we used the default parameter proposed in the MATLAB toolbox (https://github.com/stc-cqupt/letrist).

Chapter 10
Workforce Readiness and Digital Health Integration

Buddhika Senanayake
https://orcid.org/0000-0002-2278-2889
Centre for Health Services Research, The University of Queensland, Australia

Nirupama Tyagi
Centre for Health Services Research, The University of Queensland, Australia

Xiaoyun Zhou
Centre for Health Services Research, The University of Queensland, Australia

Sisira Edirippulige
Centre for Health Services Research, The University of Queensland, Australia

ABSTRACT

The benefits that digital health may offer include clinical, administrative, research, and educational. Research shows that if used in the right circumstances, digital health may increase access to healthcare services, improve clinical outcomes, safety, and quality of care. Digital health also has the potential to improve organisational efficiencies by reducing duplication and unnecessary diagnostic testing. From a healthcare consumer perspective, there is an expectation that healthcare services need to be provided in a more flexible and cost-effective way as in other spheres such as banking, commerce, and media. This is another important driver for consideration to integrate digital health in healthcare services. As digital health continues to be used in routine healthcare services, practitioners may require new knowledge, skills, and competencies to make the best use of this innovative method. Education and training relating to digital health have been recognised as a priority for developing the future healthcare workforce.

DOI: 10.4018/978-1-7998-3274-4.ch010

INTRODUCTION

Healthcare innovation over the last 50 years has resulted in much improved population health – people now live longer and experience a better quality of life than our ancestors, in part, to vastly improved medical diagnostics, treatment and management practices. The continuous challenge facing the business of healthcare is how to meet these expectations going forward; to continue to research and implement quality health improvements and importantly, to do so in a fiscally responsible manner (Dods et al., 2014). Patients often find it difficult to engage with care and care teams within this system. This is particularly relevant for the vulnerable, disadvantaged and geographically isolated people living in small communities, where there is little or no healthcare services available. Whether in a hospital or in the community, a patient's care-process can transition between multiple clinicians, particularly those who are chronically ill and therefore often in and out of the hospital. In this situation, communication is often fragmented between clinicians, teams, and organisations resulting in missing, incomplete or lost information when it is needed. This results in confusion, inefficiencies, frustration and patient risk to life. One solution to this challenge is the effective provision of health-related information and communication technology to complement and potentially improve health services. This has led to a mission for digital healthcare transformation which is achieved through exploiting existing and evolving information communication technology (ICT) of healthcare providers, and the aim is to improve productivity, efficiency, and deliver better & improved healthcare to its clients.

Digital health is defined as: 'the use of information and communication technologies (ICT) for health services, including treating patients, conducting research, educating the health workforce, tracking diseases and monitoring public health (World Health Organisation, 2016). Digital health is the use of information communication technologies in healthcare services, which includes new technologies and data deriving from such technologies. In the modern world, patients' information – their history, care plans, medication information, and test results - all of this can be digitally recorded and shared using technology. At patient-contact points, the doctor, nurse, pharmacist or allied health professional can ideally have access to the up to-date electronic patient record. Globally industries shifting towards digital service integration and knowledge driven economies. Healthcare is no different. While it is true that healthcare is lagging behind other industries, healthcare using digital health is now rapidly becoming 'business as usual.' To remain relevant, an understanding of how interconnected information communication technology (ICT) delivers and improves patient-centred care is now vital for all healthcare professionals.

Digital health is primarily about the use of information communication technology to improve healthcare and organisational efficiencies. It integrates the right technology, the right digital information and the right team on behalf of the patient at the right time. Thus, a skilled, motivated and capable workforce is an important element in this process. The digital health vision for improving healthcare has three core domains:

- Increasing access to healthcare service – telehealth, telemedicine, mobile health are all branches of digital health that have the capacity to bring healthcare to the patient, rather than the patient having to travel to healthcare
- Improving the safety and quality of care by having the right information at hand to inform clinical decision making and actively empowering and involving the patient
- Improving efficiencies in the delivery of care – reducing duplication and unnecessary diagnostic testing so, digital health is heavily focused on systems and tools that can provide decision-makers

with complete and accessible information for patients at the point of care in a secure framework. It facilitates the recording of digital data and its subsequent storage, sharing, and analysis using electronic medical records and personal health records. Digital health encompasses data, information and communication technology, and good medical practice coming together on behalf of the patient.

Technology as a Factor in the Development of Digital Health

Technology is one of the main factors in the emergence and the development of digital health. Developments in computing, the Internet and information technology, development and expansion of networks and telecommunication infrastructure, rapid adoption of technology by society, and technological innovation of medical devices, digital cameras and physiological sensors are major technological aspects that have made a significant impact on digital health.

Telehealth and Telemedicine

Telehealth, (or provision of clinical, administrative, educational and research services at a distance using information and communication technologies or ICTs), offers an alternative to traditional face-to-face delivery of healthcare services. It can offer access to services in areas where these were not traditionally available or where patients had to travel to obtain these services, and it has been shown to reduce costs for patients and clinicians, both in time and money. The renewed interest in telehealth (or telemedicine) since the early 1990s, has been chiefly driven by need, i.e. an aging population, scarcity of specialist services in areas outside metropolitan centres and the increasing complexity of diseases and their management. It has been enabled by advances in technology which supports such activities as quality videoconferencing and the sharing of diagnostic aids such as x-rays, high resolution photos, physiological data, e.g. ECG data, real-time blood pressure and oxygenation data, biochemical parameters (which can now be transmitted with a high standard of resolution).

Telehealth is defined as 'the use of information and communication technology (ICT) to deliver health services, expertise and information over distance' (Bashshur, Reardon, & Shannon, 2000). This definition includes clinical, educational, administrative and research health related activities that are carried out at a distance. Telemedicine is considered to be the use of communication and information technologies to deliver clinical care where the individuals involved are not at the same location. It also covers telecommunication to deliver non-clinical services such as research and health education promotion' (Currell, Urquhart, Wainwright, & Lewis, 2000).

There are two main approaches used in telehealth – the real-time approach and the store-and-forward approach. The real-time ('synchronous') approach means that the parties involved interact at the same time using information and communication technologies (ICTs). This involves telephone or voice over the internet, exchange of data or images (e.g. pathology images and results, images shared during a video consultation) via phone, fax, secure internet connection etc. Video consultation via a secure organisation-linked network or open source provider (i.e. Skype) is also part of the synchronous approach. The store-and-forward ('asynchronous') approach occurs when information is sent to another party and can be accessed at a later time and acted upon. It involves information (images, data, audio, video) being captured and stored ('store'), and then sent ('forward') and displayed later. Store-and forward can occur via email, messaging system, fax, mail services/couriers.

More recent developments of mobile phones and satellite communications have allowed for mobile medicine, giving easier access to patients located in remote situations and locations, especially in developing countries. m-Health (or mobile health) is becoming a fast growing field; it encompasses 'medical and public health practice supported by mobile devices, such as mobile phones, patient monitoring devices, personal digital assistants (PDAs) and other wireless devices' (World Health Organisation, 2011).

Health Informatics

The history of electronic health information exchange (health informatics) is in part matched by the evolution of telemedicine. Clinicians have sought to exploit technological development and progress to overcome everyday logistical issues they face with delivering their services (Park et al., 2013). History shows that most of the early telemedicine efforts focused on specialist diagnostic services (e.g. teleradiology, telepathology, teledermatology) that were driven by the need for specialists to enhance efficiency, better manage clinical diagnostic information and overcome distances encountered by some patients. The ability to electronically transmit text and imaged-based anatomical pathology, clinical pathology and radiology diagnostic data greatly enhanced the evolution of telemedicine.

There is lots of evidence to suggest that digital health offers a range of advantages to the stakeholders involved in healthcare.

METHODOLOGY

A thorough literature review was performed to identify facts for the research topic. The electronic databases such as "PubMed", "Google Scholar", Medline, Scopus, Emtree and "HINARI" were used to gather data. Keywords such as education and training, digital health, mHealth, health workforce, workforce readiness were entered in order to get comprehensive coverage of relevant literature. Citation information along with notes and abstracts were downloaded to Endnote X6 software. Citation and reference lists were made using Endnote X6 software in Harvard APA style –sixth edition.

The exploratory review was conducted on peer-reviewed publications published between January 2000 and December 2019. The reason for limiting searches to this narrow period was due to change in technology and teaching and learning styles rendering findings of earlier studies unsuitable for current contexts. As the study aimed to collate all evidence regarding education and training for digital health, all the potential studies that strengthen digital health in the field of learning and training were included. The review also considered any type of study (quantitative, or qualitative) if adequate information (to assess successful implementation or utilization) on the service delivered was described. Articles related to healthcare models, technical feasibility studies, case studies, letters, and published comments were excluded (inadequacy of information to reliably assess usefulness). Publications with no abstracts and non-English articles were also excluded. Grey literature was not searched.

SOLUTIONS AND RECOMMENDATIONS

Better Access

Digital health is viewed as an eloquent resolution to the inequity of healthcare access for those that dwell in underserved or geographically disadvantaged communities. This also applies to metropolitan dwellers disadvantaged by age, illness or disability. It is recognised that globally rural and remote people have poorer health, worse lifestyle habits, less access to healthcare and higher costs of health service delivery. Electronic healthcare records and telemedicine applications are viewed as a tool that will assist in 'closing the gap' of Indigenous Australian life expectancy, mental health, maternity services, paediatric services of ear, nose, and throat and aged care healthcare inequities (Dods. S et al., 2012).

Access to healthcare is one of the main rights of human beings described by the United Nations 'Universal Declaration of Human Rights.' Article 25 of the same document is about the right to have an adequate standard of living for individuals and their families; which includes food, clothing, housing and medical care (United Nations, 1948). The main driving force for digital health is that it facilitates the universal access to healthcare. All healthcare policies should actively seek to exploit digital technologies and digital health data to enhance patient care and patient outcomes.

The term 'the tyranny of distance' is an imperative expression in the field of healthcare delivery. It is often used in relation to healthcare access, particularly in the context when access to care is constrained by geography – especially – distance. Countries like Australia and Canada are prime examples where their population is affected by the tyranny of distance. Health systems of these counties are seriously challenged by the disparity of healthcare services due to distance, and they are making attempts to overcome these challenges. The introduction of telemedicine is one solution that attempted to address this challenge.

Significant telehealth research dates back to the 90's. Canada, in particular, was at the forefront of telestroke research – that is - providing stroke care at a distance. Telestroke models bring the neurologist, the remote patient, CT imaging and acute care teams together using technology – including videoconferencing to enable rapid diagnosis and the administration of clot busting therapy within the required time. This research model (now over 15 years old) is a huge telehealth. Telestroke is now integrated into clinical care models around the world. The Victorian-Health telestroke model is a notable Australian success story. Australian researchers have made significant contributions to providing mental health services by real time teleconsultation throughout South Australia.

It must always be in the best interest of the patients, not in the best interests of the technology or the technology companies. A clinical need must always be identified first and then a solution must be investigated – that may include technology. The advent of telehealth is a great example of this – the need was to improve access to care and this has been met using digital technology. Telehealth today forms an important element of health reforms. Telehealth is now evolving from its original goal- that is to increase access or provide easier access. Today telehealth is becoming a part of routine care. A new - hybrid model has been adopted where traditional face-to-face methods and telehealth is used for providing care at various settings - for example, hospitals, home, nursing homes, and primary care.

Digital health provides better access to health irrespective of the location. It is viewed as an eloquent resolution to the inequity of healthcare access for those that dwell in underserved or geographically disadvantaged communities. This also applies to metropolitan dwellers disadvantaged by age, illness or disability. It is recognised that rural and remote people have poorer health, worse lifestyle habits, less access to healthcare and higher costs of health service delivery. In particular electronic healthcare records and telemedicine applications are viewed as a tool that will assist in 'closing the gap' of marginalised community healthcare inequities (Dods et al., 2014).

Timely Access

Cost savings associated with a reduction in the unnecessary ordering of tests, services and referrals – ubiquitous electronic health records means better medication ordering and management and minimal duplication of diagnostic testing (e.g. pathology, imaging). Statistics from the Australian Digital Health Agency report that 14% of all pathology and 10% of diagnostic imaging-tests are ordered unnecessarily due to lack of access to the patients' up to date records.

Better Planning

Constant collection, 'data mining' and statistical analysis of electronic healthcare data can provide up-to-date insight into the health of the population as a whole and highlight opportunities for improvement. Vast subsets of such data is commonly measured and collected across all healthcare sectors, i.e. hospital admittance, length of stay, admitted and non-admitted patient outcomes of intervention, readmission rates, physician orders (e.g. medication, radiology, pathology, rehabilitation, referral to specialists), patient safety data (e.g. falls rates, medication errors, wrong patient-wrong procedure errors), notifiable infectious disease rates and other public health surveillance information, morbidity and mortality rates, etc.

Researchers, clinicians and organisational and government decision makers need to be able to access such health informatics data to design better planning and improve healthcare quality and advance evidence–based practices. More importantly, the collected healthcare data is made available as a national asset as they seek to unlock the significant economic value of the data it collects (Australian Government, 2013).

Better Organised Care

The business of health is aimed at improving health outcomes and quality of life. Every healthcare system strives to deliver a high standard of care. Not everyone has equitable access to the best possible care. Growing aged population, with an increased burden of chronic disease, high rates of mental illness (including dementia, depression, anxiety and stress), cancer, illegal substance, tobacco and alcohol use, musculoskeletal-related debilitation, overweight and obese individuals, are some of the health challenges for the policy makers to address. People have a right to the best possible medical care but restrictions in the health budget, lack of skilled health workforce, well-equipped, adequately funded hospitals and private practices are still formidable challenges. The use of information communication technology can improve health outcomes, reduce inefficiencies and expand the productivity of healthcare systems.

Patient Centred Care

The quality and safety of healthcare are based on two main principles. The first principle is 'First, do no harm' i.e. consider first the well-being of the patient and the second is to deliver better health and wellbeing for all, now and for future generations (Australian Medical Association, 2016).

The Australian Commission on Safety and Quality in Healthcare (ACSQHC) publishes the Safety and Quality Framework for Healthcare. This was updated in 2010 and it specifies safe, high quality healthcare needs to be consumer centred, driven by information, and organised for safety (Australian Commission on Safety and Quality in Healthcare, 2010). The provision of safe, high quality health should always be:

- Consumer centred – Providing care that is easy for patients to get when they need it.
- Driven by information – Using up-to-date knowledge and evidence to guide decisions about care
- Organised for safety – Making safety a central feature of how healthcare facilities run

Patient-centred care (or consumer driven care) is not a novel concept. The term originates from the Picker Institute in the US (established in the early 1990s) but it really gained traction following the publication of the US Institute of Medicine report in 2000 – 'To err is human: building a safer health system' (Kohn L, Corrigan J, & Donaldson M, 1999). This paper highlighted the unacceptable rates of harm that befall patients when they engage with modern healthcare services. These common 'adverse events' include medication errors, wrong surgery, wrong patient incidents, hospital-acquired infection, delays in patient-related communication that delay the best possible clinical decision making (i.e. poor clinical handover), duplication of tests (e.g. diagnostic imaging) that expose patients to unnecessary risk. Adverse events lead to less-than-optimal health outcomes for the patient – sometimes death or irreversible disability. To address this urgent issue the (US) Institute of Medicine recommended substantive patient-safety specific reform in healthcare service delivery models via patient-centred care frameworks (Committee on Quality Healthcare in America - Institute of Medicine, 2001). Patient-centred care is defined as patient-centred care is an approach to the planning, delivery and evaluation of healthcare that is grounded in mutually beneficial partnerships among healthcare providers, patients and families' (Australian Commission on Safety and Quality in Healthcare, 2011).

Patient-centred care is a healthcare model that places the patient at the centre of the care instead of the disease or illness. It considers a patient's cultural tradition, personal preferences and values, family situations, social circumstances and lifestyles as well as the clinical aspects of diagnosis, potential treatment, rehabilitation or advice on healthy behaviours. In the traditional, disease-centered model, physicians make almost all treatment decisions based largely on clinical experience and data from various medical tests. In a patient-centered model, patients become active participants in their own care and receive services designed to focus on their individual needs and preferences, in addition to advice and counsel from health professionals (Committee on Quality Healthcare in America - Institute of Medicine, 2001).

Empowered Patients: More Control to Patients Over Their Own Health

A patient-centric approach to healthcare empowers patients to be more informed and less passive or disinterested. Everyday citizens are increasingly encouraged to be actively involved and responsible in part for their healthcare outcomes and the clinical decision making process. Empowered healthcare consumers require:

- Access to high quality medical information - To become truly empowered consumers require access to high quality, credible, evidence-based information. A wealth of information is now available through various web-based portals and mobile applications. Such information is easily accessible and easily understood and greatly assists consumers to actively participate in clinical decision making regarding their current and future healthcare (Wicks, Stamford, Grootenhuis, Haverman, & Ahmed, 2014).

- An up to date personal electronic health record - Having a personal electronic health record is vital for timely, effective and up-to-date personalised care. Just like patients, healthcare teams need access to the best possible and most recent information about their patients' health status (Office for Official Publications of the European Communities, 2004). Traditionally this has been recorded in hardcopy format and stored in what is colloquially known as 'silos', i.e. the filing cabinets of GP practices, hospitals, radiology practices, pathology providers, allied health practices etc. A single electronic repository for such information, that all participants in a person's healthcare can contribute to and access, is viewed as critical for the success of many e-health innovations.

Multidisciplinary Care

These are some of the benefits of digital health. But, regardless of these known benefits, digital health has not been used widely enough. There are many challenges.

Barriers to Digital Health

Some of the benefits of integrating information and communication technology into health are expected to take years to achieve. A strategic vision thus requires a common long-term vision across all stakeholders to ensure the best possible clinical, organisational, financial, legal, ethical and quality outcomes.

There are significant barriers to digital health integration and adoption in government and clinical literature.

- Poor interoperability between current information systems – data is heterogeneous and 'siloed' in individual electronic databases and unable to be digitally exchanged (Vest & Gamm, 2010).
- Privacy and security concerns relating to the provision and scope of free and fully informed consent and the protection and controlled sharing of confidential patient information stored in electronic health records (EHRs) (Caine & Hanania, 2013).
- Evidence of e-health derived clinical quality, safety, efficacy and patient and provider satisfaction is limited and inconsistent (Black et al., 2011).
- Scalability, change management, sustainable integration and reimbursement are often problematic when integrating ICT technology and remotely provided clinical consultation into traditional work-flow practices (van Gemert-Pijnen JE et al., 2011).
- Ethical issues relating to a professional and legal duty of care - who is vicariously responsible for the patient at any given time point in the care process especially if care is provided across state, territory or country borders? (Saliba et al., 2012).

Challenges With Electronic Health Record (EHR)

In Australia, the Federal Governments My Health Record is personally controlled, and individuals can choose what health information is uploaded and who that information can then be shared with. Typically it is expected that an individual's My Health Record will contain relevant, up-to-date information so clinicians are able to access and use it to inform clinical decision making (Pearce & Bainbridge, 2014).

Individual healthcare providers receive access permission from the individual so they can upload and then view health information via My Health Record. While there are potentially many benefits there are significant barriers to its universal uptake.

Main barriers that challenge effective EHR are:

- Privacy and security issues when confidential health information is uploaded and shared.
- lack of awareness amongst the population that it exists; lack of promotion by general practitioners • current opposition to the 'opt in' and 'opt out' nature of the record – the danger that the record will not be sufficiently accurate or complete
- overcoming compatibility and connectivity issues to facilitate data sharing between the multiple legacy information systems used across the health sector
- the development and implementation of nationally agreed standards
- lack of funding and resources for technology acquisition
- resistance by patients and healthcare staff to take up ICT initiatives, challenges with computer literacy
- access to equipment and training
- lack of organisational and government leadership and direction
- (Lehnbom, Brien, & McLachlan, 2014; Liaw & Hannan, 2011).

Digital Health Transition From Research to Practice Is Slow

Lack of high quality research There are many innovative ICT solutions available with a growing evidence base that supports their clinical efficacy. However, their integration and sustained utility in routine clinical practice remain a challenge. A commonly cited barrier to the integration of digital health applications into everyday practice is the acknowledged lack of high quality and methodologically sound clinical studies (Glasgow, Phillips, & Sanchez, 2014).

Issues With Privacy, Security, and Confidentiality of Information

An effective health informatics information environment must be able to ensure that all health information specifically relating to patients is private, secure and used with consent only in appropriate and beneficial ways. Privacy-related issues are a key criticism of electronic health records, specifically to obtain adequate privacy consent from patients, and to ensure that information which is required to provide treatment for the patient is collected. The integrity of the systems that are used to access the data is critical and if the systems are breached, privacy cannot be ensured. Personal health information could potentially be leaked to unapproved persons or companies and therefore, data security issues such as the accuracy and protection of data points at entry and once entered are extremely critical (Jolly R, 2011).

But one important aspect is the lack of readiness for the workforce. The focus of this chapter is to shed light on this challenge.

WHY WORKFORCE READINESS IS IMPORTANT?

Workforce readiness can be defined as having new workplace entrants prepared to enter the workforce with the requisite knowledge, skills, abilities, and attributes in order to engage in endeavours that will be required in their respective occupations. Partnerships and alliances between educational institutions, governmental entities and employers can assist in ensuring that these new workforce entrants are sufficiently prepared to meet the challenges and opportunities they will face in the workplace.

Human Resource (HR) professionals are uniquely suited to address many of the challenges raised by workforce readiness issues. HR professionals can play a strategic role in helping employers formulate exacting standards for workforce skills, capabilities and attributes that the employer community needs. Additionally, the HR community can take the lead in coalition building to articulate the need for developing rigorous standards, which can be shared throughout the business community and serve as a basis for advocacy of workforce readiness efforts. HR professionals can bring their quantitative skills to help develop programs to improve workforce readiness and to evaluate models and pilot programs to ensure their effectiveness and adaptability in meeting current needs and their ability to anticipate future needs (El Paso Society for Human Resource Management, 2017).

How Can This Be Done?

A trained, digitally aware workforce – appropriately equipped with hardware, software and digital literacy is required (Maruthappu, Sood, & Keogh, 2014). To achieve this strategic goal, the following strategies must be put in place. Help should be available with the right support, and healthcare providers will adopt digital health technologies and services if they can be shown how to use them. A range of organisations such as the primary health networks and the regional hospital and health networks will be important partners in supporting the health and care workforce at the local level, complemented by national mechanisms (Greenhalgh, Robert, Macfarlane, Bate, & Kyriakidou, 2004).

Digital health training provided throughout training pathways: Countries must ensure that the health and care workforce is sufficiently supported and informed, with digital health embedded through all training pathways. Innovation in healthcare education is already occurring within the tertiary education sector, with pilot courses on digital health in the planning stages at many Australian universities. Increasing the capability of the university sector to evolve curricula and incorporate digital health into undergraduate and postgraduate courses will ensure students are empowered to confidently and effectively use digital technologies upon graduation (Gray K, Dattakumar A, Maeder A, Butler-Henderson K, & H., 2014).

Digital health integrated into national standards: Health and care workers increasingly need a core set of digital competencies to enable them to work safely, efficiently and effectively. More evidence is being gathered which demonstrates that failing to integrate digital health into normal workflows leads to poorer health outcomes for the Australian community. Given this evidence, integration of digital health into national workforce accreditation needs to be led by the professional associations and workforce accreditation bodies, sensitive to the needs of both technophile and technophobe health professionals (Westbrook, Woods, Rob, Dunsmuir, & Day, 2010).

Healthcare providers should have easy access to best practice guidelines, and other supporting resources, which increase their understanding of how, when and why to use digital health solutions to improve outcomes in their routine clinical practice relating to a variety of illnesses. Clinical leadership networks, professional societies and peak bodies have responsibility for guiding their members on how to embed digital health into routine clinical practice and will be supported by the Australian Digital Health Agency to gather the evidence (Cummings, Shin, Mather, & Hovenga, 2016).

A network of clinical digital health champions: A network of clinical digital health champions, who understand the benefits of digital health and encourage the upskilling of the workforce across the health system into the future, is important to build momentum and a critical mass of digital health proponents (Ingebrigtsen et al., 2014). The capture and use of high-quality data and the resulting analytics can drive changes that will lead to a safer, higher quality, more effective health system. However, to achieve this, Australia's clinicians need to have the relevant skills. Investment in clinical informatics and data analytics as core skills for the modern health workforce is a key strategy (Health Workforce Australia, 2013).

What Is the Current Status?

Facilities to education and training is limited. The availability of appropriate systematic education and training for practitioners has been highlighted as necessary for strong adoption. A literature review was conducted in 2016 to assess the delivery of education and training in telehealth, with particular focus on content, modes of delivery, types of institutions, and target clinician groups. Three hundred and eighty-eight articles were reviewed. Education and training in telehealth has been provided as both university level and vocational courses using conventional classroom-based delivery methods and e learning. Reported curriculum items included terminology, clinical applications, the evidence-base, and technological aspects. Telehealth CPD courses were also delivered by professional organisations such as health departments, or the Veterans' Health Administration (VHA). The review disclosed that Published evidence in peer-reviewed literature on telehealth education and training is limited. According to this review, a number of topics relating to telehealth have been covered by existing education programs both within tertiary and professional development levels (Edirippulige & Armfield, 2017).

There is growing evidence of the benefits of digital health for improving the performance of health systems and outcomes in developed countries. However, significant gaps remain in resource-constrained settings. Technological and socio-cultural disparities between different regions or between provinces within the same country are prevalent. Rural areas, where the promise and need are highest, are particularly deprived. In Latin America, there is an unmet need for training and building the capacity of professionals in digital health (Curioso WH, 2019). The need for training and building the capacity of healthcare professionals in digital health remains one of the most significant public health challenges (Luna, Almerares, Mayan, Gonzalez Bernaldo de Quiros, & Otero, 2014). Digital health training and research programs in this region are scarce and poorly documented. A study involving 30 Australian universities in 2012 concluded that the future health-professional workforce was not being adequately educated to achieve competence to work with eHealth (Dattakumar, Gray, Henderson, Maeder, & Chenery, 2012).

In 2018, Edirippulige and colleagues (2018) revisited eHealth education and training in Australian universities with a focus on medical schools; we aimed to explore the progress of eHealth in the Australian medical curriculum. They conducted a national interview study and interpretative phenomenological analysis with participants from all 19 medical schools in Australia. The study concluded with two main themes. First theme was the consensus on 'the importance of eHealth to current and future clinical practice'; and the second theme identified as 'there are other priorities, and no strong drivers for change' in the context of digital health. Systemic problems inhibit the inclusion of eHealth in medical education. Heads of medical institutions concerned that the curriculum is 'crowded' and with competing demands. Interestingly the accrediting bodies do not expect eHealth competence in medical graduates, and there is no external pressure for its inclusion. Unless and until accrediting bodies recognise and expect competence in eHealth, it is unlikely that it will enter in to the medical or paramedical curriculum; consequently, the future workforce will remain unprepared.

A proper health workforce trained in digital health will strengthen health systems and ensure adequate service delivery. There is growing evidence around the world of the value that well-trained personnel in digital health can offer to tackle global health challenges (Hersh, Margolis, Quiros, & Otero, 2010). Training programmes/ courses in Latin America on digital health has shown following results. The top-ranked courses were: "Introduction to Biomedical Informatics," "Data Representation and Databases," "Mobile Health," and "Security, Confidentiality, and Privacy." The research topics reported as a priority were: evaluation of health information systems, policy in health informatics, interoperability and standards, evidence-based decision making in informatics, rural telemedicine, mobile health, electronic health records, sequence analysis and gene finding, tele-education, and the analysis of cost-effectiveness in biomedical informatics (Blas et al., 2011).

Since people are central to the value-added creation of digital health services, skilled and committed human resources were identified as an essential component for the deployment of the digital health ecosystem in Latin America. Therefore, Latin American countries should invest in digital health training programs to overcome main healthcare challenges. Rodrigues proposed that systems professionals, technology products, services providers, and project teams must have superior skill levels and experience. He also proposed that efficient and robust government and academic institutions should be committed to investing in education, scientific and technological development, and public services. Some of the critical things that Latin American governments should focus on developing and implementing include developing a national vision, mission, and plan of action for the public and private sectors, and the promotion of education, training, and national planning capacity in information systems and technology (Rodrigues & Risk, 2003).

FUTURE RESEARCH DIRECTIONS

Training programs on digital health should incorporate the local context, consider the local needs, and be sensitive to the local economic, social, cultural, and organizational factors. There is a need to develop innovative intercultural and multilingual educational tools and solutions according to the health needs of populations, especially in underserved areas. Given the limited resources, the creation and strengthening of the existing networks of public and private institutions with academic centers who have experience in digital health training and research should be promoted. They should also seek to work in close collaboration with local, regional, and national governments. Partnerships with developed institutions as part of a well-planned strategy have shown encouraging results. It is essential to point out that each partnership is unique, and each program has to ensure that the curriculum is relevant to address local needs and country priorities (Curioso WH, 2019).

Skill development should be viewed as a continuous process discussed among stakeholders, including the Ministry of Health, academia, and private institutions. It is essential to inspire and encourage global decision-makers, innovators, and researchers to build together on the work already done through digital health solutions (e.g., artificial intelligence, big data analytics) and find innovative ways for public and private partnerships to improve health workforce capacity. We also want them to focus on accelerating the pace at which they can further improve the health of populations (Curioso WH, 2019).

CONCLUSION

The use of digital health in healthcare services is growing. Research evidence suggests that digital health can offer benefits to stakeholders involved in healthcare including patients, and providers. As digital health continues to be used in routine healthcare services, practitioners will require new knowledge, skills, and competencies to make the best use of this new method. However, currently there is no adequate level of education and training available relating digital health. Workforce development relating to digital health is recognised as a priority. More research must be conducted to understand the educational and training needs to address current and future educational requirements. Advanced technologies should be embedded to transform digital healthcare system which will drive the future direction of healthcare.

REFERENCES

Australian Commission on Safety and Quality in Healthcare. (2010). *Australian Safety and Quality Framework for Healthcare*. Retrieved from https://www.safetyandquality.gov.au/publications-and-resources/resource-library/australian-safety-and-quality-framework-health-care

Australian Commission on Safety and Quality in Healthcare. (2011). *Patient centred care: Improving quality and safety through partnerships with patients and consumers*. Sydney: Author.

Australian Government. (2013). *Australian Public Service Big Data Strategy*. Author.

Australian Medical Association. (2016). *AMA Code of Ethics 2004. Revised 2016*. Author.

Bashshur, R. L., Reardon, T. G., & Shannon, G. W. (2000). Telemedicine: A new healthcare delivery system. *Annual Review of Public Health, 21*, 613–637. doi:10.1146/annurev.publhealth.21.1.613

Black, A. D., Car, J., Pagliari, C., Anandan, C., Cresswell, K., Bokun, T., ... Sheikh, A. (2011). The impact of eHealth on the quality and safety of healthcare: A systematic overview. *PLoS Medicine, 8*(1), e1000387. doi:10.1371/journal.pmed.1000387 PMID:21267058

Blas, M. M., Curioso, W. H., Garcia, P. J., Zimic, M., Carcamo, C. P., Castagnetto, J. M., ... Lopez, D. M. (2011). Training the biomedical informatics workforce in Latin America: Results of a needs assessment. *BMJ Open, 1*(2), e000233. doi:10.1136/bmjopen-2011-000233 PMID:22080537

Caine, K., & Hanania, R. (2013). Patients want granular privacy control over health information in electronic medical records. *Journal of the American Medical Informatics Association, 20*(1), 7–15. doi:10.1136/amiajnl-2012-001023 PMID:23184192

Committee on Quality Healthcare in America - Institute of Medicine. (2001). *Crossing the quality chasm: a new health system for the 21st century*. Author.

Cummings, E., Shin, E. H., Mather, C., & Hovenga, E. (2016). Embedding Nursing Informatics Education into an Australian Undergraduate Nursing Degree. *Studies in Health Technology and Informatics, 225*, 329–333.

Curioso, W. H. (2019). Building Capacity and Training for Digital Health: Challenges and Opportunities in Latin America. *Journal of Medical Internet Research, 21*(12), e16513. doi:10.2196/16513 PMID:31850849

Currell, R., Urquhart, C., Wainwright, P., & Lewis, R. (2000). Telemedicine versus face to face patient care: Effects on professional practice and healthcare outcomes. *Cochrane Database of Systematic Reviews*, (2). doi:10.1002/14651858.CD002098 PMID:10796678

Dattakumar, A., Gray, K., Henderson, K. B., Maeder, A., & Chenery, H. (2012). We are not educating the future clinical health professional workforce adequately for e-health competence: Findings of an Australian study. *Studies in Health Technology and Informatics, 178*, 33–38. PMID:22797016

Dods, S., Freyne, J., Alem, L., Nepal, S., Li, J., & Jang-Jaccard, J. (2012). *Caring for the last 3%: Telehealth potential and Broadband implications for remote Australia 2012*. Academic Press.

Dods, S., Hansen, D., Boyle, J., O'Keefe, C., Alem, L., Celler, B., & Kanagasingam, Y. (2014). *A digitally-enabled health system*. Marsfield. doi:10.4225/08/584ee7360ac32

Edirippulige, S., & Armfield, N. R. (2017). Education and training to support the use of clinical telehealth: A review of the literature. *Journal of Telemedicine and Telecare, 23*(2), 273–282. doi:10.1177/1357633x16632968

Edirippulige, S., Brooks, P., Carati, C., Wade, V. A., Smith, A. C., Wickramasinghe, S., & Armfield, N. R. (2018). It's important, but not important enough: eHealth as a curriculum priority in medical education in Australia. *Journal of Telemedicine and Telecare, 24*(10), 697–702. doi:10.1177/1357633X18793282 PMID:30343657

El Paso Society for Human Resource Management. (2017). *Workforce Readiness*. Retrieved from http://www.epshrm.org/page-18065

Glasgow, R. E., Phillips, S. M., & Sanchez, M. A. (2014). Implementation science approaches for integrating eHealth research into practice and policy. *International Journal of Medical Informatics, 83*(7), e1–e11. doi:10.1016/j.ijmedinf.2013.07.002 PMID:23910896

Gray K, Dattakumar A, Maeder A, Butler-Henderson K, & H., C. (2014). Advancing eHealth education for the clinical health professions. Academic Press.

Greenhalgh, T., Robert, G., Macfarlane, F., Bate, P., & Kyriakidou, O. (2004). Diffusion of innovations in service organizations: Systematic review and recommendations. *The Milbank Quarterly, 82*(4), 581–629. doi:10.1111/j.0887-378X.2004.00325.x

Health Workforce Australia. (2013). *Health Information Workforce Report*. Author.

Hersh, W., Margolis, A., Quiros, F., & Otero, P. (2010). Building a health informatics workforce in developing countries. *Health Affairs (Project Hope), 29*(2), 274–277. doi:10.1377/hlthaff.2009.0883

Ingebrigtsen, T., Georgiou, A., Clay-Williams, R., Magrabi, F., Hordern, A., Prgomet, M., ... Braithwaite, J. (2014). The impact of clinical leadership on health information technology adoption: Systematic review. *International Journal of Medical Informatics, 83*(6), 393–405. doi:10.1016/j.ijmedinf.2014.02.005 PMID:24656180

Jolly, R. (2011). The e health revolution—easier said than done (P. o. Australia Ed.). Parliamentary Library, Parliament of Australia.

Kohn, L., Corrigan, J., & Donaldson, M. (1999). *To err is human: building a safer health system* (N. A. Press, Ed.). Washington, DC: Committee on Quality of Healthcare in America, Institute of Medicine.

Lehnbom, E. C., Brien, J. E., & McLachlan, A. J. (2014). Knowledge and attitudes regarding the personally controlled electronic health record: An Australian national survey. *Internal Medicine Journal, 44*(4), 406–409. doi:10.1111/imj.12384 PMID:24754689

Liaw, S. T., & Hannan, T. (2011). Can we trust the PCEHR not to leak? *The Medical Journal of Australia, 195*(4), 222. doi:10.5694/j.1326-5377.2011.tb03287.x PMID:21843131

Luna, D., Almerares, A., Mayan, J. C. III, Gonzalez Bernaldo de Quiros, F., & Otero, C. (2014). Health Informatics in Developing Countries: Going beyond Pilot Practices to Sustainable Implementations: A Review of the Current Challenges. *Healthcare Informatics Research, 20*(1), 3–10. doi:10.4258/hir.2014.20.1.3 PMID:24627813

Maruthappu, M., Sood, H. S., & Keogh, S. B. (2014). The NHS Five Year Forward View: Transforming care. *The British Journal of General Practice, 64*(629), 635–635. doi:10.3399/bjgp14X682897 PMID:25452525

Office for Official Publications of the European Communities. (2004). *E-Health, Making Healthcare Better for European Citizens: An Action Plan for a European E-health Area*. Author.

Park, S., Parwani, A., Aller, R., Banach, L., Becich, M., Borkenfeld, S., ... Pantanowitz, L. (2013). The history of pathology informatics: A global perspective. *Journal of Pathology Informatics, 4*(1), 7–7. doi:10.4103/2153-3539.112689

Pearce, C., & Bainbridge, M. (2014). A personally controlled electronic health record for Australia. *Journal of the American Medical Informatics Association, 21*(4), 707–713. doi:10.1136/amiajnl-2013-002068 PMID:24650635

Rodrigues, R. J., & Risk, A. (2003). eHealth in Latin America and the Caribbean: Development and policy issues. *Journal of Medical Internet Research, 5*(1), e4–e4. doi:10.2196/jmir.5.1.e4 PMID:12746209

Saliba, V., Legido-Quigley, H., Hallik, R., Aaviksoo, A., Car, J., & McKee, M. (2012). Telemedicine across borders: A systematic review of factors that hinder or support implementation. *International Journal of Medical Informatics, 81*(12), 793–809. doi:10.1016/j.ijmedinf.2012.08.003 PMID:22975018

United Nations. (1948). *Universal Declaration of Human Rights*. Author.

Van Gemert-Pijnen, J. E., Nijland, N., van Limburg, M., Ossebaard, H. C., Kelders, S. M., Eysenbach, G., & Seydel, E. R. (2011). A Holistic Framework to Improve the Uptake and Impact of eHealth Technologies. *Journal of Medical Internet Research, 13*(4). doi:10.2196/jmir.1672

Vest, J. R., & Gamm, L. D. (2010). Health information exchange: Persistent challenges and new strategies. *Journal of the American Medical Informatics Association, 17*(3), 288–294. doi:10.1136/jamia.2010.003673 PMID:20442146

Westbrook, J. I., Woods, A., Rob, M. I., Dunsmuir, W. T., & Day, R. O. (2010). Association of interruptions with an increased risk and severity of medication administration errors. *Archives of Internal Medicine*, *170*(8), 683–690. doi:10.1001/archinternmed.2010.65 PMID:20421552

Wicks, P., Stamford, J., Grootenhuis, M. A., Haverman, L., & Ahmed, S. (2014). Innovations in e-health. *Quality of Life Research: An International Journal of Quality of Life Aspects of Treatment, Care and Rehabilitation*, *23*(1), 195–203. doi:10.100711136-013-0458-x PMID:23852096

World Health Organisation. (2011). mHealth: New horizons for health through mobile technologies. Author.

World Health Organisation. (2016). *Global diffusion of eHealth: Making universal health coverage achievable*. Report of the third global survey on eHealth. Retrieved from Geneva: https://apps.who.int/iris/bitstream/10665/252529/1/9789241511780-

KEY TERMS AND DEFINITIONS

eHealth: The use of information and communications technology in support of health and health-related fields.

Electronic Health Record: Is a digital version of a patient's paper chart. It is real-time, patient-centered records that make information available instantly and securely to authorized users.

Health Informatics: The interdisciplinary study of the design, development, adoption, and application of IT-based innovations in healthcare services delivery, management, and planning.

Health System: All activities whose primary purpose is to promote, restore, and maintain health.

mHealth: Medical and public health practice supported by mobile devices, such as mobile phones, patient monitoring devices, personal digital assistants (PDAs), and other wireless devices.

Telehealth: Use of telecommunication techniques for the purpose of providing telemedicine, medical education, and health education over a distance.

Telemedicine: The delivery of healthcare services, where distance is a critical factor, by all healthcare professionals using information and communication technologies for the exchange of valid information for diagnosis, treatment and prevention of disease and injuries, research and evaluation, and for the continuing education of healthcare providers, all in the interests of advancing the health of individuals and their communities.

Chapter 11
Process Analytics Model Approach in Healthcare:
The Technological Perspective

S. Santhosh Kumar
Department of Computer Science, Alagappa University, India

A. Sumathi
Department of CSE, SRC, SASTRA University (Deemed), India

ABSTRACT

Process analytics involves the relationship between the doctor, diagnostic centers and patient. The primary advantages of using process analytics in healthcare are expert guidance, global medical assistance, and possible alternate treatment mechanisms. The secondary advantages are the analysis of the same type of disease complications and the creation of a disease-based healthcare data repository. This chapter focuses on the process model-based approach for healthcare analytics. The two emerging techniques Big data and IoT are needed to be incorporated with the process model for storing and analyzing the healthcare data. The first category assists administrators with identifying areas to streamline operations and concretely increase savings. Research and development are crucial aspects of healthcare, providing new innovative solutions and treatments that can be properly tracked, measured, and analyzed.

BACKGROUND

Today a small town is having chemical labs and test labs with computer facility. The doctor gives the subscription to the patient based on the test report given by the lab. But the hospital and doctor are not maintainging the patients data consistently. The patient history can be analysed manually with technical assistance. The same method is followed for all other tests like CT Scan, MRI, ECG, etc. The leading hospital consists of patient personal information and his treatment history alone. For comparing any two test reports like Blood sugar with the Eye scan report. The doctor has to compare both manually, more-

DOI: 10.4018/978-1-7998-3274-4.ch011

over, the patient has to keep his medical records in each time of the visit. It is one of the most complex tasks and not possible to maintain the overall medical records for a long time.

In certain cases, the doctor may need for patients' teenage treatment history while treating him at the age of '50s. The disease like tuberculosis, cancer occurs due to the lifestyle habits of a person in the his early age (Amer, 2018; Lee, 2019; d'Angelo et al., 2019).

The following aspects must be considered

- There is a need for digitization of the medical history of a person since from his birth.
- There is a need to integrate the multiple resources of data stored in different devices.
- There is a need to monitor a patient from remote places i.e. houses and hospitals with the use of technology.

INTRODUCTION

Data has become one of the most valuable assets in the world. Data has its value and it can be changed when it is used for business applications. The growth of the Internet and the digitization of real-world processes lead to digital transmission (Meeker, & Wu, 2018; Angus & Westbrook, 2018; Pereira & Pereira, 2015; Contreas, 2018; Kuziemsky et al., 2019; Pendse et al., 2019). The storage becomes more centralized which is also secured as personalized one. Email, smart phone, Laptops, Desktops and all other electronic devices are connected with the internet and it generates large amounts of data every day. The secured centralized storage called cloud storage provides sophisticated efficient use of data once it is stored (Batrouni et al., 2018; Zhong et al., 2018). The stored data can be accessed and modified with any electronic devices from anywhere in the world. The use of technologies in all fields has become paperless, cost-efficient and instant access to data to all of its users. Exchange of information through the digital medium is a time-saving and it gives solutions for division making the problem-solving.In the healthcare industry, healthcare data is computerized and stored separately in magnetic disks. The patient records are stored as files and manual work is needed more in the system. The digitization and storing all sources of data in a single location or possible to Interco melt one another when it is needed will do magics in analysis and decision making. This chapter discusses the role of the Internet of Things and Big Data in healthcare Digitalization (Khan & Salah, 2018; Srinivasan et al., 2019; Sowmya et al., 2019; Bilami & Sahraoui, 2020; Oussous et al., 2018).

The Healthcare analytics is a service-oriented architecture which helps to store, analyze and manage the patient records whenever it is needed (Mehta & Pandit, 2018; Manogaran & Lopez, 2018; Carvalho et al., 2019; Fernandez-Luque et al., 2019). It gives the present biography of a human with their historical healthcare information. It is very useful for remote medical assistance, decision making, possible treatment methods, etc., The outcomes of healthcare analytics lead to increased healthcare and critical care. The vast growth of data, internet, and technology leads to generate and combine the data in the second which is useful for many purposes. In the medical industry decision making and treatment methodology are leading factors of patient survival. The drug and treatment procedure is the common procedure that will be positive only when proper medicine is given or treatment procedure followed.

HEALTHCARE ANALYSIS

The digitized medical data or health record can be used for analysis. The analysis can be done as a manual process with the use of any computerized devices. The analysis is a manual process where the doctor performs decision making for a patient by analyzing his records with current data. The healthcare analysis has the following drawbacks:

- It requires processes of the data.
- It requires human support in each level of digitization of data.
- It delays the decision-making process during critical conditions.
- It gives a poor or worst performance in healthcare support activities.

HEALTHCARE ANALYTICS

It is an automated version of healthcare analysis which performed all operations automatically. The human interaction is much less in the present system. For that, time can be obtained and analyzed automatically with the used of emerging technologies like IoT and Big Data.

The healthcare analytics executes the output based on the analysis of input data. It is an automated self-decision making system that enables the patient, hospital, and physician can perform those tasks through automatic made where the overall inter-process can be done by the computers. This automatic system alerts and sends a notification whenever the needed. The benefits of healthcare analytics are:

- Increased use of electronic devices.
- Self-automated and decision making
- Cost-efficient and Time-consuming

BIG DATA

When the patients are monitored using a Digital monitoring system (Polyakova et al., 2019; Chattopadhyay, Das, & Das, 2019). Te very large volume of data is to be stored every day. Once the data is stored, the next complex thing is searching the data in large data storage.When the current data is compared with the historical data, then the big data technique is needed. For spot analysis and decision making. The patient may have his medical history in three hospitals which are in different locations, the big data enabled to integrate all the databases and predicts the results by comparing with current input data.

The basic properties of big data are:

Velocity: To healthcare analysis, then data retrieval, comparison, and transformation of data should be done in the stipulated time, the big data works in a dynamic environment which gives better solutions with time efficiency.

Variety: As discussed earlier (or) as noted above, the data collected from different devices and manual inputs are stored and compared dynamically. The big data techniques are used to store, analyze and modify the data in the database.

Volume: The volume of data is one of the remarkable features of Big data. The volume of data could affect the performance of data analysis. The volume of data needs a dynamic storage facility.

Cloud Storage

Cloud Storage is a service which used to store the data dynamically and can able to access the data from anywhere. Then cloud storage provides better solutions for healthcare analysis and healthcare death maintenance. The patient, hospital-physician can have cloud storage to store the data, digitization of data.

The cloud storage application/benefits lead to

- Less use of computer resources
- Reduced hardware maintenance
- Reduced storage space in physical devices
- Dynamic usage of data from any place
- Cost-efficient and time consumption.

Big Data and Its Importance in Healthcare

Big data is an integration of different databases dynamically. The internet nature of Big data has different forms of data. The major classifications are:

Structured: The data is stored in a formatted during creation, updation and process are called Structured data. The text, file, excel and test reports with indicators are structured. But the data need to be restructured when the transformation is required, The healthcare data is partial structure. The metrics used for standard tests produce structured reports.

Unstructured: The data is not available in an informal nature during creation, updation, and process is called Unstructured data. The patient input, physician instructions hrz case history discharge summary contains important data in an unstructured format.The Data transformation easy with Unstructured data.

Semistructured: Semistructured data is a combination of Structured and unstructured data. The healthcare data is always Semistructured during exchanging information between various stakeholders. Any Structured or Unstructured data can be used as Semistructured data.

Big Data Concepts

There are different existing concepts used in big data. Each concept has its applications. The collective use of existing techniques in big data results in better performance and outcomes in healthcare industry. The most important concepts which are involved in big data are discussed below:

Batch Processing: It is one of the hardware processing technique which is used to integrate the different kinds of data from large databases. Each time the overall databases are mapped into a single process and give the results are delivered to the requested system.

Data Mining: To find similar and unknown hidden patterns from the healthcare databases, big data uses data mining techniques are used to extract, integrate, transform and analyze the data from large heterogeneous databases.

Cluster Computing: The set of loosely coupled systems combined called cluster which works as a single computer for a particular process or tsks. The healthcare systems are loosely coupled in nature and need to be integrated during process timeThe The overall process integration combined into a single process which response as a single output to the responder.

Data Lake: It refers to the repository of data in the original format. It is also like a metadata repository for a set of relevant domains. The repositories are referred to using XML and other coding techniques to access the required information. The use of data mining technologies can transform the original format to application formats.

ETL: Extraction of data and transform it into requested from to Load the data for the application use is one of the needed domain ask of Big data frame work. For that enrichment of original data, Shaping the original data with added things are the needed tasks in ETL (Biswas et al., 2019; Gao, 2019; Sachin et al., 2019; Passos et al., 2019).

Data Science: Big data requires the integration of many large databases. The incorporation of different databases in different domains needs lexical linkage between the databases. In the case of healthcare analytics, the biological databases, drug data repositories, hospital databases are to be combined with lexical relationships or under one umbrella. Computational techniques like Data visualization, machine learning and statistics are incorporated with another.

Data Analysis: Data Analysis is the preliminary step in healthcare Analytics. The data analysis technique can be used as a manual process for analyzing data using existing techniques. The data analysis can be performed by database administrators, business analyst and by users.

Business Intelligence: The overall bigdata applications are associated with business objectives. The business goals are desired as business objectives during application development and later it is called applications or features of the product. Business Intelligence gives the overall enterprise view of the product.

Hadoop: It is a Java supported open-source framework developed by the Apache group which is used as a support platform for the integration of big data tools and devices (Thind & Simon, 2019; Raj & D'Souza, 2019).

Map Reduce: It is a specific tool to support the integration of data warehouses and various large databases. It supports heterogeneous data and operating environment.

Python: It is an open-source programming language that supports dynamic and simple code generation features. It supports multi-paradigm programming and object-oriented program support. It handles meta-objects by doing meta-programming and logic programming concepts.

INTERNET OF THINGS

Internet of Things is the connection of wearable devices with the use of the Internet is one of winning jargon in the present Eva. The IoT opened and a new pathway to the technological world by interconnecting any devices in the world. IoT is one of the buzz word in the business sector which plays the cruse to efficient business activities. Like the same, the healthcare industry is also regenerated by using IoT is medical processes. For example, an IoT enabled glucometer and insulin can avoid the patient to consult the doctor in person and aslo the doctor can adjust the insulin level from remote places. The advantages of the use of IoT technology is countless and will give very positive outcomes like

- Increased life system
- Improved medical assistance
- Improved patient care with 24*7 support from remote patient monitoring

- Expert guidance
- Identification of critical condition and early prediction of diseases.
- Dynamic medical assistance based on the present condition of a patient.

Input

IoT uses sensors, devices as input sources. The Gps enabled devices with internet facility are used to send or received data.

Process

The output received from the sensors and other devices are stored in the databases and also in cloud storage. The healthcare system monitors a patient periodically. It stores every output generated by the electronic device. The data collected is stored in a location and the notification will be sent to the hospital and physician immediately if anything happens critically. For processing data for analysis, the determining, database query techniques are used. Apart from the diagnosis, the data-based application like searching, integrating of data can be done using computation techniques.

Output

The result of the analysis is considered as the output which can be either input for next level diagnosis or treatment outcome. Based on the out the input and next treatment procedure will be analyzed by the physician.

IoT DEVICES USED IN HEALTHCARE

The use of specialised IOT enabled devices are essential part of IOT health monitoring and management. These devices are internet connected, ups enabled had interconnected with other devices. The normal medical equipments and other devices can also used as a IOT device in healthcare analytics.

Biosensors

The biometric sensors or biosensors are used to get the inputs from the patient as finger print face, voice, blood. Temperature, heart beat as input. Each biometric inputs needs relevant sensors, inputs device which is internets and ups enabled. There are two major types of sensors in biometric operations. The physiological sensors are used to gets the physical identity of a person are the behavioural sensors are used to gets the external identity of a person like keystroke, signature and voice.

Neural and Brain Sensors

Latest research outcomes in IOT produced devices to sense the activity of brain and neural activities of a person. It is very useful to monitor the mental health to a person. The inputs taken from the sensors are analyzed to adjust the treatment method and drug dosage levels. The patient in critical condition due to accident or acute illness cases are analysed using neural sensors will gives the current status of brain. The other devices are also used as IOT enabled devices to monitor and manage the patient in hospital and remote patient monitoring. The normal temperature devices are used to monitor the temperature level of patient, environment and other external devices are used to provide child care, old age people assistance etc.

BUSINESS MODEL IN HEALTHCARE

In general business models are used to develop, process and outcomes based on the current needs with a business strategy. According healthcare perspective, business models are used to simplify the internal process of patient care and analytics with use of edging technologies like IOT, big data and cloud. In business process model will gives economic, paper less and improved medical assistance is positive outcomes. The process analytics has become the leading automation techniques which has been introduced in many application areas. In healthcare analytics there are different perspectives.

The Patient Perspective

The patient needs quick medical assistance during critical/emergency conditions. The medical assistance with less cost, reduced transportation and 24x7 medical care are the prior needs of each patient.

The patient needs medical data repository had advanced medical from the experts in the world are the additional requirements. The use of digital documentation in cloud environment or by the hospitals of a patient in the form of electronic records could be the primary step for healthcare analytics.

The Physician Perspective

The medical practioners had physicians are lack in monitoring the patients to predict the critical condition. The doctor gets attention only the patient report himself physically to the hospital during normal and pathetic conditions. The remote monitoring of a patient simplifies the work of the physician to support give medical assistance to the patient in the time. The healthcare system reduces the physical visiting time of a patient during his normal conditions and also possible/enables to give physical & remote support when the condition is critical.

The Organisation Perspective

Any organization in the existing medical sector is facing many constraints in giving good medical assistance to the patients. Even though private organisations are having higher medical assistance, the linkage gap and miscommunication and in lack of monitoring of a patient condition, the overall process gets failure. To encourage the 24X7 medical assistance in a hospital like ICU, CCU, Emergency unit to the patient. Which requires more manpower, infrastructure and other environmental support. It results the medical assistance is higher cost which could not be affordable by all the people. The other significant failures like unavailability specialised expert/doctor, lack of medical equipment support drug unavailability are leading factors of total death in hospitals.

In a simple example we explain, when the ambulance is remotely connected with the nearby hospital with IOT & technical support, the condition of the patient in a ambulance cloud be automatically known by the nearby hospital and the management team can arrange all the supportive medical assistance before the patient arrived to hospital. The use of EHI can give the previous medical history of a patient. Which results increased life saving possibility of the patient. The overall process could be easy, cost effective and occurs in need of the hour.

ONTOLOGY

The role of ontology in healthcare is must and if plays significant role in both data exchange and visualization (Subramaniyaswamy et al., 2019; Moreno-Conde et al., 2019). The ontology helps to understand the same information n different perspectives by different people. The data visualization, building relationships among data, data transformation are the building blocks in healthcare analytics. The ontology makes it possible to build data repositories with linguistic and lexical relationships. It helps to build high level relationships among large databases in different domains.

CONCLUSION

The process analytics in healthcare is one of the integrations of data, process and decision making. The healthcare sector needs a lot of computational support in all staged levels of healthcare. According to WHO, the increase of the old age population leads to the scarcity of manual medical support and assistance. There is a need of the hour of the automated healthcare system to monitor and maintain the patients from different places. The earlier investment for the establishment of IoT and Big Data supported the healthcare system can be high. But the benefits are everlasting and hence these emerging technology will give the dramatic change in the healthcare industry.

REFERENCES

Amer, I. A. A. M. (2018). *Measurement of Quality of Life of Free Flap Transfer in Reconstrucion of the Head and Neck Tumor Defects after Ablative Surgery in Asturias, Spain Thesis* (Doctoral dissertation). Oviedo University.

Angus, A., & Westbrook, G. (2018). Top 10 Global Consumer Trends for 2018. *Euromonitor International, 61*, 29–76.

Banerjee, S., Hemphill, T., & Longstreet, P. (2018). Wearable devices and healthcare: Data sharing and privacy. *The Information Society, 34*(1), 49–57. doi:10.1080/01972243.2017.1391912

Batrouni, M., Finch, S., Wilson, S., Bertaux, A., & Nicolle, C. (2018, October). Intelligent Cloud Storage Management for Layered Tiers. In *International Conference on Cooperative Design, Visualization and Engineering* (pp. 33-43). Springer. 10.1007/978-3-030-00560-3_5

Bilami, A., & Sahraoui, S. (2020). Mechanisms to secure communications in the IoT. In Securing the Internet of Things: Concepts, Methodologies, Tools, and Applications (pp. 498-521). IGI Global. doi:10.4018/978-1-5225-9866-4.ch027

Biswas, N., Chattapadhyay, S., Mahapatra, G., Chatterjee, S., & Mondal, K. C. (2019). A New Approach for Conceptual Extraction-Transformation-Loading Process Modeling. *International Journal of Ambient Computing and Intelligence*, *10*(1), 30–45. doi:10.4018/IJACI.2019010102

Carvalho, J. V., Rocha, Á., Vasconcelos, J., & Abreu, A. (2019). A health data analytics maturity model for hospitals information systems. *International Journal of Information Management*, *46*, 278–285. doi:10.1016/j.ijinfomgt.2018.07.001

Chattopadhyay, S., Das, T. K., & Das, A. (2019). *Digital Learning and Training Methodology in Study of Health Monitoring in Resco System.* Available at SSRN 3377635

Chaudhry, J. (2018, April). Securing Healthcare Data Using Biometric Authentication. *Security and Privacy in Communication Networks: SecureComm 2017 International Workshops, ATCS and SePrIoT, Niagara Falls, ON, Canada, October 22–25, 2017 Proceedings*, *239*, 123.

Contreras, D. L. (2018). A workflow and protocol describing the field to digitization process for new project-based fossil leaf collections. *Applications in Plant Sciences*, *6*(2), e1025. doi:10.1002/aps3.1025 PMID:29732256

d'Angelo, M., Castelli, V., Catanesi, M., Antonosante, A., Dominguez-Benot, R., Ippoliti, R., ... Cimini, A. (2019). PPARγ and Cognitive Performance. *International Journal of Molecular Sciences*, *20*(20), 5068. doi:10.3390/ijms20205068 PMID:31614739

Duggal, R., Brindle, I., & Bagenal, J. (2018). *Digital healthcare: regulating the revolution.* Academic Press.

Fernandez-Luque, L., Aupetit, M., Palotti, J., Singh, M., Fadlelbari, A., Baggag, A., & Al-Thani, D. (2019). Health Lifestyle Data-Driven Applications Using Pervasive Computing. In *Big Data, Big Challenges: A Healthcare Perspective* (pp. 115–126). Cham: Springer. doi:10.1007/978-3-030-06109-8_10

Gao, C. (2019). *Research on the Application of Big Data in Security Information Collection.* Academic Press.

Khan, M. A., & Salah, K. (2018). IoT security: Review, blockchain solutions, and open challenges. *Future Generation Computer Systems*, *82*, 395–411. doi:10.1016/j.future.2017.11.022

Kim, J., Campbell, A. S., de Ávila, B. E. F., & Wang, J. (2019). Wearable biosensors for healthcare monitoring. *Nature Biotechnology*, 1. PMID:30804534

Kuziemsky, C. E., Eynakchi, R., Jibb, L., & Stacey, D. (2019). Digital Process Innovation for Patient Centred Cancer Symptom Management. In ITCH (pp. 250-255). Academic Press.

Lee, K. (2019). Epidemiology is ecosystem science. *Synthese*, 1–29.

Manogaran, G., & Lopez, D. (2018). Health data analytics using scalable logistic regression with stochastic gradient descent. *International Journal of Advanced Intelligence Paradigms, 10*(1-2), 118–132. doi:10.1504/IJAIP.2018.089494

Meeker, M., & Wu, L. (2018). *Internet trends 2018.* Academic Press.

Mehta, N., & Pandit, A. (2018). Concurrence of big data analytics and healthcare: A systematic review. *International Journal of Medical Informatics, 114*, 57–65. doi:10.1016/j.ijmedinf.2018.03.013 PMID:29673604

Moreno-Conde, A., Parra-Calderón, C. L., Sánchez-Seda, S., Escobar-Rodríguez, G. A., López-Otero, M., Cusso, L., ... Albertí-Ibarz, M. (2019). ITEMAS ontology for healthcare technology innovation. *Health Research Policy and Systems, 17*(1), 47. doi:10.118612961-019-0453-y PMID:31046786

Oussous, A., Benjelloun, F. Z., Lahcen, A. A., & Belfkih, S. (2018). Big Data technologies: A survey. *Journal of King Saud University-Computer and Information Sciences, 30*(4), 431–448. doi:10.1016/j.jksuci.2017.06.001

Passos, N. R., Rodrigues, A. F., Macedo, H. T., Prado, B. O., da Silva, G. J., & Matos, L. N. (2019, May). Open Data Extraction, Transformation, and Loading as a Tool for Supporting 2018 Elections' Voters. In *Proceedings of the XV Brazilian Symposium on Information Systems* (p. 23). ACM. 10.1145/3330204.3330232

Pendse, S., Benson, J. J., Maurya, P., & Miller, M. J. (2019). *U.S. Patent Application No. 15/725,630.* US Patent Office.

Pereira, R., & Pereira, E. G. (2015). Future internet: Trends and challenges. *International Journal of Space-Based and Situated Computing, 5*(3), 159–167. doi:10.1504/IJSSC.2015.070952

Polyakova, A. G., Loginov, M. P., Serebrennikova, A. I., & Thalassinos, E. (2019). *Design of a socio-economic processes monitoring system based on network analysis and big data.* Academic Press.

Raj, A., & D'Souza, R. (2019). *A Review on Hadoop Eco System for Big Data.* Academic Press.

Sachin, S., Goyal, S. K., Avinash, S., & Kamal, K. (2019). Nuts and Bolts of ETL in Data Warehouse. In *Emerging Trends in Expert Applications and Security* (pp. 1–9). Singapore: Springer. doi:10.1007/978-981-13-2285-3_1

Shuwandy, M. L., Zaidan, B. B., Zaidan, A. A., & Albahri, A. S. (2019). Sensor-based mHealth authentication for real-time remote healthcare monitoring system: A multilayer systematic review. *Journal of Medical Systems, 43*(2), 33. doi:10.100710916-018-1149-5 PMID:30612191

Sowmya, B. J., Shetty, C., Cholappagol, N. V., & Seema, S. (2019). IOT and Data Analytics Solution for Smart Agriculture. In *The Rise of Fog Computing in the Digital Era* (pp. 210–237). IGI Global. doi:10.4018/978-1-5225-6070-8.ch010

Srinivasan, C. R., Rajesh, B., Saikalyan, P., Premsagar, K., & Yadav, E. S. (2019). A review on the different types of Internet of Things (IoT). *Journal of Advanced Research in Dynamical and Control Systems, 11*(1), 154–158.

Subramaniyaswamy, V., Manogaran, G., Logesh, R., Vijayakumar, V., Chilamkurti, N., Malathi, D., & Senthilselvan, N. (2019). An ontology-driven personalized food recommendation in IoT-based healthcare system. *The Journal of Supercomputing*, *75*(6), 3184–3216. doi:10.100711227-018-2331-8

Thind, J. S., & Simon, R. (2019, June). Implementation of Big Data in Cloud Computing with optimized Apache Hadoop. In *2019 3rd International conference on Electronics, Communication and Aerospace Technology (ICECA)* (pp. 997-1001). IEEE. 10.1109/ICECA.2019.8821854

Wu, W., & Haick, H. (2018). Healthcare Monitoring: Materials and Wearable Devices for Autonomous Monitoring of Physiological Markers. *Advanced Materials*, *30*(41), 1870309. doi:10.1002/adma.201870309 PMID:29498115

Zhong, H., Zhu, W., Xu, Y., & Cui, J. (2018). Multi-authority attribute-based encryption access control scheme with policy hidden for cloud storage. *Soft Computing*, *22*(1), 243–251. doi:10.100700500-016-2330-8

Chapter 12
Investigating Diabetic Subjects on Their Correlation With TTH and CAD:
A Statistical Approach on Experimental Results

Rohit Rastogi
https://orcid.org/0000-0002-6402-7638
Dayalbagh Educational Institute, Agra, India & ABES Engineering College, Ghaziabad, India

Devendra K. Chaturvedi
https://orcid.org/0000-0002-4837-2570
Dayalbagh Educational Institute, Agra, India

Parul Singhal
ABES Engineering College, Ghaziabad, India

Mayank Gupta
Tata Consultancy Services, Noida, India

ABSTRACT

Digital technology is modernizing healthcare. Large volumes of data refer to big data by digitising health information that can quickly be processed by machines. Digital healthcare analysis is the ability to diagnose and suggest ways to reduce costs; provide quality patient care and outcomes, available 24/7; reach to patients located in vast distant geographical areas; and avert preventable diseases. Artificial intelligence (AI) is an autonomous real-time machine system in comparison to natural information analyzed by humans. Diabetes is a serious, under-reported, life-threatening disease affecting millions of people of all ages, and researchers have identified it to be a major public health problem that is approaching epidemic proportions globally. The purpose of this study is to investigate diabetes analysis from CAD and other diseases using the latest advanced digital technologies to analyze information extracted from IoT and big data and stress correlation (TTH) on human health.

DOI: 10.4018/978-1-7998-3274-4.ch012

INTRODUCTION

Machine Vision

Machine Vision is the in which computer has the ability to display and use one or more video cameras, analog-to-digital (ADC), and digital signal processing (DSP). The obtained data is controlled by computer or robot. The scene of a machine is similar in complexity to speech recognition. Each visual sensitivity and resolution system has two important features.

- Sensitivity is the ability of a device to detect weaknesses in weak light or invisible wavelengths.
- Resolution is how much the device can differ between objects. In general, resolution tends to limit the field of view. The sensitivity depends on the transparency. All other factors remain constant, reducing sharpness sensitivity and reducing sensitivity resolution.

The human eye is sensitive to electromagnetic radiation in the 390-770 nm range. Video cameras are sensitive to a wide range of wavelengths. Some of the vision systems in this device work with infrared wavelengths, ultraviolet light or x-rays.

The sight requires a computer with an advanced processor. In detail, high-resolution cameras require large amounts of random access memory (RAM) and AI programming. Equipment venues are used in various medical and industrial applications.

Here's an example:

- Electronic component analysis
- Identify signature
- optical character recognition
- Handwriting recognition
- Finding Object
- pattern recognition
- Content inspection
- make money
- Medical image analysis

The term device often refers to industrial computer programs, but computer terms are often used to describe digital computers, data processing and any kind of technology for which some of them are recorded.

Components of Machine Vision System are different but in most cases there are many factors. These elements are as follows:

- Digital or analog camera to capture images
- Instruments for digitizing images like camera interfaces
- Processor

When these three components are connected to the device, it is known as a smart camera. The car's visual system can be obtained from smart cameras equipped with the following add-ons.

- Input / output hardware
- Lens
- Light sources such as LED lights and halogen bulbs
- Image processing program
- Sensors to detect and access images
- Parts category

General Application

- Product inspection
- Visual inventory control and management of barcode reading, counting, interface store etc.
- The food and beverage industry uses automotive vision systems to monitor quality.

In the medical field, machine vision systems are used in medical imaging and inspection methods.

Medical Imaging

Medical imaging refers to those techniques and processes that are used to treat images of different parts of the human body for diagnostic purposes and for the treatment of digital health. The term medical imaging includes various radiography methods.

- X-ray
- Fluorescence microscope
- Magnetic Resonance Imaging (MRI)
- Medical ultrasound or ultrasound
- Endoscopy
- Elastography
- Tactical imaging
- Thermograph

Medical photography and applied imaging techniques for positron emission tomography (PET)

Medical imaging involves measurement and recording techniques that not only generate images, but also data that is often displayed in charts and maps.

This includes electroencephalograms (EEGs), magneto encephalography (MEGs), electrocardiograms (EKGs).

Medical Imaging Usage in Digital Health

Medical imaging is important for all medical settings and all levels of medicine. Medical imaging enables physicians to make more accurate diagnoses and appropriate treatment decisions. Without medical imaging, both diagnosis and treatment in digital health can't be very accurate at all levels.

Biomedical Image and Analysis

Biomedical imaging measures the human body at various scales (microscope, macro scope, etc.) (Martin et al., 2018). They are measured by various imaging methods (e.g. CT scanners, ultrasound devices etc) and physical properties of the human body (wireless density, x-ray turbidity etc). These images are interpreted by specialists (such as radiologists) to perform clinical work (such as diagnosis) and have a major impact on physician decisions.

Figure 1. Medical imaging example (upper left to lower right): MRI multiple brain distribution: T1 weight, reverse T1 recovery and FLAIR T2 channel; MRI total wrist; flat heart ultrasound; X-ray chest; MRI heart MRI (Martin et al., 2018)

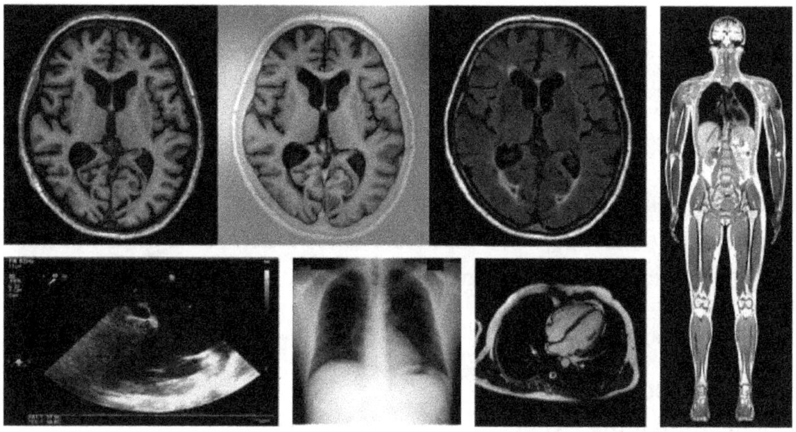

Biomedical images are usually 3D images, sometimes with additional dimensions (4D) and / or multiple channels (4-5D) (e.g. multi-dimensional MR images). As a clinical protocol for stratification of image acquisition methods (e.g., patients on the back not bent), changes in biomedical images are very different from normal images (e.g., photographs). In the analysis, we intend to identify nuances (eg, some small areas show abnormal findings).

Big Data and IoT

As the name implies, Big data represents large amounts of data. But that's not all. In addition to quantity, IBM data scientists have recognized large data to show diversity, speed and accuracy.

Big data is the result of a variety of resources, including social media, transactions, organizational content, sensors, and mobile devices. I immediately point out that a large amount of data is being collected. Every 60 seconds, a 72-hour video is uploaded to YouTube, 216,000 posts are sent, and 204 million emails are sent. With confidence, the collected data should be in good time constantly updated in real time. Large-scale data analysis is of great value to companies and individuals that use it. (McAfee et al., 2012; Tsai et al., 2013)

On the other hand, the Internet of Things (IoT) transforms "things" into smart objects every day. Transport container with sensors that interconnect with the refrigerator, watch, thermostat, car, internet for data collection and transmission. This information, when combined with information from other sources and other large data above, can be large data (Murdoch et al., 2013; Tenhunen et al., 2015).

Artificial Intelligence (AI) and Machine Learning (ML)

Artificial Intelligence: The term AI includes two words: "Artificial" and "Intelligent." Artificial means human-made things and abnormalities, and intelligence means the ability to understand and think. There is a misconception that artificial intelligence is a system, but this is not a system.

AI runs on the system. AI has many definitions, but the definitions are as follows. So this is the intelligence that we want to add to them all the capabilities of the device, including humans (Gabbe et al., 2018; Chaturvedi et al., 2012).

Machine Learning: A learning device that can be learned without the device with its own explicit program. It is an AI application that allows the system to automatically learn and improve the experience. You can now combine the application inputs and outputs to create an application. A simple definition of machine learning is that "machine learning" learns from E's experience. If class work learners measured by P are improved by experience, then T classes and performance measures P.

Use of Machine Intelligence in Digital Healthcare

Here are the top 10 applications of machine learning in healthcare

- Learning care in the healthcare is one of the things that is seen in the gradual acceptance of the healthcare industry. Google has recently launched a machine learning algorithm to detect cancerous tumors in mammography, and Stanford researchers have used deep learning to identify skin cancer. The Learning Machine (ML) currently has various responsibilities in health management. ML helps healthcare analyze and analyze thousands of different data points, providing timely risk assessment, accurate resource allocation, and other applications.
- With the increasing use of autonomous learning in healthcare, it will be possible to support millions of patients in the future without data, analysis and innovation coming together. Soon it will spread to find ML-based programs that contain real-time patient data from multiple medical systems in multiple countries, which will increase the effectiveness of new treatment options. It was not available before (Kasper et al., 2015).
- Disease Identification and Diagnosis: One of the major ML programs in healthcare is diagnosing and diagnosing diseases that are otherwise difficult to diagnose. It can include anything from cancers that are difficult to obtain in the early stages and difficult to become other genetic conditions.
- Drug Discovery and Production: One of the clinical applications of machine learning is the early detection of drugs. It also includes R & D technologies such as next-generation sequencing and medical accuracy to help find alternatives to the treatment of multi factorial diseases.
- Currently, machine learning techniques include unmatched learning that can identify data patterns without prediction.

- Imaging medical detection: Machine learning and deep learning are both responsible for a ground-breaking technology called computer vision. The findings were approved by Microsoft for the Inner Eye initiative, which works with image recognition tools for image analysis. As car learning becomes more familiar and its explanatory ability increases, it is expected that more sources of diverse medical images that are part of this AI based diagnostic process will be seen.
- There are many lesions, cancers, etc that can't be simplified using complex equations. ML-based algorithms are used in various instances in the hand, making it easy to find and find variables. The most common applications of ML in medical image analysis is to classify objects such as lesions into categories such as normal or abnormal, lesions or non-lesions (Tenhunen et al., 2015).

Use of Digital Healthcare to Diagnose and Cure Diseases Using Big Data and IoT

The main problem is that all patients, especially in remote areas, can't receive medical treatment or treatment in critical situations. It has had unpleasant consequences for people with regard to hospital and doctor services. Today, these problems are mostly solved by using new technologies that use IoT devices to monitor healthcare.

- Health Tracking: Massive Data and Analytics beyond the Internet (IoT) is a revolution that can track user statistics and information. In addition to helpless feet that can help the patient sleep, heart rate, exercise, gait etc, there are new medical innovations that can control the patient's blood pressure, pulse oximeter, glucose monitor etc.
- Cost savings: Large amounts of data are the best way to save the cost of hospitals that are more or less of this book. Predictive analytics helps solve this problem by helping to predict admission rates and assigning employees. This reduces hospital investment and actually helps maximize the investment potential. The insurance industry can prevent patients from being hospitalized by securing hygienic trackers in wearables. (Plant et al., 2018; Felman et al., 2016)
- Higher Risk Support: If all hospital records are digitized, this is complete information that you can understand about many patient patterns. Return these patients to the hospital to identify their chronic problems. Such understanding will help to provide better care for such professionals and insights to rectify corrective actions to reduce their frequent visits. This is a great way to maintain a list of at-risk patients and provide them with professional care.

Diabetes and Its Types

Diabetes (DM) has been identified as a series of pancreas due to insulin cleansing and / or abnormal exercise. Due to insulin deficiency, blood sugar levels increase and hyperglycemia is caused by carbohydrate, fat and protein. DM, who has affected over 200 one million people worldwide. The possibility of diabetes is expected to increase in the following few years. DM can be split into many different characters. Yet, according to the disease (Brazier et al., 2018).

There are two main types of clinics, type-1 diabetes (T1D) and type-2 diabetes (T-2D). The most common form of T2D diabetes is considered 95% of all diabetes patients, mainly due to insulin resistance T2D, lifestyle factors, physical activity, dietary habits and congenital heart disease (Rastogi et al., 2018). Due to the devastation of the T1D effective system, it is visible from planarians, pancreases beta cells intestlezes. T1D affects about 10% of diabetes patients worldwide, 10% of which eventually develop Idiopathic diabetes.

Gestational diabetes, endocrine disorders, type-2 diabetes mellitus, neuritis, mitochondria, and pregnancy are based on the specifications of other types of DM and the onset of insulin hygiene.

Complications

The long-term complications of diabetes gradually increase. The more diabetes, less glycemic control, the risk of more complications, the complications of diabetes are also safe. Potential complications are:

- Cardiovascular Disease: Diabetes increases the risk of cardiovascular attacks such as chest pain (angina), heart attack, stroke and arterial stenosis (atherosclerosis), such as coronary artery disease. If you have diabetes, you may experience heart disease or stroke.
- Neuropathy (extra sugar content): This can strengthen the walls of small blood vessels (capillaries) especially on the leg.
- There is a risk of burning, numbness, burning or pain. It usually starts with your finger and spreads slowly. If left untreated, you can lose all your organs.
- Damage to the gastrointestinal tract can cause nausea, vomiting, diarrhea or constipation. For men, this can lead to erectile dysfunction.
- Kidney disease (nephropathy): There are millions of brightly colored mass (glomeruli) in the kidney, which filter the blood. Diabetes can damage this delicate filtration system. Serious injury can lead to kidney failure or irreversible kidney disease, which may require dialysis or kidney transplantation.
- Eye damage (retinopathy): Diabetes damage the retinal blood vessels (diabetic retinopathy) and cause blindness. Disease increases the risk of developing physical conditions such as cataracts and glaucoma. Because untreated residues are reduced and vaccinated, rarely the treatment of serious infections occurs. After all, these are infectious breaks.
- Skin condition: Due to skin problems including bacterial and fungal infections, diabetes can occur.
- Deafness: Deafness in people with diabetes is more common.
- Alzheimer's disease: Type 2 diabetes can increase the risk of dementia such as Alzheimer's disease. Your blood glucose control is weak, it seems more dangerous. Although there are many ways in which these anomalies can be related, there is no evidence to show them.
- Depression: Symptoms of depression are common among people with type 1 and 2 diabetes. Depression can affect diabetes management (Masis et al., 2019).
- Pregnancy diabetes complications: Most women suffering from gestational diabetes have a healthy baby. However, losing control or decreasing blood sugar can be a problem for you and your baby.
- The complications of the child can be due to pregnancy associated with diabetes.
- Hypertrophy: excessive glucose can pass through the placenta. This will make your child very big Very large babies may need to be born (Vyas et al., 2018).
- Hypoglycemia: Children with gestational diabetes can develop glucose (hypoglycemia) after birth due to high insulin production. Fast feeding and sometimes intravenous glucose solutions can restore blood sugar level of the normal child.
- Type 2 diabetes: The mother of gestational diabetes is at risk of obesity and type 2 diabetes.
- Gestational diabetes can cause the death of the child before and after birth.

Diabetes and Headache

Not everyone diabetic will experience a headache. Those who have recently been diagnosed with diabetes tend to have headaches because they are still trying to control their blood sugar and use a diet.

For people with diabetes, headaches are usually due to changes in blood sugar levels.

A headache can indicate that your blood sugar is high, and your doctor calls it hyperglycemia. Instead, blood sugar levels may be very low, a doctor called it hypoglycemia. Changes in blood sugar levels are more likely to cause headaches for diabetics. (Cancer Research U.K., 2019; Abdelhamid et al., 2014)

Obesity

Obesity is a medical condition that affects health if an individual has an excess amount of body fat or is very overweight. Doctors usually indicate that obese people are obese.

Body Mass Index (BMI) is a device used by physicians to assess whether a person is eligible for weight, age, or height. The combination of average and weight is between 25 and 29.9, and BMI indicates that the person is overweight. More than 30 BMIs indicate that a person may be suffering from obesity.

Eating too much can increase weight and cause obesity. People who use a diet that primarily consists of whole grains, water, fruit, and vegetables, are also at risk of being overweight.

However, while maintaining a healthy weight, people are exposed to more diverse diets. Fresh foods and beans contain fiber, which can make people feel better and helps promote healthy digestion (Saini et al., 2018).

Coronary Artery Disease (CAD)

If coronary artery disease is too limited, cardiovascular disease (CHD) or coronary artery disease will progress. Coronary arteries are blood vessels that carry oxygen and blood to the heart.

CHD produces cholesterol in the arterial wall. These plaques cause arterial stenosis and reduce blood flow to the heart. Thrombosis can sometimes disrupt the bloodstream and cause serious health problems. CHD can cause angina. This is a type of chest pain associated with heart disease. Angina can cause the following feelings across the chest:

- Squeeze
- Pressure
- Weight
- Tightening
- Burn
- Painful (Yadav et al., 2018).

Treatment

There is no cure for CHD. However, there are ways in which one can manage the situation. Treatment includes changing your lifestyle, including quitting smoking, eating a healthy diet, and regular exercise.

However, there are people who need to receive medicine and treatment.

- Medicine: Doctor talks about medicine. There are various drugs for the treatment of cardiovascular disease.
- The following are the drugs that people can use to reduce the risk and impact of CHD:
- Beta-blockers: Physicians may prescribe beta-blockers to lower blood pressure &heart rate, especially for people who have had a previous heart attack. Sprays, Nitroglycerin Patches or pills: This increases arteries, increases blood pressure in the heart, and relieves chest pain.

Insulin

Insulin is a chemical messenger that allows cells to carry glucose and glucose from sources. The pancreas is the abdomen, and the main cause of insulin size in pancreatic cells called hormone components is the physical formation of blood glucose (Duke Univ. Medical Center, 2019).

When this happens, blood sugar stays in the blood and cells can't absorb it and can not convert it into energy. The problem with insulin: The immune system attacks the islets and some people do not produce insulin.

This is the introduction of T1D, and people with this type of diabetes need regular insulin to survive. In some people, especially overweight, obese or inactive people, insulin is not effective at transmitting glucose and can't enhance its effectiveness. Insulin inhibition affects tissues.

Type 2 diabetes occurs when insulin islets do not show insulin resistance. Because insulin is isolated in the early 20th century and cannot be manufactured alone or as an insulin supplement, insulin cannot withstand it.

Hypertension (HTN)

Hypertension (HBP) is a long-term medical condition in which blood pressure in the veins rises.

- Complications: Coronary artery disease, stroke.
- Other names: arterial hypertension, high blood pressure.
- Diagnostic method: resting blood pressure.
- Treatment: lifestyle change, addiction.

Prevention

Type 1 diabetes can't be stopped. However, choosing a healthy lifestyle to prevent diabetes, type 2 diabetes, and gestational diabetes can also prevent it.

- Eat Healthy Foods: Choose low-calorie and low-calorie foods and increase fiber. Focus on fruits, vegetables and whole grains. I am trying to avoid fatigue.
- More physical activity: The goal of average physical activity is 30 minutes in the day. If you are riding a bike, then extend your session to smaller sessions throughout the day if you are not focusing on long practice.
- Losing extra weight Lose weight 200 pounds (90.7 kg) and 7% of body weight (for example, 14 pounds (6.4 pounds) loses. You can reduce the risk of diabetes.

- However, do not try to lose weight during pregnancy. Talk about increasing weight during pregnancy. To keep your weight healthy, focus on continuous change in your diet and exercise habits. Inspire yourself by remembering the benefits of losing weight such as healthy mind, more energy and more confidence.
- Sometimes medication is also an option. Oral diabetes drugs such as metformin (eg, glucophage, glutasezza) may reduce the risk of type 2 diabetes, but you need to choose a healthy lifestyle. Check your blood glucose levels at least once a year to ensure that you do not develop type 2 diabetes (Aggarwal et al., 2018; Singh et al., 2018).

LITERATURE REVIEW

According to researchers, Sugar intake may increase in an hour at night from being monitored over a digital device such as a smart phone or a tablet (Singhal et al., 2019). The research teams at the University of Strasbourg and the University of Amsterdam examined the effects of light blue (light emitted by the device) and its effect on blood sugar regulation. Artificial light is already High risk of developing type 2 diabetes other health conditions, but it is expected to occur because it disrupts the daily functioning of the body.

The researchers at the University of Strasbourg and the University of Amsterdam in their study found that, measuring the food intake and glucose tolerance the following day, by be exposing male rats to water-blue light for one hour at night. The mice specimen used in this experimental study were monitored daily, meaning that they were awake during the day and slept at night

As a result, the following day, the animals were given the choice of a balanced diet (rodent food), water, pork and water. The researchers have found that blue light is an hour even enough to eat more sugar at night. Because the retina is sensitive to the neglected light of the device and sends information to the part of the brain that controls appetite, researchers explained that this may have a relationship to the study. Their findings suggests that people who use digital devices such as smart phones, tablets and laptops at night are susceptible to sweet snacks.

Anayanci Masís-Vargas (Singh et al., 2019) reported that restricting the time spent in front of the screen at night has been the best way to protect yourself from the harmful effects of blue light, and the author suggests that touching the equipment at night, if necessary may be lead to other impacts. They used night time programs and device features that recommend orange and blue screens, or the use of commercially available clear blue filters. The findings were presented to the Respiratory Society in the Netherlands (SSIB). British studies have shown new findings for cancer patients which suggests that people with obesity, hypertension & CAD are more likely to smoke, than those who currently having two smoke in the United Kingdom. Charitable agencies and government organisations will use the findings to better understand and deal with obesity among young people (Chaturvedi et al., 2017).

According to researchers, about a third of adults in the United Kingdom are obese, Smoking is still the leading cause of cancer prevention in the country, and the risk of illness is more than obesity. Analysis of cancer research in the United Kingdom has shown that overweight and obesity are the main causes of four different types of cancer In the United Kingdom, more weight than smoking causes about 1,900 cases of colon cancer. The same pattern of anxiety is related to kidney cancer (1,400 times in a year in the UK), ovary (460) and liver (180).

This week's Cancer research in the UK was conducted to raise awareness about the link between obesity and cancer. Excessive fat cells in the body can cause further division, which can lead to damage and send signals over time, which can increase the risk of cancer. This campaign shows smoking and obesity that it helps people develop healthy habits rather than dealing with tobacco. Because of the decline in smoking rates and the rise in obesity, they clearly have threat that these children can't be our generations, but when the government establishes politics, and when it is in the sand, the nation's health is in crisis.

Mitchell (Chaturvedi et al., 2013) head of the UK said, cancer research I have a record that leads to "I found.

We need to get rid of childhood obesity, and now interfere with the elimination of the epidemic. They still have an opportunity to save lives. Scientists already recognize obesity as having 13 different types of cancer, but the mechanisms are not well understood. Therefore, the fact that excess fat can lead to cancer needs to be further examined. The charity is trying to reduce government ambition by 2030, halve childhood obesity and reduce climbers at 9 pm to create unwanted advertisements on television and the Internet. Restrict promotional offers for unhealthy and easy-to-drink food.

Linda Bald said, there is no specific drug to reduce CAD, hypertension & obesity, a UK cancer prevention expert, "but smoking has been sharply reduced year by year due to advertising and environmental bans. Because it is necessary to work on smoking with a high smoking rate, it is suitable for obesity now. Our world does not facilitate health, so we need government action to resolve it, but replace unwanted food for healthier choices or reduce the risk of cancer it's all that helps.

In the United Kingdom, there are approximately 13.4 million obese non-smokers (BMI 30+), 630,000 overweight smokers, and 1.5 million smokers and obese adults. Obesity is higher than the number of people who smoke 2: 1. In the United Kingdom, there are about 14.9 million obese adults, and about 29 percent of the adult population in the United Kingdom has cancer information.

The Cancer Research team combines the adult population estimated, (2017) (18+) from the National Bureau of Statistics with adult data from the occurrence of obesity in the 2017 Health Survey, (2017), Health Survey survey (16+) Estimate this estimate by: Wales National Survey, (2017) and Northern Ireland Health Assessment, (2017) Brown, Lamb gay, (2018) etc.: Percentage of cancers associated with dangerous risk factors in the United Kingdom, Wales, Scotland, Northern Ireland and the UK, (2015) (25 BMI of over 30 + body and overweight defined as fat)

Health studies show two years of new data from Duke to reduce the risk of fatal diseases such as diabetes and heart disease, and recovery is always seen. The random findings of adults who are currently gaining weight with healthy weight or consuming only about at 300 calories a day (Saxena et al., 2018), the level of markers such as good cholesterol, blood pressure, glucose etc. will be greatly improved. Adults under the age of 50 were on the 11th July list of Lennesty's diabetes and endocrinology.

The test, which is part of a continuing project with the National Institute of Health called CALERIE, highlights the hypothesis of the researchers. It is a mere weight loss leading to this improvement, but it is part of a complex metabolic change. Eat fewer calories than consumed calories.

William E. Crouss, (2014) author of this study, said, "He is Duke's cardiologist and medical professor." We collect blood, muscles, and other specimens from these participants, and we keep saying that this metabolic signal or magic molecule may be. There is something about calorie restriction; some of the mechanisms we do not yet understand show the results of these improvements. According to him, during the in the first month of study, participants ate three meals a day and reduced their daily calorie intake to help train their new diet.

Kloes said. "People can do this fairly comfortably by reducing their volume so that they will see little advice from anywhere, or perhaps to drink after dinner." This is what we used in this study It has been suggested that as many changes as can be made in this country, the burden of diabetes and heart disease can be reduced. "Various food programs, including cultural environment and other requirements, participants participated in the group and personal counseling session for the first six months of study. In addition, members of Control Group continued their regular diet and every six months the researchers visited.

They got results, Participants were asked to maintain their calorie intake for more than 25 years. Their ability is diverse, and the average calorie deficiency for all participants is around 12%. However, they were able to lose 10% of the weight, 71% of which were fat. There are many advances in markers that measure the risk of developing metabolic disorders. There are many advances in markers that measure the risk of developing metabolic disorders. Two years later, participants also showed a decrease in biomarker which shows the old swelling. It is also associated with heart disease, cancer and cognitive decline.

Kraus said. "People can easily ease their little discretion here and there, or perhaps reduce their quantity, like snacking after dinner". Can reduce the burden of diabetes and heart disease, which we have in this country ". This study was conducted by the National Institute for Aging, Institute of Gastrointestinal Allergy (NIH Assistance U01AG022132, U01AG020478, U01AG020487, and U01AG020480) and the NIH Comprehensive Clinical Research Center. (Saxena et al., 2018)

RESEARCH METHODOLOGY

Our Experimental Results, Interpretation, and Discussion

Experimental Setup

The Subjects chosen under investigation were suffering from Diabetes as informed by their Health Insurance Providers without disclosing any Personal Information (PI) or Sensitive Personal Information (SPI) by Law. To identify each case uniquely, sample ids like S1, S2 etc. has been allotted to the subjects. We have collected this big data and studied the people; we have studied their tension level and helped them to cure it. In this chapter, we did our best to analyses the Diabetes with CAD and other Diseases. Sample Data from lab tests and medical reports has been collected for the following characteristics:

- Gender
- Age
- Diabetes Type
- Subject on Insulin
- Subject having Obesity
- Subject having CAD
- Subject having HTN
- Subject suffering from TTH / Migraine.

Our area of interest is on TTH/ Migraine parameter. The study focuses on finding the role of diabetes in causing TTH and what are the peculiar probabilities/ pattern which do/can lead subject to TTH.

We are interested to check the pattern and behavior of data trend of subjects suffering with CAD (Coronary Artery Disease).To find the pattern and relationship on different parameters; we first, analyzed the collected sample data. The Tableau software was used for the analysis.

About the Study and Analysis

In the present Analysis, we have collected the possible sample of thirty random Indian subjects and they were deeply scrutinized under various medical parameters. These subjects were suffering from diabetes and their various other symptoms were recorded. It was checked whether there is possibility of other diseases with diabetes. Patients with Diabetes Type-I and II were investigated and those who were and who were not consuming Insulin also participated in study.

The results show the correlation of different other diseases like obesity, hypertension, CAD etc. with TTH and its direct prediction of happening these issues in future course of life. The Age and gender parameters were also taken care of and detained analysis was executed in reflection to it.

RESULTS AND DISCUSSION

The overall age group with number of subject having TTH and CAD or not is plotted in below grouped stacked column chart. It can be observed that very few cases are observed for TTH for the males below 60 but the number increased dramatically as age goes beyond 60. This signifies old age men are having highest probability among all segregation having TTH and CAD. It also shows a direct correlation of TTH and CAD as per increasing age group. (shown in Figure 3)

Figure 2. TTH-CAD distribution among subjects as per age groups

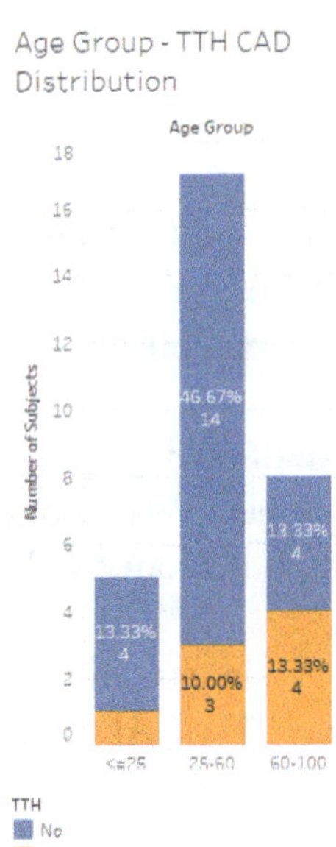

Figure 3. TTH-CAD distribution among subjects as per gender groups

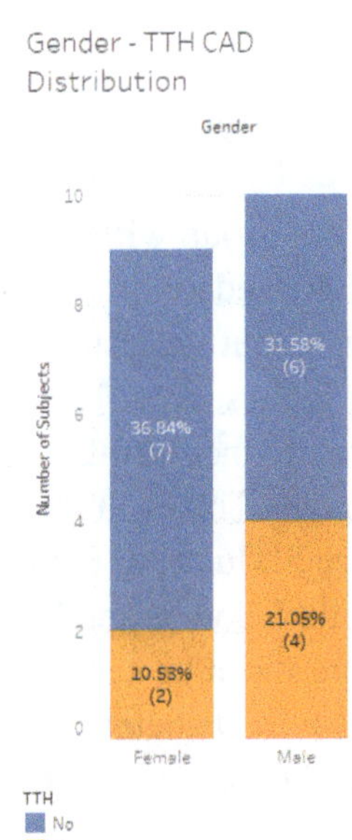

In the collected sample, total 31.58% subjects are reported of having TTH and CAD. This number becomes significant as it is saying that out 4 diabetic patients 1 is suffering from TTH-CAD. Diabetic patients are generally reported of having TTH due to stress and mental demotivation caused due to problems like Diabetes.

On analyzing this ratio distribution within the gender, it has been found that males are more prone to TTH and consequently to CAD than as compared to females. Around 10.9% more males are reported having TTH than females. On detailed look into the data and subjected to discussion it has been found that sampled males are working at office environment while females are less working so there is possibility of work stress which is causing more frequent headache (shown in Figure 4)

Figure 4. TTH-CAD distribution among subjects as per age groups in terms of presence of CAD in different genders

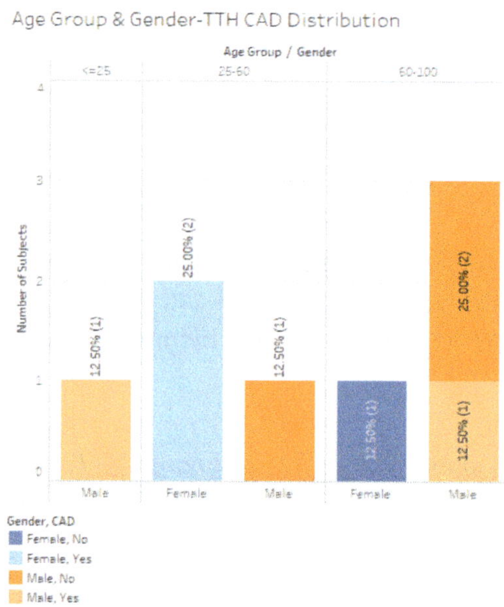

The overall age group with gender and number of subject having TTH and CAD or not is plotted in below grouped stacked column chart. It can be observed that very few cases are observed for TTH for the males below 60 but the number increased dramatically as age goes beyond 60. This signifies old age men are having highest probability among all segregation having TTH.

Also, for females increasing trends of TTH can be observed up to age of 60 beyond that case of TTH and CAD decreases. This is in line with the overall pattern of diabetic subject variation with age group. (shown in Figure 5). In order to visualize this pattern keenly, above graph is plotted only for TTH with CAD subjects and below graph is obtained:

In conclusion, it can be said that TTH-CAD cases increasing with age in case of males and not following the pattern of Diabetes variation with age while in case of female TTH-CAD pattern variation is same as diabetes i.e., increasing trend up to age of 60 then decreasing. (shown in Figure 6)

Figure 5. TTH-CAD distribution among subjects as per age groups in terms of presence of CAD

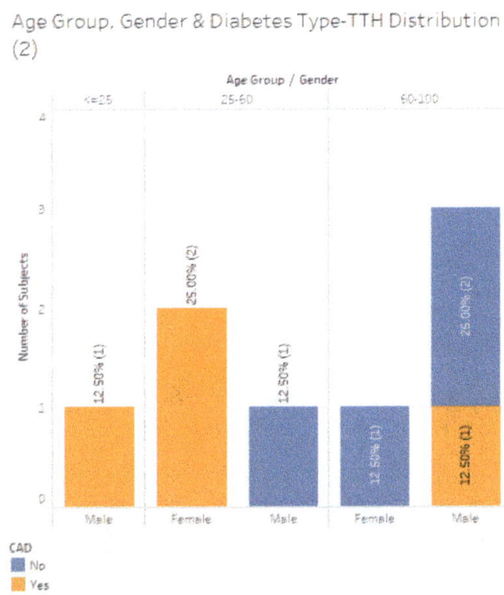

Table 1. The summary data for the diseases TTH & CAD as per type 1 & 2 diabetes

Diabetes Type	TTH	% of Total Number of Subjects	% of Total Number of Subjects within each diabetic type	Number of Subjects
Type- I	Yes	12.5%	100%	1
Type- I	No	0%	0%	0
Type- II	Yes	37.5	42.85%	3
Type- II	No	50%	57.15%	4

(shown in Figure 7)In order to gain more in-sight and to know the role of diabetic type in causing the TTH-CAD, a stacked bar relationship of diabetes type and TTH is plotted and it has been observed that Type-I diabetic is almost no contribution in TTH and CAD. In other words subject suffering from Type-I is reported very less about TTH and CAD too. It can be justified as Type-I subjects are of younger age groups so they are able to cope up with tense situation or it might be the case they do not have such a significant level of tension with coronary disease that can cause the TTH and CAD(As per Table 1). But the number increases significantly for type-II diabetes patient. The summary data of various are as:

TTH Cannot Be

In surge of finding the different co-existence of illness causing TTH or not, it has been seen the person who is on insulin and having Coronary Arteriosclerosis Disease (CAD)but No Hyper Blood Pressure (HTN) are safe from TTH. In the samples subjects are found to be of 25-60 age group from both the genders who falls under these parameters. In such combination male dominance can be easily seen. 2/3 of the population is male of this combination. (shown in Figure 8)

Figure 6. TTH-CAD distribution w.r.t. presence of diabetes type-I and II among subjects

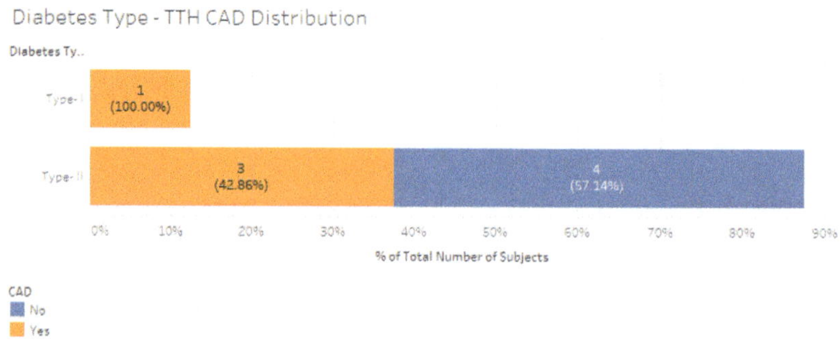

Figure 7. Correlation of diabetes with TTH and possibility of CAD, HTN, obesity etc. diseases with insulin Consumption

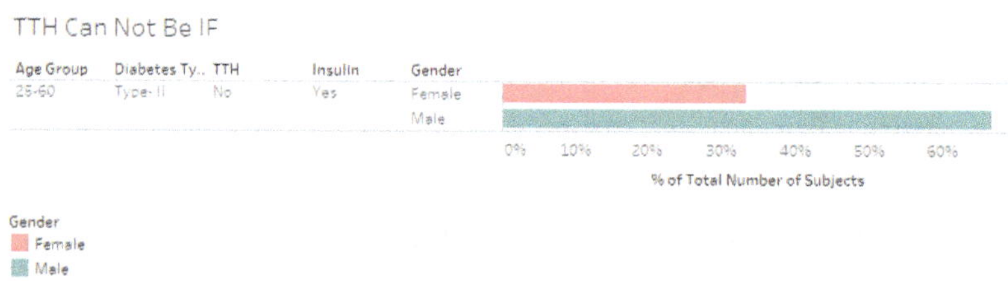

Such subjects are found to be sufferer of Type-II diabetes so they are insulin consumers. Subjects do not of issues related with digestion systems as they were reported to have no obesity problems. So, it can be concluded if patients are not having problems related with blood pressure then even of having CAD then also they cannot have TTH. This signifies that subjects if control on their hyper tensions and blood pressure then can save themselves from TTH even having cardiac illness. When drill down in detail in the data it has been found ratio of female has been less in such categories because problem of depression is not reported in females. While male patients are equally distributed among between depression and not depression. So we can say such category subjects are equally divided in three groups: female, Male having depression and Male not having depression. In the sample collected it has been seen female are having negligible depression that can be one of the major reason of overall TTH is lesser in female as compare to males.

Figure 8. Summary chart of analytical data for correlation of diabetes with TTH and possibility of CAD, HTN, obesity etc. diseases with insulin consumption

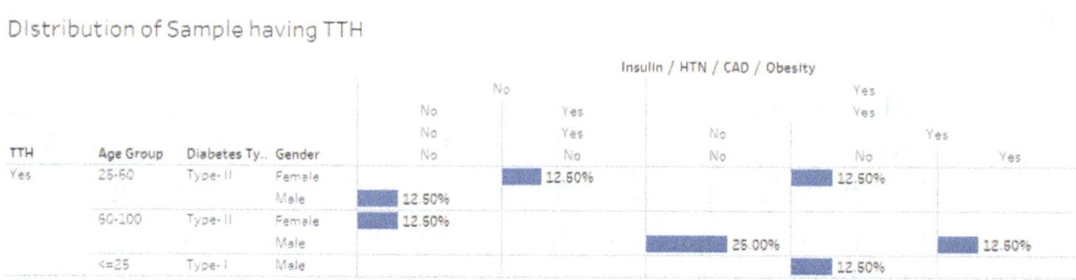

When analyzing the sample having TTH, an interesting result can be seen that the ratio of old age male having TTH is maximum that can be easily seen in Age group gender distribution study but this graph shows they are insulin consumer and they are having hyper blood pressure. So, it can be concluded clearly that if old age male is having hypertension and sufferer of type-II diabetes then he must be having TTH. On deeper look it shows that there is 1:3 ratio is further found for such males having CAD and not having CAD and same ratio is found for obesity as well. (shown in Figure 9)

Overall if TTH subjects are generally having HTN. 6 out of 8 Subjects which are reported of having TTH are having HTN as well i.e. 75% of the TTH subjects. These numbers clearly signifies HTN has a relation with the TTH. If a subject is having Diabetes and HTN then one day or the other there are very high chances of occurring TTH as well and probability further gets increased if subject is male.

NOVELTY IN THE PRESENTED WORK

The Internet can communicate, interact and identify anytime, anywhere to make life more difficult and easy. This is one of the existing trends and innovations in recent technological advances.

IoT-based solutions are experiencing explosive growth in a variety of areas, including healthcare systems, using cloud computing, connectivity, and large amounts of data. In the healthcare sector, for example, IoT monitors IoT functionality for stunning and sustained heart rate monitors (HR), recording HR data from Pulse-Glasses embedded in Android smart phones seamlessly stored in the cloud.

Mass data analysis in healthcare: Today, there are a large number of disparate resources such as social networks, the Internet, and healthcare systems. The use of several technology trends, such as the expansion of smart devices, is the Internet. Of things and the spread of cloud computing. In general, healthcare systems provide specialized data that is difficult to store, process, and interpret . These data are structured, semi-structured and Unstructured (Rachel et al., 2018), it is impossible to manage it with traditional database management. As a result, the use of large amounts of data in health systems is highly required. Good data can be used to improve medical quality with past medical data, and can now improve medical quality (Plant et al., 2016). There are many machine learning techniques used to analyze sensor data in health systems. These technologies help improve the work of healthcare workers, monitor healthcare and make the system more accurate. The aim of our research is to prevent and treat diabetes and improve the lives of all people with diabetes. By improving the classification method.

Given the availability of the above information, more attention is being paid to the healthcare industry and more research is being done to target data to improve healthcare. Health data is becoming increasingly complex with medical staff, medical records, medical records, clinical records, medical imaging, cyber physical systems, medical internet related issues, genetic data and systems. Significant increase in support clinical and clinical decisions.

New types of data from sources such as social networking services and genomic data are used to build personalized personal care systems. Therefore, different types of health data from different sources, fields, and technologies, the nature of their disorder is a proper analysis. All analytical research needs to overcome these obstacles to mining data and generate meaningful insights to save lives.(Felman et al., 2018; Min et al., 2018)

FUTURE RESEARCH DIRECTIONS ALONG WITH POSSIBLE LIMITATIONS

We have found from our sample analysis our sample is not susceptible to sex. It can be used to analyze large sample samples in the future. We can easily find changes in TTH with changes in other diseases in a subject separate from the diseases mentioned, such as obesity, cancer and heart attack, etc (Yadav, V. et al., 2018). Using Tableau S / W for large collections. This type of TTH and both types of diabetes depend on a variety of factors such as age, gender, type of diabetes, insulin issue, obesity, subject to CAN and subject from TTH / migraine, etc. (Cancer research, U.K., 2019; Vyas et al., 2018; Tsai et al., 2013).

Because the sample size is smaller than the conclusion, it should study larger samples for patients with type 1 diabetes living in different areas. With the help of technology, it is necessary to create a system for the creation and analysis of large-scale diabetes data and to predict the potential risks based on it. Predictive analysis is a process that incorporates various data mining techniques, machine learning algorithms, and statistics that integrate current and historical data sets to gain insights and predict future risks.

Do not miss symptoms that may be due to low or high blood sugar, hypoglycemia or lack of knowledge about dehydration. When checking your blood sugar level, make sure that your blood sugar level is set to glucose if your symptoms do not match your reading system or if you suspect that your reading is incorrect. This study is not intended for pregnant women, dialysis patients, or cancer patients.

SOLUTIONS AND RECOMMENDATION

The researchers sought to include information such as age, gender, insulin factors, and relationships with diabetic patients. Issues for diabetes required further details under this title to provide health insurers further disclosure about personal information (PI) or sensitive personal information (SPI) which are subject to the framework for legal health legislations. Finally, TTH-CAD cases can vary with age in men, and the lack of patterns of diabetes changes with age, but noting sharp distinction for changes in TTH-CAD patterns in women are similar to diabetes, i.e. the rate of increase to 60 years of age and subsequent decline rates in specific gender patterns were notably reported. This data has highlighted the need for the researchers to focus on such issues based on gender differentiations that can unravel important and unique information on how diabetes can impact different people based on gender. Hence in our study we draw attention to such issues to investigate deeper on data based on different gender patterns.

It can be observed that very few cases are observed for TTH for the males below 60 but the number get increased dramatically as age goes beyond 60. This signifies old age men are having highest probability among all segregation having TTH and CAD. It also shows a direct correlation of TTH and CAD as per increasing age group.

The overall age group with gender and number of subject having TTH and CAD or not is plotted in the grouped stacked columnar chart. It can be observed that very few cases are observed for TTH for the males below 60 but the number get increased dramatically as age goes beyond 60. This signifies old age men are having highest probability among all segregation having TTH (Gulati et al., 2018).

Also, for females increasing trends of TTH can be observed up to age of 60 beyond that case of TTH and CAD decreases. This is in line with the overall pattern of diabetic subject variation with age group. It can be justified as Type-I subjects are of younger age groups so they are able to cope up with tense situation or it might be the case they do not have such significant level of tension with coronary disease that can cause the TTH and CAD. But the number increases significantly for type-II diabetes patient.

In the samples subjects are found to be of 25-60 age groups from both genders who falls under these parameters. In such combination male dominance can be easily seen. 2/3 of the population is male of this combination. When analyzing the sample having TTH, an interesting result can be seen that the ratio of old age male having TTH is maximum that can be easily seen in Age group gender distribution study but this graph shows they are insulin consumer and they are having hyper blood pressure. So, it can be concluded clearly that if old age male is having hypertension and sufferer of type-II diabetes then he must be having TTH. On deeper look it shows that there is 1:3 ratio is further found for such males having CAD and not having CAD and same ratio is found for obesity as well.

Design goals include comprehensive health analysis of the entire patient ecosystem. Not only can this system provide careful and timely care, a diagnostic recommendation that works for the same thing, it can also predict possible medical illnesses.

CONCLUSION

In the present Analysis, we have collected the possible sample of thirty random Indian subjects and they were deeply scrutinized under various medical parameters. These subjects were suffering from diabetes and their various other symptoms were recorded. It was checked whether there is possibility of other diseases with diabetes. Patients with Diabetes Type-I and II were investigated and those who were and who were not consuming Insulin also participated in study. The results shows the correlation of different other diseases like obesity, hypertension, CAD etc. with TTH and its direct prediction of happening these issues in future course of life. The Age and gender parameters were also taken care of and detained analysis was executed in reflection to it. In the collected sample, total 31.58% subjects are reported of having TTH and CAD (Yadav et al., 2018). This number becomes significant as it is saying that out 4 diabetic patient 1 is suffering from TTH-CAD (Mcafee et al., 2012) and (Abdelhamid et al. 2014; Brazier et al., 2018). Diabetic patients are generally reported of having TTH due to stress and mental demotivation caused due to problems like Diabetes (Cancer Research U.K., 2019; Rastogi et al., 2918).

On analyzing this ratio distribution within the gender, it has been found that males are more prone to TTH and consequently to CAD than as compare to females. Around 10.9% more males are reported having TTH than females. On detailed look into the data and subjected to discussion it has been found that sampled males are working at office environment while females are less working so there is possibility of work stress which is causing more frequent headache.

In conclusion, it can be said that TTH-CAD cases increasing with age in case of males and not following the pattern of Diabetes variation with age while in case of female TTH-CAD pattern variation is same as diabetes i.e increasing trend up to age of 60 then decreasing.

In order to gain more in-sight and to know the role of diabetic type in causing the TTH-CAD, a stacked bar relationship of diabetes type and TTH is plotted and it has been observed that Type-I diabetic is almost no contribution in TTH and CAD. In other words subject suffering from Type-I is reported very less about TTH and CAD too. In surge of finding the different co-existence of illness causing TTH or not, it has been seen the person who is on insulin and having Coronary Arteriosclerosis Disease (CAD) but No Hyper Blood Pressure (HTN) are safe from TTH. (Saxena et al., 2018; Chaturvedi et al., 2012)

Overall if TTH subjects are generally having HTN. 6 out of 8 Subjects which are reported of having TTH are having HTN as well i.e. 75% of the TTH subjects. These numbers clearly signifies HTN has a relation with the TTH. If a subject is having Diabetes and HTN then one day or the other there are very high chances of occurring TTH as well and probability further gets increased if subject is male.

This research provides updates on new Machine learning algorithms, optimization algorithms, and intelli gent health applications. Discuss important issues such as privacy, pre-surveys, real projects, and links between data analysis and healthcare staff. These issues are essential for healthcare development, otherwise it is difficult to release machine learning algorithms and optimize in actual operation.

As a result, humans are expected to increasingly receive healthcare plans in the coming decades. To protect future patient health and access to future health services, it is necessary to ensure that health services are economically sustainable and sustainable. (Singhal et al., 2019)

Evidence was found for accelerating research efforts aimed at developing artificial intelligence tools to prevent and prevent complications associated with diabetes. Our findings suggest that artificial intelligence technology is constantly being established as being suitable for use in clinical practice as well as diabetes management itself. As a result, these methods are powerful tools for improving the quality of life of patients.

ACKNOWLEDGMENT

We would like to thanks seniors of ABES Engineering College, Ghaziabad, Dayalbagh Educational Institute, Agra and experts from Tata Consultancy Services for their extraordinary support in this research process. The Infrastructure and research samples by different labs have been collected. We pay our sincere thanks to all direct and indirect supporters.

REFERENCES

Abdelhmid Salih, M. S., & Abraham, A. (2014). *Novel Ensemble Decision Support and Healthcare Monitoring System. International Journal of Computer Information Systems and Industrial Management Applications.*

Agrawal, A., Rastogi, R., Chaturvedi, D. K., Sharma, S., & Bansal, A. (2018). Audio Visual EMG & GSR Biofeedbac Analysis for Effect of Spiritual Techniques on Human Behavior and Psychic Challenges. *Proceedings of the 12th INDIACom,* 252-258.

American Diabetes Association. (2011). Standards of medical care in diabetes. *Diabetes Care, 34*(S11) 61. . doi:10.2337/dc11-S011

American Diabetes Association. (2018). *Dietary supplements.* https://www.diabetes.org/living-with-diabetes/treatment-and-care/medication/other-treatments/herbs-supplements-and-alternative-medicines/talking-to-your-health-care-provider.html

Brazier, Y. (2018). What is obesity and what causes it? *Medical News Today.* https://www.medicalnewstoday.com/articles/323551.php

Cancer Research UK. (2019). Obese people outnumber smokers two to one. *Science Daily.* www.sciencedaily.com/releases/2019/07/190702211335.htm

Chaturvedi, D. K. (2012). Human Rights and Consciousness. *International Seminar on Prominence of Human Rights in the Criminal Justice System (ISPUR 2012), Proceedings of Organized Ambedkar Chair, Dept. of Contemporary Social Studies & Law, Dr. B.R. Ambedkar University, Agra,* 33.

Chauhan, S., Rastogi, R., Chaturvedi, D. K., Arora, N., & Trivedi, P. (2017). Framework for Use of Machine Intelligence on Clinical Psychology to study the effects of Spiritual tools on Human Behavior and Psychic Challenges. *Proceedings of NSC-2017(National system conference).*

Cunningham, F. G. (2014). *Diabetes mellitus* (24th ed.). New York, NY: The McGraw-Hill Companies. http://accessmedicine.mhmedical.com

Duke University Medical Center. (2019). Even in svelte adults, cutting about 300 calories daily protects the heart. Researchers seeking a signal in metabolism or a 'magic molecule' to explain this. *Science Daily.* www.sciencedaily.com/releases/2019/07/190711183758.htm

Felman, A. (2018). An overview of insulin. *Medical News Today.* https://www.medicalnewstoday.com/articles/323760.php

Gabbe, S. G. (2018). Diabetes mellitus complicating normal pregnancy. In *Obstetrics: Normal and Problem Pregnancy* (7th ed.). Saunders Elsevier. https://www.clinicalkey.com

Gulati, M., Rastogi, R., Chaturvedi, D. K., Satya, S., Arora, N., & Singhal, P. (2018). Statistical Resultant Analysis of Spiritual & Psychosomatic Stress Survey on Various Human Personality Indicators. *The International Conference proceedings of ICCI 2018.*

Gulati, M., Rastogi, R., Chaturvedi, D. K., Sharma, P., Yadav, V., Chauhan, S., . . . Singhal, P. (2019). Statistical Resultant Analysis of Psychosomatic Survey on Various Human Personality Indicators: Statistical Survey to Map Stress and Mental Health. In *Handbook of Research on Learning in the Age of Transhumanism* (pp. 363-383). Hershey, PA: IGI Global. doi:10.4018/978-1-5225-8431-5.ch022

Gupta, M., Rastogi, R., Chaturvedi, D. K., Satya, S. A., Verma, H., Singhal, P., & Singh, A. (2019). Comparative Study of Trends Observed During Different Medications by Subjects under EMG & GSR Biofeedback. *IJITEE, 8*(6S), 748-756. https://www.ijitee.org/download/volume-8-issue-6S/

Kasper, D. L. (2015). Diabetes mellitus: Diagnosis, classification and pathophysiology. In *Harrison's Principles of Internal Medicine* (19th ed.). New York, NY: McGraw-Hill Education. http://accessmedicine.mhmedical.com

Kuo, T., Sahama, A. W., Kushniruk, E., Borycki, M., & Grunwell, D. K. (2014). Health big data analytics: Current perspectives, challenges and potential solutions. *Int. J. Big Data Intell., 1*(2), 114–126.www.techrepublic.com/article/understanding-the-differences-between-ai-machine-learning-and-deep-learning

Marrie, R.A., Patel, R., Figley, C.R., Kornelsen, J., Bolton, J.M., Graff, L., … Fisk, J.D. (2019). Diabetes and anxiety adversely affect cognition in multiple sclerosis. *Multiple Sclerosis and Related Disorder Satellites, 27*(1), 164-170.

Martin, R., Ira Ktena, S. & Pawlowski, N. (2018). An Introduction to Biomedical Image Analysis with Tensor Flow and DLT. *Imperial College London, 29*(1), 82-85.

Masís Vargas, A. (2019). *Society for the Study of Ingestive Behavior. Blue light at night increases the consumption of sweets in rats. Science Daily.*

Masís Vargas, A. (2019). *One hour of device screen time at night could lead to increased sugar consumption*. Society for the Study of Ingestive Behavior (SSIB).

McAfee, A., Brynjolfsson, E., Davenport, T.H., Patil, D.J., & Barton, D. (2012). Big data: the management revolution. *Harvard Bus Rev, 90*(1), 60-68.

Minn, R., & Morrow, E. S. (2018). Natural medicines in the clinical management of diabetes. *Natural Medicines.* https://naturalmedicines.therapeuticresearch.com

Murdoch, T. B., & Detsky, A. S. (2013). The inevitable application of big data to healthcare. *Journal of the American Medical Association, 309*(13), 1351–1352. doi:10.1001/jama.2013.393 PMID:23549579

Nall, R. (2018). An overview of diabetes types and treatments. *Medical News Today.* https://www.medicalnewstoday.com/articles/323627.php

Nordqvist, C. (2019). What to know about coronary heart disease. *Medical News Today*. https://www.medicalnewstoday.com/articles/184130.php

Panch, T., Szolovits, P., & Atun, R. (2018, December). Artificial intelligence, machine learning and health systems. *Journal of Global Health, 8*(2), 020303. doi:10.7189/jogh.08.020303 PMID:30405904

Plant, L., Noriega, B., Sonti, A., Constant, N., & Mankodiya, K. (2016). Smart E-textile gloves for quantified measurements in movement disorders. *Proceedings of the IEEE MIT Undergraduate Research Technology Conference (URTC)*, 1–4. 10.1109/URTC.2016.8284077

Rastogi, R., Chaturvedi, D. K., Arora, N., Trivedi, P., & Mishra, V. (2017). Swarm Intelligent Optimized Method of Development of Noble Life in the perspective of Indian Scientific Philosophy and Psychology. *Proceedings of NSC-2017(National system conference).*

Rastogi, R., Chaturvedi, D. K., Satya, S., Arora, N., Yadav, V., Chauhan, S., & Sharma, P. (2018). SF-36 Scores Analysis for EMG and GSR Therapy on Audio, Visual and Audio Visual Modes for Chronic TTH. In Proceedings of the ICCIDA-2018. Springer.

Saini, H., Rastogi, R., Chaturvedi, D. K., Satya, S., Arora, N., Verma, H., & Mehlyan, K. (2018). Comparative Efficacy Analysis of Electromyography and Galvanic Skin Resistance Biofeedback on Audio Mode for Chronic TTH on Various Indicators. In *Proceedings of ICCIIoT- 2018*. Elsevier.

Saini, H., Rastogi, R., Chaturvedi, D. K., Satya, S. N., Gupta, M., & Verma, H. (2019). An Optimized Biofeedback EMG and GSR Biofeedback Therapy for Chronic TTH on SF-36 Scores of Different MMBD Modes on Various Medical Symptoms. In Hybrid Machine Intelligence for Medical Image Analysis, Studies Comp. Intelligence. Springer Nature Singapore, Pte Ltd. doi:10.1007/978-981-13-8930-6_8

Saxena, M., Sharma, M., Sain, M.K., Bohra, G., & Sinha, R. (2018). Yagya reduced level of indoor Electro-Magnetic Radiations (EMR). *Interdisciplinary Journal of Yagya Research, 1*(2), 231-239.

Saxena, M., Kumar, B., & Matharu, S. (2018). Impact of Yagya on Particulate Matters. *Interdisciplinary Journal of Yagya Research, 1*(1), 1-8.

Saxena, M., Sengupta, B. & Pandya, P. (2008). Controlling the Microflora in Outdoor Environment: Effect of Yagya. *Indian Journal of Air Pollution Control, 8*(2), 30 – 36.

Sharma, A., Rastogi, R., Chaturvedi, D. K., Satya, S., Arora, N., Trivedi, P., ... Singh, A. (2019). *Intelligent Analysis for Personality Detection on Various Indicators by Clinical Reliable Psychological TTH and Stress Surveys. In Proceedings of CIPR 2019 at Indian Institute of Engineering Science and Technology*. Springer-AISC Series.

Sharma, P., Rastogi, R., Chaturvedi, D. K., Satya, S., Arora, N., Yadav, V., & Chauhan, S. (2018). *Analytical Comparison of Efficacy for Electromyography and Galvanic Skin Resistance Biofeedback on Audio-Visual Mode for Chronic TTH on Various Attributes. In Proceedings of the ICCIDA-2018. Springer.*

Singh, A., Rastogi, R., Chaturvedi, D. K., Satya, S., Arora, N., Sharma, A., & Singh, A. (2019). Intelligent Personality Analysis on Indicators in IoT-MMBD Enabled Environment. In *Multimedia Big Data Computing for IoT Applications: Concepts, Paradigms, and Solutions.* Springer. doi:10.1007/978-981-13-8759-3_7

Singh, P., Rastogi, R., Chaturvedi, D. K., Arora, N., Trivedi, P., & Vyas, P. (2018). Study on Efficacy of Electromyography and Electroencephalography Biofeedback with Mindful Meditation on Mental health of Youths. *Proceedings of the 12th INDIACom,* 84-89.

Singh, V., Rastogi, R., Chaturvedi, D. K., Satya, S., Arora, N., Sirohi, H., . . . Verma, P. (2018). Which One is Best: Electromyography Biofeedback Efficacy Analysis on Audio, Visual and Audio- Visual Modes for Chronic TTH on Different Characteristics. In *Proceedings of ICCIIoT-2018.* Elsevier.

Singhal, P., Rastogi, R., Chaturvedi, D. K., Satya, S., Arora, N., Gupta, M., . . . Gulati, M. (2019). Statistical Analysis of Exponential and Polynomial Models of EMG & GSR Biofeedback for Correlation between Subjects Medications Movement & Medication Scores. *IJITEE, 8*(6S), 625-635. https://www.ijitee.org/download/volume-8-issue-6S/

Tenhunen, H. (2015). Smart e-health gateway: bringing intelligence to Internet-of-Things-based ubiquitous healthcare systems. In *Proceedings of the Annual IEEE Consumer Communications and Networking Conference*. IEEE.

Tsai, H. C., Cohly, H., & Chaturvedi, D. K. (2013). Towards the Consciousness of the Mind, Towards a Science of Consciousness. *Dayalbagh Conference Proceeding, 1*(1), 20-29.

Vyas, P., Rastogi, R., Chaturvedi, D. K., Satya, S., Arora, N., & Singh, P. (2018). Statistical Analysis for Effect of Positive Thinking on Stress Management and Creative Problem Solving for Adolescents. *Proceedings of the 12th INDIACom*, 245-251.

Yadav, V., Rastogi, R., Chaturvedi, D. K., Satya, S., Arora, N., & Bansal, I. (2018). Intelligent Analysis for Detection of Complex Human Personality by Clinical Reliable Psychological Surveys on Various Indicators. *The national Conference on 3rd MDNCPDR-2018 at DEI.*

Yadav, V., Rastogi, R., Chaturvedi, D. K., Satya, S., Arora, N., Gupta, M., . . . Sharma, P. (2019). Chronic TTH Analysis by EMG & GSR Biofeedback on Various Modes and Various Medical Symptoms Using IoT. In Advances in ubiquitous sensing applications for healthcare. Book-Big Data Analytics for Intelligent Healthcare Management.

Yadav, V., Rastogi, R., Chaturvedi, D.K., Satya, S., Arora, N., Yadav, V., Sharma, P., & Chauhan, S. (2018). Statistical Analysis of EMG & GSR Biofeedback Efficacy on Different Modes for Chronic TTH on Various Indicators. *Int. J. Advanced Intelligence Paradigms, 13*(1), 251-275. Doi:10.1504/IJAIP.2019.10021825

Compilation of References

Abdelhmid Salih, M. S., & Abraham, A. (2014). *Novel Ensemble Decision Support and Healthcare Monitoring System. International Journal of Computer Information Systems and Industrial Management Applications.*

Adam, K., Snyder, J., Crooks, V. A., & Johnston, R. (2015). Tourism discourse and medical tourists' motivations to travel. *Tourism Review*, *70*(2), 85–96. doi:10.1108/TR-04-2014-0015

Adeyemi, O. A. (2017). *Organizational change and how it effects healthcare employees: A study on employee resistance to change in electronic medical record implementation* (Doctoral dissertation). Colorado Technical University. ProQuest Dissertations & Theses Global database. (10602795 D.M.)

ADHA. (2019). What is digital health? *Australian Digital Health Agency*. https://www.digitalhealth.gov.au/get-started-with-digital-health/what-is-digital-health

Agag, G. M., & El-Masry, A. A. (2017). Why do consumers trust online travel websites? Drivers and outcomes of consumers trust towards online travel websites. *Journal of Travel Research*, *56*(3), 347–36. doi:10.1177/0047287516643185

Agarwal, R., Guodong, G., DesRoches, C., & Jha, A. K. (2010). The Digital Transformation of Healthcare: Current Status and the Road Ahead. *Information Systems Research*, *21*(4), 796–809.

Agarwal, R., Gupta, A. K., & Kraut, R. (2008). The Interplay between Digital and Social Networks. *Information Systems Research*, *19*(3), 243–252.

Agarwal, R., Gao, G., Des Roches, C., & Jha, A. K. (2010). Research commentary—The digital transformation of healthcare: Current status and the road ahead. *Information Systems Research*, *21*(4), 796–809. doi:10.1287/isre.1100.0327

Agrawal, A., Rastogi, R., Chaturvedi, D. K., Sharma, S., & Bansal, A. (2018). Audio Visual EMG & GSR Biofeedbac Analysis for Effect of Spiritual Techniques on Human Behavior and Psychic Challenges. *Proceedings of the 12th INDIACom,* 252-258.

Aguilera, A. (2015). Digital Technology and Mental Health Interventions: Opportunities and Challenges. *Arbor*, *191*(771), a210. doi:10.3989/arbor.2015.771n1012

Agut, S., Grau, R., & Peiró, J. M. (2003). Competency needs among managers from Spanish hotels and restaurants and their training demands. *International Journal of Hospitality Management*, *22*(3), 281–295. doi:10.1016/S0278-4319(03)00045-8

Alaimo, C., & Kallinikos, J. (2017). Computing the Everyday: Social Media as Data Platforms. *Information Society*, *33*(4), 175–191.

Allman, S. (2009). Leadership vs. Management. *Successful Meetings, 58*(11), 12.

Alnidawy, A. A. B. (2015). The Effect of Identifying Training Needs on the Effectiveness of the Training Process and Improving the Individual and Organizational Performance: Applied Study in the Jordanian Health Sector. *International Journal of Business Administration*, *6*(4), 48.

Amer, I. A. A. M. (2018). *Measurement of Quality of Life of Free Flap Transfer in Reconstrucion of the Head and Neck Tumor Defects after Ablative Surgery in Asturias, Spain Thesis* (Doctoral dissertation). Oviedo University.

American Diabetes Association. (2011). Standards of medical care in diabetes. *Diabetes Care, 34*(S11) 61. . doi:10.2337/dc11-S011

American Diabetes Association. (2018). *Dietary supplements*. https://www.diabetes.org/living-with-diabetes/treatment-and-care/medication/other-treatments/herbs-supplements-and-alternative-medicines/talking-to-your-health-care-provider.html

Anderson, C., & Robey, D. (2017). Affordance Potency: Explaining the Actualization of Technology Affordances. *Information and Organization*, *27*(2), 100–115.

Anderson, M., & Anderson, S. L. (2019). How Should AI Be Developed, Validated, and Implemented in Patient Care? *AMA Journal of Ethics*, *21*(2), E125–E130. doi:10.1001/amajethics.2019.125 PMID:30794121

Andrews, L., Gajanayake, R., & Sahama, T. (2014). The Australian general public's perceptions of having a personally controlled electronic health record. *International Journal of Medical Informatics*, *83*(12), 889–900. doi:10.1016/j.ijmedinf.2014.08.002 PMID:25200198

Angus, A., & Westbrook, G. (2018). Top 10 Global Consumer Trends for 2018. *Euromonitor International*, *61*, 29–76.

Anonymous. (2017). Physicians optimistic about digital health. *Physician Practice Perspectives*, *36*(1), 6–8.

Antheunis, M. L., Tates, K., & Nieboer, T. E. (2013). Patients' and health professionals' use of social media in healthcare: Motives, barriers and expectations. *Patient Education and Counseling*, *92*(3), 426–431. doi:10.1016/j.pec.2013.06.020 PMID:23899831

Antropova, N., Huynh, B. Q., & Giger, M. L. (2017). A deep feature fusion methodology for breast cancer diagnosis demonstrated on three imaging modality datasets. *Medical Physics*, *44*(10), 5162–5171. doi:10.1002/mp.12453 PMID:28681390

Arbab Kash, B., Spaulding, A., Johnson, C. E., & Gamm, L. (2014). Success factors for strategic change initiatives: A qualitative study of healthcare administrators' perspectives. *Journal of Healthcare Management*, *59*(1), 65–81. doi:10.1097/00115514-201401000-00011 PMID:24611428

Archer, N., Fevrier-Thomas, U., Lokker, C., McKibbon, K. A., & Straus, S. E. (2011). Personal Health records: A scoping review. *Journal of the American Medical Informatics Association*, *18*(4), 515–522. doi:10.1136/amiajnl-2011-000105 PMID:21672914

Atchison, T. A. (1999). Managing change. *Frontiers of Health Services Management*, *16*(1), 3–29. doi:10.1097/01974520-199907000-00002 PMID:10557432

Atienza, A. A., Zarcadoolas, C., Vaughon, W., Hughes, P., Patel, V., Chou, W.-Y., & Pritts, J. (2015). Consumer Attitudes and Perceptions on mHealth Privacy and Security: Findings from a Mixed-Methods Study. *Journal of Health Communication*, *20*(6), 673–679. doi:10.1080/10810730.2015.1018560 PMID:25868685

Australia's National Digital Health Strategy. (2019). https://conversation.digitalhealth.gov.au/sites/default/files/adha-strategy-doc-2ndaug_0_1.pdf

Australian Commission on Safety and Quality in Healthcare. (2010). *Australian Safety and Quality Framework for Healthcare*. Retrieved from https://www.safetyandquality.gov.au/publications-and-resources/resource-library/australian-safety-and-quality-framework-health-care

Australian Commission on Safety and Quality in Healthcare. (2011). *Patient centred care: Improving quality and safety through partnerships with patients and consumers*. Sydney: Author.

Australian Commission on Safety and Quality in Healthcare. (2011). *Patient-centred care: Improving quality and safety through partnerships with patients and consumers*. Retrieved from Sydney: https://www.safetyandquality.gov.au/wp-content/uploads/2012/03/PCC_Paper_August.pdf

Australian Digital Health Agency (ADHA). (2019). *MyHRC*. Available from https://www.myhealthrecord.gov.au/for-you-your-family/what-is-'MyHRC'

Australian Digital Health Agency. (2018a). *My health record opt-out period extended to 31 January 2019*. Available from https://www.myhealthrecord.gov.au/news-and-media/my-health-record-stories/opt-out-period-extended-january-2019

Australian Digital Health Agency. (2018b). *Annual Report 2017-2018*. Available from https://www.digitalhealth.gov.au/about-the-gency/publications/reports/annual-report/Annual_Report_Australian_Digital_Health_Agency_2017-2018_Online.pdf

Australian Government. (2013). *Australian Public Service Big Data Strategy*. Author.

Australian Government. (2016a). *Welcome to 'MyHRC'*. Available from https://myhealthrecord.gov.au/internet/mhr/publishing.nsf/content/home

Australian Government. (2016b). *'MyHRC's Rule 2016*. Available from https://www.legislation.gov.au/Details/F2016C00607

Australian Government. (2019a). *Health Portfolio Additional Estimates Statements 2018-19*. Department of Health. Available from https://www.health.gov.au/resources/publications/health-portfolio-budget-statements-2018-19

Australian Government. (2019b). *Impact of digital health on the safety and quality of healthcare*. Available from https://www.oaic.gov.au/privacy/other-legislation/my-health-record/

Australian Government. (2019c). *My Health Record Statistics*. Available from https://www.myhealthrecord.gov.au/sites/default/files/my_health_record_dashboard_-_28_july_2019.pdf?v=1565831963

Australian Health Minister's Conference. (2008). *National e-Health Strategy Summary*. Melbourne: Australian Government.

Australian Medical Association. (2016). *AMA Code of Ethics 2004. Revised 2016*. Author.

Aziz, L. (2007). *Managing change in healthcare information technology projects: the role of the project manager*. Project Management Institute.

Baker, C., Charlebois, M., Lopatka, H., Moineau, G., & Zelmer, J. (2016). Influencing Change: Preparing the Next Generation of Clinicians to Practice in the Digital Age. *Healthcare Quarterly*, *18*(4), 5–7. doi:10.12927/hcq.2016.24569 PMID:27009699

Baldwin, J. L., Singh, H., Sittig, D. F., & Giardina, T. D. (2017). Patient portals and health apps: Pitfalls, promises, and what one might learn from the other. *Health Care*, *5*(3), 81–85. PMID:27720139

Banerjee, S., Hemphill, T., & Longstreet, P. (2018). Wearable devices and healthcare: Data sharing and privacy. *The Information Society*, *34*(1), 49–57. doi:10.1080/01972243.2017.1391912

Bashshur, R. L., Reardon, T. G., & Shannon, G. W. (2000). Telemedicine: A new healthcare delivery system. *Annual Review of Public Health, 21*(1), 613–637. doi:10.1146/annurev.publhealth.21.1.613 PMID:10884967

Batrouni, M., Finch, S., Wilson, S., Bertaux, A., & Nicolle, C. (2018, October). Intelligent Cloud Storage Management for Layered Tiers. In *International Conference on Cooperative Design, Visualization and Engineering* (pp. 33-43). Springer. 10.1007/978-3-030-00560-3_5

Bauer, J. C. (2002). Rural America and the digital transformation of healthcare: new perspectives on the future...third annual Southern Illinois Healthcare/Southern Illinois University Health Policy Institute, Rural Healthcare: Current Issues and Future Directions, May 31 and June 1, 2001. *Journal of Legal Medicine, 23*(1), 73–83. doi:10.1080/019476402317276678 PMID:11957332

BBC. (2018, July 20). *Singapore personal data hack hits 1.5m, health authority says.* Available from https://www.bbc.com/news/world-asia-44900507

Benbasat, I., & Zmud, R. W. (2003). The Identity Crisis within the Is Discipline: Defining and Communicating the Discipline's Core Properties. *MIS Quarterly, 27*(2), 183–194.

Bender, J. L., Jimenez-Marroquin, M., & Jadad, A. R. (2011). Seeking support on Facebook: A content analysis of breast-cancer group. *Journal of Medical Internet Research, 13*(1), e16. doi:10.2196/jmir.1560 PMID:21371990

Bennis, W., Sample, S. B., & Asghar, R. (2015). *The art and adventure of leadership.* San Francisco: John Wiley & Sons Inc.

Bernardi, R. (2016). How Do Online Communities of Patients Aggregate on Twitter? An Affordance Perspective. Icis, 1–19.

Betbeze, P. (2016). *Get comfortable with bundles.* www.healthleadersmedia.com

Bilami, A., & Sahraoui, S. (2020). Mechanisms to secure communications in the IoT. In Securing the Internet of Things: Concepts, Methodologies, Tools, and Applications (pp. 498-521). IGI Global. doi:10.4018/978-1-5225-9866-4.ch027

Birru, M. S., Monaco, V. M., Charles, L., Drew, H., Njie, V., Bierria, T., ... Steinman, R. A. (2004). Internet usage by low-literacy adults seeking health information: An observational analysis. *Journal of Medical Internet Research, 6*(3), e25. doi:10.2196/jmir.6.3.e25 PMID:15471751

Biswas, N., Chattapadhyay, S., Mahapatra, G., Chatterjee, S., & Mondal, K. C. (2019). A New Approach for Conceptual Extraction-Transformation-Loading Process Modeling. *International Journal of Ambient Computing and Intelligence, 10*(1), 30–45. doi:10.4018/IJACI.2019010102

Black, A. D., Car, J., Pagliari, C., Anandan, C., Cresswell, K., Bokun, T., ... Sheikh, A. (2011). The impact of eHealth on the quality and safety of healthcare: A systematic overview. *PLoS Medicine, 8*(1), e1000387. doi:10.1371/journal.pmed.1000387 PMID:21267058

Blas, M. M., Curioso, W. H., Garcia, P. J., Zimic, M., Carcamo, C. P., Castagnetto, J. M., ... Lopez, D. M. (2011). Training the biomedical informatics workforce in Latin America: Results of a needs assessment. *BMJ Open, 1*(2), e000233. doi:10.1136/bmjopen-2011-000233 PMID:22080537

Blau, P. M. (1964). *Exchange and Power in Social Life.* New York: John Wiley.

Bodenheimer, T. (2002). Patient Self-Management of Chronic Disease in Primary Care. *Jama, 288*(19), 2469.

Bodenheimer, T., & Sinsky, C. (2014). From triple to quadruple aim: Care of the patient requires care of the provider. *Annals of Family Medicine, 12*(6), 573–576. doi:10.1370/afm.1713 PMID:25384822

Bonomi, S. (2016). *The Electronic Health Record: A Comparison of Some European Countries*. Available from: https://www.researchgate.net/publication/303364932_The_Electronic_Health_Record_A_Comparison_of_Some_European_Countries

Bookman, M. Z., & Bookman, K. R. (2007). *Medical-tourism in Developing Countries*. New York: Palgrave Macmillan. doi:10.1057/9780230605657

Boone, C. (2018). What is sustainability? *ASU School of Sustainability*. Retrieved from https://schoolofsustainability.asu.edu/about/what-is-sustainability/)

Bourgeois, R., & Stacy, A. (2007). The impact of information technology on small, medium, and large hospitals: Quality, safety, and financial metrics (PhD dissertation). The University of Texas at Arlington. ProQuest Central; ProQuest Dissertations & Theses Global database. (3288889)

Bowersox, D. J., Closs, D. J., & Drayer, R. W. (2005). The digital transformation: Technology and beyond. *Supply Chain Management Review*, *9*(1), 22–29.

Boyd, J. S., LoPresti, C. M., Core, M., Schott, C., Mader, M. J., Lucas, B. P., ... Colon-Molero, A. (2019). Current use and training needs of point-of-care ultrasound in emergency departments: A national survey of VA hospitals. *The American Journal of Emergency Medicine*, *37*(9), 1794–1797. doi:10.1016/j.ajem.2019.02.043 PMID:30878406

Bozic, K. (2016). *Transition to value based healthcare*. The Knee Society.

Bracy, C. (2016). *The healthcare value creation equation.* https://www.aaos.org/AAOSNow/2016/Apr/Managing/managing5/

Brandrud, A. S., Schreiner, A., Hjortdahl, P., Helljesen, G. S., Nyen, B., & Nelson, E. C. (2011). Three success factors for continual improvement in healthcare: An analysis of the reports of improvement team members. *BMJ Quality &amp. Safety*, *20*(3), 251–259. doi:10.1136/bmjqs.2009.038604 PMID:21209149

Bratan, T., Stramer, K., & Greenhalgh, T. (2010). 'Never heard of it' – Understanding the public's lack of awareness of a new electronic patient record. *Health Expectations*, *13*(4), 379–391. doi:10.1111/j.1369-7625.2010.00608.x PMID:20579117

Brazier, Y. (2018). What is obesity and what causes it? *Medical News Today.* https://www.medicalnewstoday.com/articles/323551.php

Brockes, C., Grischott, T., Dutkiewicz, M., & Schmidt-Weitmann, S. (2017). Evaluation of the Education "Clinical Telemedicine/e-Health" in the Curriculum of Medical Students at the University of Zurich. *Telemedicine Journal and e-Health*, *23*(11), 899–904. doi:10.1089/tmj.2017.0011 PMID:28498779

Brolan, C. E., Forman, L., Dagron, S., Hammonds, R., Waris, A., Latif, L., & Ruano, A. L. (2017). The right to health of non-nationals and displaced persons in the sustainable development goals era: Challenges for equity in universal healthcare. *International Journal for Equity in Health*, *16*(1), 14. doi:10.118612939-016-0500-z PMID:28219374

Brown, D. (2007). Horizon scanning and the business environment -- the implications for risk management. *BT Technology Journal*, *25*(1), 208–214. doi:10.100710550-007-0022-8

Bryant, A. (2014). *An interpretative phenomenological analysis of student engagement in learning at the middle level* (Education Doctoral Theses Paper). Northeastern University. Retrieved from https://repository.library.northeastern. edu/files/neu:336553

Buhalis, D., & Law, R. (2008). Progress in information technology and tourism management: 20 years on and 10 years after the Internet-the state of eTourism research. *Tourism Management*, *29*(4), 609–623. doi:10.1016/j.tourman.2008.01.005

Bumpass, D., & Samora, J. (2016). *Price transparency in healthcare: the other half of the value equation.* https://www.aaos.org/AAOSNow/2015/Jan/advocay/advocay1/?ssopc=1

Burns, R. L. (2015). Medical-tourism opportunities and challenges: Illustration from US-India trade. *International Journal of Healthcare Management, 8*(1), 15–26. doi:10.1179/2047971914Y.0000000091

Burzler, N. (2018). *Most Popular Social Networks Worldwide 2018.* Academic Press.

Buvat, J., Crummener, C., Kar, K., Sengupta, A., Solis, B., Aboud, C., & Aoufi, E. H. (2018). *The digital culture challenge: Closing the employee-leadership gap.* Academic Press.

Byra, M. (2018). Discriminant analysis of neural style representations for breast lesion classification in ultrasound. *Biocybernetics and Biomedical Engineering, 38*(3), 684–690. doi:10.1016/j.bbe.2018.05.003

Caine, K., & Hanania, R. (2013). Patients want granular privacy control over health information in electronic medical records. *Journal of the American Medical Informatics Association, 20*(1), 7–15. doi:10.1136/amiajnl-2012-001023 PMID:23184192

Calvillo, J., Román, I., & Roa, L. M. (2015). How technology is empowering patients? A literature review. *Health Expectations, 18*(5), 643–652. doi:10.1111/hex.12089

Cancer Research UK. (2019). Obese people outnumber smokers two to one. *Science Daily.* www.sciencedaily.com/releases/2019/07/190702211335.htm

Carman, K. L., Dardess, P., Maurer, M., Sofaer, S., Adams, K., Bechtel, C., & Sweeney, J. (2013). Patient and family engagement: A framework for understanding the elements and developing interventions and policies. *Health Affairs, 32*(2), 223–231. doi:10.1377/hlthaff.2012.1133 PMID:23381514

Carvalho, J. V., Rocha, Á., Vasconcelos, J., & Abreu, A. (2019). A health data analytics maturity model for hospitals information systems. *International Journal of Information Management, 46*, 278–285. doi:10.1016/j.ijinfomgt.2018.07.001

Center for Control Diseases and Prevention. (2016). *Health United States, 2016 with special feature in medical technology.* Retrieved from https://www.cdc.gov/nchs/hus/index.htm

Chanda, R. (2002). Trade in Health Services. *Bulletin of the World Health Organization, 80*(2), 158–163. PMID:11953795

Chang, B., Bakken, S., Brown, S., Houston, T., Kreps, G., Kukafka, R., . . . Stavri, Z. (2004). Bridging the digital divide: reaching vulnerable populations. *JAMIA, 11*, 448-457.

Chang, C., & Lin, C. (2011). LIBSVM : A Library for Support Vector Machines. *ACM Transactions on Intelligent Systems and Technology, 2*(3), 1–39. doi:10.1145/1961189.1961199

Charmaz, K. (2008). Grounded Theory as an Emergent Method. Handbook of Emergent Methods, (3), 155–170.

Charmaz, K. (2006). *Constructing Grounded Theory: A Practical Guide through Qualitative Analysis* (Vol. 10). Academic Press.

Chattopadhyay, S., Das, T. K., & Das, A. (2019). *Digital Learning and Training Methodology in Study of Health Monitoring in Resco System.* Available at SSRN 3377635

Chaturvedi, D. K. (2012). Human Rights and Consciousness. *International Seminar on Prominence of Human Rights in the Criminal Justice System (ISPUR 2012), Proceedings of Organized Ambedkar Chair, Dept. of Contemporary Social Studies & Law, Dr. B.R. Ambedkar University, Agra,* 33.

Chaudhry, J. (2018, April). Securing Healthcare Data Using Biometric Authentication. *Security and Privacy in Communication Networks: SecureComm 2017 International Workshops, ATCS and SePrIoT, Niagara Falls, ON, Canada, October 22–25, 2017 Proceedings*, *239*, 123.

Chauhan, S., Rastogi, R., Chaturvedi, D. K., Arora, N., & Trivedi, P. (2017). Framework for Use of Machine Intelligence on Clinical Psychology to study the effects of Spiritual tools on Human Behavior and Psychic Challenges. *Proceedings of NSC-2017(National system conference).*

Cheng, E. W., & Ho, D. C. (2001). The influence of job and career attitudes on learning motivation and transfer. *Career Development International*, *6*(1), 20–28. doi:10.1108/13620430110381007

Chhanabhai, P., & Holt, A. (2007). Consumers are ready to accept the transition to online and electronic records if they can be assured of the security measures. *General Medicine (Los Angeles, Calif.)*, *9*(1), 8. PMID:17435617

Chin, W. W. (2010). How to Write Up and Report PLS Analyses. In V. E. Vinzi, W. W. Chin, J. Henseler, & H. Wang (Eds.), *Handbook of Partial Least Squares Concepts, Methods and Applications* (pp. 650–690). Berlin: Springer-Verlag. doi:10.1007/978-3-540-32827-8_29

Choy, K., & Schlagwein, D. (2016). Crowdsourcing for a Better World: On the Relation between IT Affordances and Donor Motivations in Charitable Crowdfunding. *Information Technology and People*, *29*(1), 221–247.

Chretien, K. C., Azar, J., & Kind, T. (2011). Physicians on Twitter. *Journal of the American Medical Association*, *305*(6), 566–568. doi:10.1001/jama.2011.68 PMID:21304081

Chung, N., & Koo, C. (2015). The use of social media in travel information search. *Telematics and Informatics*, *32*(2), 215–229. doi:10.1016/j.tele.2014.08.005

Clark, N. M., Gong, M., & Kaciroti, N. (2001). A model of self-regulation for control of chronic disease. *Health Education & Behavior*, *28*(6), 769–782. doi:10.1177/109019810102800608 PMID:11720277

Clark, N. M., Rosenstock, I., Hassan, H., Wasilewski, Y., Evans, D., Feldman, C., & Mellins, R. (1998). The effect of health beliefs and feelings of self-efficacy on self-management behavior of children with a chronic disease. *Patient Counseling and Education*, *11*(2), 131–139. doi:10.1016/0738-3991(88)90045-6

Clark, N. M., Starr-Schneidkraut, N. J., & Windsor, R. A. (1994). Management of asthma by patients and families. *American Journal of Respiratory and Critical Care Medicine*, *149*(2), 554–556. doi:10.1164/ajrccm/149.2_Pt_2.S54 PMID:8298769

Cohn, D., & Caumont, A. (2016). *10 demographic trends that are shaping the U.S. and the world.* Retrieved from https://www.pewresearch.org/fact-tank/2016/03/31/10-demographic-trends-that-are-shaping-the-u-s-and-the-world/

Cohn, K. H. (2015). Training for physician engagement. *Talent Development*, *69*(5), 58–62.

Coile, R. C. Jr. (2000). The digital transformation of healthcare. *Physician Executive*, *26*(1), 8. PMID:10788126

Collins, A., Medhekar, A., Wong, H. Y., & Cobanoglu, C. (2019). Factors influencing outbound medical travel from the USA. *Tourism Review*, *74*(3), 463–479. doi:10.1108/TR-06-2018-0083

Commins, J. (2014). Addressing physician engagement. *HealthLeaders, 17,* 8-10.

Committee on Quality Healthcare in America - Institute of Medicine. (2001). *Crossing the quality chasm: a new health system for the 21st century.* Author.

Commonwealth of Australia. (2012). *'MyHRC's Act 2012 (Australia).* Available from https://www.legislation.gov.au/Series/C2012A00063

Commonwealth of Australia. (2015). *'MyHRC's Regulation 2012 (Australia).* Available from https://www.legislation.gov.au/Details/F2016C00093

Connell, J. (2015). From medical-tourism to transnational healthcare? An epilogue for the future. *Social Science & Medicine, 124*, 398–401. doi:10.1016/j.socscimed.2014.11.015 PMID:25467883

Contreras, D. L. (2018). A workflow and protocol describing the field to digitization process for new project-based fossil leaf collections. *Applications in Plant Sciences, 6*(2), e1025. doi:10.1002/aps3.1025 PMID:29732256

Cope, J. (2011). Entrepreneurial learning from failure: An interpretative phenomenological analysis. *Journal of Business Venturing, 26*(6), 604–623. doi:10.1016/j.jbusvent.2010.06.002

Cormany, D., & Baloglu, S. (2011). Medical travel facilitator websites: An exploratory study of web page contents and services offered to the prospective medical-tourist. *Tourism Management, 32*(4), 709–716. doi:10.1016/j.tourman.2010.02.008

Coughlin, S. S., Stewart, J. L., Young, L., Heboyan, V., & DeLeo, G. (2018). Health Literacy and Patient Web Portals. *International Journal of Medical Informatics, 113*(1), 43–48. doi:10.1016/j.ijmedinf.2018.02.009 PMID:29602432

Cox, D., & Pinto, N. (2011). Beyond simple features: A large-scale feature search approach to unconstrained face recognition. In *2011 IEEE International Conference on Automatic Face and Gesture Recognition and Workshops, FG 2011* (pp. 8–15). 10.1109/FG.2011.5771385

Creswell, J. W. (2014). *Research Design: Qualitative, Quantitative, and Mixed Methods Approaches* (4th ed.). Thousand Oaks, CA: SAGE Publications.

Cripps, H., & Standing, C. (2012). *Building patient trust in electronic health records, Australian eHealth Informatics and Security Conference.* Edith Cowan University Research Online. https://ro.ecu.edu.au/cgi/viewcontent.cgi?referer=https://www.google.com.au/&httpsredir=1&article=1002&context=aeis

Crooks, V. A., Turner, L., Snyder, J., Johnston, R., & Kingsbury, P. (2011). Promoting medical-tourism in India: Messages, images, and the marketing of international patient travel. *Social Science & Medicine, 72*(5), 726–732. doi:10.1016/j.socscimed.2010.12.022 PMID:21310519

Csurka, G., Dance, C. R., Fan, L., Willamowski, J., & Bray, C. (2004). Visual categorization with bags of keypoints. In *Proceedings of the ECCV International Workshop on Statistical Learning in Computer Vision* (pp. 59–74). 10.1234/12345678

Cummings, E., Shin, E. H., Mather, C., & Hovenga, E. (2016). Embedding Nursing Informatics Education into an Australian Undergraduate Nursing Degree. *Studies in Health Technology and Informatics, 225*, 329–333.

Cunningham, F. G. (2014). *Diabetes mellitus* (24th ed.). New York, NY: The McGraw-Hill Companies. http://accessmedicine.mhmedical.com

Curioso, W. H. (2019). Building Capacity and Training for Digital Health: Challenges and Opportunities in Latin America. *Journal of Medical Internet Research, 21*(12), e16513. doi:10.2196/16513 PMID:31850849

Currell, R., Urquhart, C., Wainwright, P., & Lewis, R. (2000). Telemedicine versus face to face patient care: Effects on professional practice and healthcare outcomes. *Cochrane Database of Systematic Reviews*, (2): Cd002098. doi:10.1002/14651858.Cd002098 PMID:10796678

d'Angelo, M., Castelli, V., Catanesi, M., Antonosante, A., Dominguez-Benot, R., Ippoliti, R., ... Cimini, A. (2019). PPARγ and Cognitive Performance. *International Journal of Molecular Sciences, 20*(20), 5068. doi:10.3390/ijms20205068 PMID:31614739

Dadgar, M., & Joshi, K. D. (2018). The Role of Information and Communication Technology in Self-Management of Chronic Diseases: An Empirical Investigation through Value Sensitive Design. *Journal of the Association for Information Systems*, *19*(2), 86–112.

Dameri, R. P. (2012). Defining an evaluation framework for digital cities implementation. In *Information Society (i-Society), 2012 International Conference on* (pp. 466-470). IEEE.

Dattakumar, A., Gray, K., Henderson, K. B., Maeder, A., & Chenery, H. (2012). *We are not educating the future clinical health professional workforce adequately for e-health*. Academic Press.

Dattakumar, A., Gray, K., Henderson, K. B., Maeder, A., & Chenery, H. (2012). We are not educating the future clinical health professional workforce adequately for e-health competence: Findings of an Australian study. *Studies in Health Technology and Informatics*, *178*, 33–38. PMID:22797016

Daubechies, I. (1992). *Ten Lectures on Wavelets*. Ten Lectures on Wavelets; doi:10.1137/1.9781611970104

Davis, F. D. (1989). Perceived usefulness, perceived ease of use, and user acceptance of information technology. *MIS Quarterly, 13*(3), 319-340. Retrieve from http://www.jstor.org/stable/249008

Davis, F. D. (1989). Perceived usefulness, perceived ease of use, and user acceptance of information technology. *MIS quarterly*, 319-340. competence: Findings of an Australian study. *Studies in Health Technology and Informatics*, *178*, 33–38.

Deloitte. (2010). *How digital technologies is transforming health and social care*. Available from https://www2.deloitte.com/content/dam/Deloitte/uk/Documents/life-sciences-health-care/deloitte-uk-connected-health.pdf

Demšar, J. (2006). Statistical Comparisons of Classifiers over Multiple Data Sets. *Journal of Machine Learning Research*, *7*, 1–30. doi:10.1016/j.jecp.2010.03.005

Department of Health & Human Services. (2016). *Care for People with Chronic Conditions: Guide for the Community Health*. Author.

Department of Health. (2012). *Integrated Chronic Disease Prevention*. World Health Organization.

Department of Health. (2016, March). MyHRC. Canberra: Australian Government. Available from https://myhealthrecord.gov.au/internet/mhr/publishing.nsf/

Dess, G., McNamara, G., Eisner, A., & Hyun, S. (2019). *Strategic management: Creating competitive advantages* (9th ed.). McGraw-Hill Education.

Diab, S. M., & Ajlouni, M. T. (2015). The influence of training on employee's performance, organizational commitment, and quality of medical services at Jordanian private hospitals. *International Journal of Business and Management*, *10*(2), 117. doi:10.5539/ijbm.v10n2p117

Dods, J., Alem, L., & Nepal, S. (2012). *Caring for the last 3%: Telehealth potential and Broadband implications for remote Australia. CSIRO ICT Centre*.

Dods, S., Freyne, J., Alem, L., Nepal, S., Li, J., & Jang-Jaccard, J. (2012). *Caring for the last 3%: Telehealth potential and Broadband implications for remote Australia 2012*. Academic Press.

Dods, S., Hansen, D., Boyle, J., O'Keefe, C., Alem, L., Celler, B., & Kanagasingam, Y. (2014). *A digitally-enabled health system*. Marsfield. doi:10.4225/08/584ee7360ac32

DowJones. (2016). Press Release: New Study Reveals High Confidence in Digital Transformation Success Despite Major Challenges. *Dow Jones Institutional News*.

Dugani, S. M. D. P., Duke, T. M. D., & Kissoon, N. M. (2016). Transforming health through sustainable development. *Canadian Medical Association. Journal, 188*(10), E213-E214.

Duggal, R., Brindle, I., & Bagenal, J. (2018). *Digital healthcare: regulating the revolution.* Academic Press.

Duke University Medical Center. (2019). Even in svelte adults, cutting about 300 calories daily protects the heart. Researchers seeking a signal in metabolism or a 'magic molecule' to explain this. *Science Daily.* www.sciencedaily.com/releases/2019/07/190711183758.htm

Dyrda, L. (2018, February). Hospital Transaction and valuation issue. *Backer's Hospital Review.* Retrieved from https://www.beckershospitalreview.com/hospital-transactions-and-valuation/healthcare-transactions-in-the-era-of-megamergers-and-vertical-integration-q-a-with-jeff-swearingen.html

Dzenowagis, J., Kelley, E., Kluge, H., & Ganesh, V. (2018). *Digital technologies: shaping the future of primary healthcare.* WHO Headquarters. https://www.who.int/docs/default-source/primary-health-care-conference/digital-technologies.pdf?sfvrsn=3efc47e0_2

Economist. (2005). *Cherry picking profitable operations from general service hospitals.* https://economistsview.typepad.com/economistsview/2005/06/cherrypicking_p.html

ECRI. (2011). *AHRQ Healthcare horizon scanning system protocol and operations manual.* Prepared by ECRI Institute under Contract No. HHSA290201000006C. Rockville, MD: Agency for Healthcare Research and Quality.

Edejer, T. T.-T. (2000). Disseminating health information in developing countries: The role of the internet. *BMJ (Clinical Research Ed.), 321*(7264), 797–800. doi:10.1136/bmj.321.7264.797 PMID:11009519

Edirippulige, S., & Armfield, N. R. (2017). Education and training to support the use of clinical telehealth: A review of the literature. *Journal of Telemedicine and Telecare, 23*(2), 273–282. doi:10.1177/1357633X16632968 PMID:26892005

Edirippulige, S., Armfield, N. R., & Smith, A. C. (2012). A qualitative study of the careers and professional practices of graduates from an e-health postgraduate programme. *Journal of Telemedicine and Telecare, 18*(8), 455–459. doi:10.1258/jtt.2012.gth107 PMID:23209263

Edirippulige, S., Brooks, P., Carati, C., Wade, V. A., Smith, A. C., Wickramasinghe, S., & Armfield, N. R. (2018). It's important, but not important enough: eHealth as a curriculum priority in medical education in Australia. *Journal of Telemedicine and Telecare, 24*(10), 697–702. doi:10.1177/1357633X18793282 PMID:30343657

Edirippulige, S., Samanta, M., & Armfield, N. R. (2018). Assessment of Self-Perceived Knowledge in e-Health Among Undergraduate Students. *Telemedicine Journal and e-Health, 24*(2), 139–144. doi:10.1089/tmj.2017.0056 PMID:28708457

Edirippulige, S., Smith, A. C., Armfield, N. R., Bensink, M., & Wootton, R. (2012). Student perceptions of a hands-on practicum to supplement an online eHealth course. *Journal of Medical Internet Research, 14*(6), e182–e182. doi:10.2196/jmir.2029 PMID:23246840

Edirippulige, S., Smith, A. C., Wickramasinghe, S., & Armfield, N. R. (2018). Examining the Influence of E-Health Education on Professional Practice. *Journal of Medical Systems, 42*(11), 215. doi:10.100710916-018-1084-5 PMID:30276486

Eisenhardt, K. M. (1989). Building Theories from Case Study Research. *Academy of Management Review, 14*(4), 532–550.

El Paso Society for Human Resource Management. (2017). *Workforce Readiness.* Retrieved from http://www.epshrm.org/page-18065

Elf, M., Flink, M., Nilsson, M., Tistad, M., von Koch, L., & Ytterberg, C. (2017). The care of value-based healthcare for people living with complex long-term conditions. *BMC Health Services Research, 17*(24), 1-6.

Ellahham, S., Ellahham, N., & Simsekler, M. C. E. (2019). Application of Artificial Intelligence in the Healthcare Safety Context: Opportunities and Challenges. *American Journal of Medical Quality*, *§§§*, 1062860619878515. PMID:31581790

Emerson, R. M. (1976). Social exchange theory. *Annual Review of Sociology*, *2*(0), 335–362. doi:10.1146/annurev.so.02.080176.002003

Erhan, D., Courville, A., Bengio, Y., & Vincent, P. (2010). Why does unsupervised pre-training help deep learning? Journal of Machine Learning Research. doi:10.1145/1756006.1756025

European Commisssion. (2004). *E-Health, Making Healthcare Better for European Citizens: An Action Plan for a European E-health Area*. Retrieved from https://ec.europa.eu/digital-single-market/en/news/e-health-making-healthcare-better-european-citizens-action-plan-european-e-health-area

Eysenbach, G. (2008). Medicine 2.0. Social networking, collaboration, participation, apomediation, and openness. *Journal of Medical Internet Research*, *10*(3), e22. doi:10.2196/jmir.1030 PMID:18725354

Faddis, A. (2018). The digital transformation of healthcare technology management. *Biomedical Instrumentation & Technology*, *52*(s2), 34–38. doi:10.2345/0899-8205-52.s2.34 PMID:29775387

Fadel, K. J. (2012). User Adaptation and Infusion of Information Systems. *Journal of Computer Information Systems*, *52*(3), 1–10.

Faraj, S., & Azad, B. (2012). The Materiality of Technology: An Affordance Perspective. Materiality and Organizing: Social Interaction in a Technological World, 237–258.

Farzandipour, M., Sadoughi, F., Ahmadi, M., & Karimi, I. (2010). Security requirements and solutions in electronic health records: Lessons learned from a comparative study. *Journal of Medical Systems*, *34*(4), 629–642. doi:10.100710916-009-9276-7 PMID:20703917

Fassaert, T., van Dulmen, S., Schellevis, F., & Bensing, J. (2007). Active listening in medical consultations: Development of the Active Listening Observation Scale (ALOS-global). *Patient Education and Counseling*, *68*(3), 258–264. doi:10.1016/j.pec.2007.06.011 PMID:17689042

Fayard, A.-L., & Weeks, J. (2014). Affordances for Practice. *Information and Organization*, *24*(4), 236–249.

Felman, A. (2018). An overview of insulin. *Medical News Today*. https://www.medicalnewstoday.com/articles/323760.php

Fernández-Alemán, J. L., Carrión Señor, I., Lozoya, P. L. O., & Toval, A. (2013). Security and privacy in electronic health records: A systematic literature review. *Journal of Biomedical Informatics*, *46*(3), 541–562. doi:10.1016/j.jbi.2012.12.003 PMID:23305810

Fernandez-Luque, L., Aupetit, M., Palotti, J., Singh, M., Fadlelbari, A., Baggag, A., & Al-Thani, D. (2019). Health Lifestyle Data-Driven Applications Using Pervasive Computing. In *Big Data, Big Challenges: A Healthcare Perspective* (pp. 115–126). Cham: Springer. doi:10.1007/978-3-030-06109-8_10

Fernando, J., & Dawson, L. (2009). The health information system security threat lifecycle: An informatics theory. *International Journal of Medical Informatics*, *78*(12), 815–826. doi:10.1016/j.ijmedinf.2009.08.006 PMID:19783203

Fichman, R. G., Kohli, R., & Krishnan, R. (2011). The Role of Information Systems in Healthcare: Current Research and Future Trends. *Information Systems Research*, *22*(3), 419–428.

Filkins, B. L., Kim, J. Y., Roberts, B., Armstrong, W., Miller, M. A., Hultner, M. L., ... Steinhubl, S. R. (2016). Privacy and security in the era of digital health: What should translational researchers know and do about it? *American Journal of Translational Research*, *8*(3), 1560–1580. PMID:27186282

Fisher, J., & Clayton, M. (2012, 2Q). Who gives a tweet: assessing patients' interest in the use of social media for health-care. *World Views on Evidence-Based Nursing,* 100-108.

Fragidis, L., & Chatzoglou, P. (2018). Implementation of a Nationwide Electronic Health Record (EHR): The International Experience in 13 Countries. *International Journal of Health Care Quality Assurance*, *31*(2), 116–13. doi:10.1108/IJHCQA-09-2016-0136 PMID:29504871

Freshman, B., & Rubino, L. (2002). Emotional intelligence: A core competency for healthcare administrators. *The Health Care Manager*, *20*(4), 1–9. doi:10.1097/00126450-200206000-00002 PMID:12083173

Friedman, T. L. (2007). *The world is flat, A brief history of the twenty-first century* (2nd rev ed.). Farrar, Straus, and Giroux Publisher.

Fry, C. L., Spriggs, M., Arnold, M., & Pearce, C. (2014). Unresolved ethical challenges for the Australian Personally Controlled Electronic Health Record (PCEHR) system: Key informant interview findings. *AJOB Empirical Bioethics*, *5*(4), 30–36. doi:10.1080/23294515.2014.919972

Gabbe, S. G. (2018). Diabetes mellitus complicating normal pregnancy. In *Obstetrics: Normal and Problem Pregnancy* (7th ed.). Saunders Elsevier. https://www.clinicalkey.com

Gao, C. (2019). *Research on the Application of Big Data in Security Information Collection*. Academic Press.

Gardenswartz, L., Rowe, A., Digh, P., & Bennett, M. (2003). *The global diversity desk reference: Managing an international workforce*. Pfeiffer.

Gardner, P. J. (2009). Organizational change: All we want is better projects-why so difficult? *AACE International Transactions*, PM.03.01-PM.03.25.

George, B. P., & Henthorne, T. L. (2009). The incorporation of telemedicine with medical-tourism: A study of consequences. *Journal of Hospitality Marketing & Management*, *18*(5), 512–522. doi:10.1080/19368620902950097

Georgeff, M. (2014). RACGP - Digital Technologies and Chronic Disease Management. Australian Family Physician, 842–6.

Georgiou, A., & Prgomet, M. (2018). E-Health: Developing trust, confidence, quality and sustainability. *The HIM Journal*, *4*(2), 59–61. doi:10.1177/1833358318808064 PMID:30392402

Gibson, J. J. (1986). 04-JJ Gibson-Ch8-Affordances. Chapter Eight The Theory of Affordances, 127–136.

Gill, M. J. (2014). The Possibilities of Phenomenology for Organizational Research. *Organizational Research Methods*, *17*(2), 118–137. doi:10.1177/1094428113518348

Gill, R. (2003). Change Management or Change Leadership. *Journal of Change Management*, *3*(4), 307–318. doi:10.1080/714023845

Ginsburg, P., Loera-Brust, A., Brandt, C., & Durak, A. (2018). *The opportunities and challenges of data analytics in healthcare.* Report Produced by Artificial Intelligence and Emerging Technologies Initiative.

Gioia, D. A., Corley, K. G., & Hamilton, A. L. (2013). Seeking Qualitative Rigor in Inductive Research: Notes on the Gioia Methodology. *Organizational Research Methods*, *16*(1), 15–31.

Glasgow, R. E., Phillips, S. M., & Sanchez, M. A. (2014). Implementation science approaches for integrating eHealth research into practice and policy. *International Journal of Medical Informatics*, *83*(7), e1–e11. doi:10.1016/j.ijmedinf.2013.07.002 PMID:23910896

Gleason, A. W. (2015). mHealth-Opportunities for Transforming Global Healthcare and Barriers to Adoption. *Journal of Electronic Resources in Medical Libraries, 12*(2), 114–125. doi:10.1080/15424065.2015.1035565

Goh, J. M., Gao, G. G., & Agarwal, R. (2011). Evolving Work Routines : Adaptive Routinization of Information Technology in Healthcare. *Information Systems Research.*

Goldberg, S. (2002a). *Building the Evidence for a standardized Mobile Internet (wireless) Environment.* Internal Inet Documentation. Ontario, Canada: Inet.

Goldberg, S. (2002b). *HTA Presentation Rendering Component Summary.* Internal Inet documentation. Ontario, Canada: Inet.

Goldberg, S. (2002c). *HTA Quality Assurance Component Summary.* Internal Inet documentation. Ontario, Canada: Inet.

Goldberg, S. (2002d). *Wireless POC Device Component Summary.* Internal Inet documentation. Ontario, Canada: Inet.

Gray K, Dattakumar A, Maeder A, Butler-Henderson K, & H., C. (2014). Advancing eHealth education for the clinical health professions. Academic Press.

Gray, M. (2018). Value based Healthcare. *BMJ, 356*, 1-2.

Gray, K., Dattakumar, A., Maeder, A., Butler-Henderson, K., & Chenery, H. (2014). *Advancing ehealth education for the clinical health professions: Final report 2014*. Academic Press.

Greenes, R. A., & Shortliffe, E. H. (1990). Medical informatics. An emerging academic discipline and institutional priority. *Journal of the American Medical Association, 263*(8), 1114–1120. doi:10.1001/jama.263.8.1114

Greenhalgh, T. (2009). Chronic Illness: Beyond the Expert Patient. BMJ, 338, 629–631.

Greenhalgh, T., Robert, G., Macfarlane, F., Bate, P., & Kyriakidou, O. (2004). Diffusion of innovations in service organizations: Systematic review and recommendations. *The Milbank Quarterly, 82*(4), 581–629. doi:10.1111/j.0887-378X.2004.00325.x

Greenlalgh, T., Hinder, S., Stramere, K., Bratan, T., & Russell, J. (2010). Adoption, non-adoption, and abandonment of a personal electronic health record: Case study of HealthSpace. *Biomedical Journal, 341*, c5814. PMID:21081595

Griffis, H. M., Kilaru, A. S., Kilaru, A. S., Werner, R., Asch, D. A., Hershey, J. C., & … . (2014). Use of Social Media across US Hospitals: Descriptive Analysis of Adoption and Utilization. *Journal of Medical Internet Research, 16*(11), e264. doi:10.2196/jmir.3758 PMID:25431831

Gulati, M., Rastogi, R., Chaturvedi, D. K., Sharma, P., Yadav, V., Chauhan, S., . . . Singhal, P. (2019). Statistical Resultant Analysis of Psychosomatic Survey on Various Human Personality Indicators: Statistical Survey to Map Stress and Mental Health. In *Handbook of Research on Learning in the Age of Transhumanism* (pp. 363-383). Hershey, PA: IGI Global. doi:10.4018/978-1-5225-8431-5.ch022

Gulati, M., Rastogi, R., Chaturvedi, D. K., Satya, S., Arora, N., & Singhal, P. (2018). Statistical Resultant Analysis of Spiritual & Psychosomatic Stress Survey on Various Human Personality Indicators. *The International Conference proceedings of ICCI 2018.*

Guo, U., Chen, L., & Mehta, P. H. (2017). Electronic health record innovations: Helping physicians – One less click at a time. *The HIM Journal, 43*(3), 140–144. doi:10.1177/1833358316689481 PMID:28671038

Gupta, M., Rastogi, R., Chaturvedi, D. K., Satya, S. A., Verma, H., Singhal, P., & Singh, A. (2019). Comparative Study of Trends Observed During Different Medications by Subjects under EMG & GSR Biofeedback. *IJITEE, 8*(6S), 748-756. https://www.ijitee.org/download/volume-8-issue-6S/

Gutiérrez-Ibarluzea, I., Chiumente, M., & Dauben, H.-P. (2017). The life cycle of health technologies. Challenges and ways forward. *Frontiers in Pharmacology, 8*, 14–14. doi:10.3389/fphar.2017.00014 PMID:28174538

Haas, S., Wohlgemuth, S., Echizen, I., Sonehara, N., & Müller, N. (2011). Aspects of privacy for electronic health records. *International Journal of Medical Informatics, 80*(2), 26–31. doi:10.1016/j.ijmedinf.2010.10.001 PMID:21041113

Haddad, P., Schaffer, J. L., & Wickramasinghe, N. (2015). Evaluating Business Value of IT in Healthcare: Three Clinical Practices from Australia and the US. In *EHealth-enabled Health: Proceedings of the 15th World Congress on Health and Biomedical Informatics* (*Vol. 216*, p. 183). IOS Press.

Hadeel, A., & Sandhu, K. (2021). PLS Model Performance for Factors Influencing Students Acceptance of Elearning Analytics Recommender. *International Journal of Virtual and Personal Learning Environments.*

Hall, D. (2011). Debate: Innovative teaching to enhance critical thinking and communication skills in healthcare professionals. *The Internet Journal of Allied Health Sciences and Practice, 9*(3), 7.

Halvorson, G. C. (2013). The culture to cultivate. *Harvard Business Review.* PMID:24730168

Hambleton, S., & Aloizos, J. (2019). Australia's digital health journey. *The Medical Journal of Australia, 210*(6), S5–S6. doi:10.5694/mja2.50039 PMID:30927473

Han, H., & Hwang, J. (2018). Growing competition in the healthcare tourism market and customer retention in medical clinics: New and experienced travellers. *Current Issues in Tourism, 21*(6), 680–702. doi:10.1080/13683500.2015.1104292

Hanna, L., Gill, S. D., Newstead, L., Hawkins, M., & Osborne, R. H. (2017). Patient perspectives on a personally controlled electronic health record used in regional Australia: 'I can be like my own doctor'. *The HIM Journal, 46*(1), 42–48. doi:10.1177/1833358316661063 PMID:27486184

Hartnell, C. (2012). Leadership and organizational culture: An integrative view of leaders as culture creators and culture as social context (PhD dissertation). Arizona State University. ProQuest Dissertations & Theses Global database. (3504099)

Hassan, H., Asad, S., & Hoshino, Y. (2016). Connecting the Post-Training Task and Contextual Performance with the Essentials of Training Program and Characteristics of Trainees. *International Journal of Business and Management, 11*(4), 11. doi:10.5539/ijbm.v11n4p48

Hawn, C. (2009). Take two aspirins and tweet me in the morning: How Twitter, Facebook and other social media are reshaping healthcare. *Health Affairs, 28*(2), 361–368. doi:10.1377/hlthaff.28.2.361 PMID:19275991

Health Information Management Association of Australia Limited (HIMAA). (2019). *Educational Services for Health Information Professionals.* Available from http://himaa2.org.au/education/?q=node/2

Health Workforce Australia. (2013). *Health Information Workforce Report.* Author.

Heckemann, B., Zeller, A., Hahn, S., Dassen, T., Schols, J. M. G. A., & Halfens, R. J. G. (2015). The effect of aggression management training programmes for nursing staff and students working in an acute hospital setting. A narrative review of current literature. *Nurse Education Today, 35*(1), 212–219. doi:10.1016/j.nedt.2014.08.003 PMID:25200511

Hemsley, B., Georgiou, A., Carter, R., Hill, S., Higgins, I., van Vlient, P., & Balandin, S. (2016). Use of the 'MyHRC' by people with communication disability in Australia: A review to inform the design and direction of future research. *The HIM Journal, 45*(3), 107–115. doi:10.1177/1833358316652060 PMID:27269277

Hemsley, B., McCarthy, S., Adams, S., Georgiou, A., Hill, S., & Balandin, S. (2017). Legal, ethical, and rights issues in the adoption and use of the "MyHRC' by people with communication disability in Australia. *Journal of Intellectual & Developmental Disability, 43*(4), 506–514. doi:10.3109/13668250.2017.1294249

Hemsley, B., Rollo, M., Georgiou, A., Balandin, S., & Hill, S. (2018). The health literacy demands of electronic personal health records (e-PHRs): An integrative review to inform future inclusive research. *Patient Education and Counseling, 101*(1), 2–15. doi:10.1016/j.pec.2017.07.010 PMID:28864052

Hero, J., Blendon, R., Zaslavsky, A., & Campbell, A. (2016). Understanding what makes Americans Dissatisfied with their healthcare system: an international comparison. *Health Affairs, 35*(3), 502-509.

Herscovitch, L. (2004). *Resistance to organizational change: Toward a multidimensional conceptualization* (Doctoral dissertation). The University of Western Ontario. ProQuest Dissertations & Theses Global database. (NQ96828)

Hersh, W., Margolis, A., Quiros, F., & Otero, P. (2010). Building a health informatics workforce in developing countries. *Health Affairs (Project Hope), 29*(2), 274–277. doi:10.1377/hlthaff.2009.0883

Hill, C. W., & Hult, T. M. (2018). *Global business today* (10th ed.). McGraw-Hill Education.

Ho, S. Y., Guo, X., & Vogel, D. (2019). Opportunities and Challenges in Healthcare Information Systems Research: Caring for Patients with Chronic Conditions. *Communications of the Association for Information Systems*, (44), 852–873. doi:10.17705/1CAIS.04439

Househ, M., Borycki, E., & Kushniruk, A. (2014). Empowering Patients through Social Media: The Benefits and Challenges. *Health Informatics Journal, 20*(1), 50–58.

Hsu, J., Huang, J., Kinsman, J., Fireman, B., Miller, R., Selby, J., & Ortiz, E. (2005). Use of e-health services between 1999 and 2002 a growing digital divide. *Journal of the American Medical Informatics Association, 12*(2), 164–171. doi:10.1197/jamia.M1672 PMID:15561786

Huang, H., Zhang, S., Feng, T., Zhu, J., Zheng, Z., Tao, Y., & Qian, B. (2017). Questionnaire analysis of clinical research capacity and training needs for physicians at university hospitals. *Chinese Journal of Medical Science Research Management, 30*(4), 293–299.

Huang, J., & Ling, C. X. (2005). Using AUC and accuracy in evaluating learning algorithms. *IEEE Transactions on Knowledge and Data Engineering*. doi:10.1109/TKDE.2005.50

Husain, M. Y., Mokhtar, S. B., Ahmad, A. A., & Mustapha, R. (2010). Importance of employability skills from employers' perspective. *Procedia: Social and Behavioral Sciences, 7*, 430–438. doi:10.1016/j.sbspro.2010.10.059

Iliashenko, O., Bikkulova, Z., & Dubgorn, A. (2019). Opportunities and challenges of artificial intelligence in healthcare. In *E3S Web of Conferences* (Vol. 110, p. 02028). EDP Sciences. doi:10.1051/e3sconf/201911002028

Ingebrigtsen, T., Georgiou, A., Clay-Williams, R., Magrabi, F., Hordern, A., Prgomet, M., ... Braithwaite, J. (2014). The impact of clinical leadership on health information technology adoption: Systematic review. *International Journal of Medical Informatics, 83*(6), 393–405. doi:10.1016/j.ijmedinf.2014.02.005 PMID:24656180

Institute for Healthcare Improvement. (2012). *The IHI Triple Aim*. Retrieved from http://www.ihi.org/Engage/Initiatives/TripleAim/Pages/default.aspx

Institute of Medicine. (2001). *Crossing the Quality Chasm: A New Health System for the 21st Century*. Washington, DC: The National Academies Press.

International Council of Nurses. (2005). *Summary- Global shortage of registered nurses*. Author.

Isika, N. U., Mendoza, A., & Bosua, R. (2016). The Use of Social Media by Adults with Chronic Illness: Analysing the Support Mechanisms of Four Social Media Platforms. In *The 27th Australasian Conference on Information Systems* (Vol. 1). Academic Press.

Iyawa, G. E., Herselman, M., & Botha, A. (2016). Digital Health Innovation Ecosystems: From Systematic Literature Review to Conceptual Framework. *Procedia Computer Science*, *100*, 244–252. doi:10.1016/j.procs.2016.09.149

Jain, E., & Yadav, A. (2017). Marketing and Technology: Role of Technology in Modern Marketing. *IOSR Journal of Business and Management*, *19*(5), 49–53. doi:10.9790/487X-1905064953

Jha, A. K., Doolan, D., Grandt, D., Scott, T., & Bates, D. W. (2008). The use of health information technology in seven nations. *International Journal of Medical Informatics*, *77*(12), 848–854. doi:10.1016/j.ijmedinf.2008.06.007 PMID:18657471

Jiang, F., Jiang, Y., Zhi, H., Dong, Y., Li, H., Ma, S., ... Wang, Y. (2017). Artificial intelligence in healthcare: Past, present and future. *Stroke and Vascular Neurology*, *2*(4), e000101. doi:10.1136vn-2017-000101 PMID:29507784

Jiju, A., Snee, R., & Hoerl, R. (2017). Lean Six Sigma: Yesterday, today and tomorrow. *International Journal of Quality & Reliability Management*, *34*(7), 1073–1093. doi:10.1108/IJQRM-03-2016-0035

John, S., Larke, R., & Kilgour, M. (2018). Applications of social media for medical-tourism marketing: An empirical analysis. *Anatolia*, *13*(2), 1–13. doi:10.1080/13032917.2018.1473261

Jolly, R. (2011). The e health revolution—easier said than done (P. o. Australia Ed.). Parliamentary Library, Parliament of Australia.

Joseph, T. (2019). *Digital Tools for the Future of Healthcare Providers*. Available from https://www.fingent.com/blog/digital-tools-for-the-future-of-healthcare-providers

Kallenberg, M., Petersen, K., Nielsen, M., Ng, A. Y., Diao, P., & Igel, C. … Lillholm, M. (2016). Unsupervised Deep Learning Applied to Breast Density Segmentation and Mammographic Risk Scoring. *IEEE Transactions on Medical Imaging*. doi:10.1109/TMI.2016.2532122 PMID:26915120

Kallinikos, J. (2002). Reopening the Black Box of Technology. ICIS, 287–294.

Kallinikos, J. (2012). Form, Function, and Matter: Crossing the Border of Materiality. In Materiality and Organizing: Social Interaction in a Technological World (Vol. 1, pp. 45–66). doi:10.1093/acprof:oso/9780199664054.003.0004

Kallinikos, J., Leonardi, P. M., & Nardi, B. A. (2012). The Challenge of Materiality: Origins, Scope, and Prospects. *Materiality and Organizing: Social Interaction in a Technological World.*

Kampmeijer, R., Pavlova, M., Tambor, M., Golinowska, S., & Groot, W. (2016). The use of e-health and m-health tools in health promotion and primary prevention among older adults: A systematic literature review. *BMC Health Services Research*, *16*(S5), 290. doi:10.118612913-016-1522-3 PMID:27608677

Kane, G. C. (2015). How digital transformation is making healthcare safer, faster and cheaper. *MIT Sloan Management Review*, *57*(1), 0.

Kane, G. C., Alavi, M., Labianca, Giuseppe, J., & Borgatti, S. P. (2014). What's Different about Social Media Networks? A Framework and Research Agenda. MIS Quarterly, 38(1), 274–304.

Kannala, J., & Rahtu, E. (2012). BSIF: Binarized statistical image features. In *21st International Conference on Pattern Recognition (ICPR)* (pp. 1363–1366). Academic Press.

Kaplan, A. M., & Haenlein, M. (2010). Users of the World, Unite! The Challenges and Opportunities of Social Media. *Business Horizons*, *53*(1), 59–68.

Kaplan, R., & Porter, E. (2011). *How to solve the cost crisis in healthcare.* Harvard Business Review Reprint R1109B.

Karahanna, E., Xu, S. X., Xu, Y., & Zhang, N. (2018). The needs–affordances–features perspective for the use of social media. *MIS Quarterly*, *42*(3), 737–756. doi:10.25300/MISQ/2018/11492

Kasper, D. L. (2015). Diabetes mellitus: Diagnosis, classification and pathophysiology. In *Harrison's Principles of Internal Medicine* (19th ed.). New York, NY: McGraw-Hill Education. http://accessmedicine.mhmedical.com

Kelly, S. (2016). Creating a culture of continuous improvement and sustainable management systems at Abbott Diagnostics Longford. *Global Business and Organizational Excellence*, *36*(1), 6–24. doi:10.1002/joe.21753

Kerai, P., Wood, P., & Martin, M. (2014). A pilot study on the views of elderly regional Australians of personally controlled electronic health records. *International Journal of Medical Informatics*, *83*(3), 201–209. doi:10.1016/j.ijmedinf.2013.12.001 PMID:24382474

Khan, M. A., & Salah, K. (2018). IoT security: Review, blockchain solutions, and open challenges. *Future Generation Computer Systems*, *82*, 395–411. doi:10.1016/j.future.2017.11.022

Khan, M. J., Chelliah, S., & Haron, M. S. (2016). International patients; Travel decision-making process- A conceptual framework. *Iranian Journal of Public Health*, *45*(2), 134–145. PMID:27114978

Kietzmann, J. H., Hermkens, K., McCarthy, I. P., & Silvestre, B. S. (2011). Social Media? Get Serious! Understanding the Functional Building Blocks of Social Media. *Business Horizons*, *54*(3), 241–251.

Kim, J., Campbell, A. S., de Ávila, B. E. F., & Wang, J. (2019). Wearable biosensors for healthcare monitoring. *Nature Biotechnology*, 1. PMID:30804534

Kim, K., & Kwon, N. (2010). Profile of e-patients: Analysis of their cancer information-seeking from a national survey. *Journal of Health Communication*, *15*(7), 712–733. doi:10.1080/10810730.2010.514031 PMID:21104502

Kim, M. I., & Johnston, K. B. (2002). Personal Health Records: Evaluation of Functionality and Utility. *Journal of the American Medical Informatics Association*, *9*(2), 171–180. doi:10.1197/jamia.M0978 PMID:11861632

Kitsiou, A., Galanis, P., Bilali, A., Vraka, I., & Theodorou, M. (2016). Training needs of nurses in public hospitals in Cyprus. *Nursing Care & Research/Nosileia kai Ereuna*, (46).

Kluge, E.-H. W. (2008). Ethical aspects of future healthcare: Globalization of markets and differentiation of societies-ethical challenges. *Studies in Health Technology and Informatics*, *134*, 77–87. PMID:18376035

Kohn, L., Corrigan, J., & Donaldson, M. (1999). *To err is human: building a safer health system* (N. A. Press, Ed.). Washington, DC: Committee on Quality of Healthcare in America, Institute of Medicine.

Konijn, E. A., Veldhuis, J., & Plaisier, X. S. (2013). YouTube as a Research Tool: Three Approaches. *Cyberpsychology, Behavior and Social Networking*, *16*(9), 695–701.

Korda, H., & Itani, Z. (2013). Harnessing social media for health pormotion and behaviour change. *Health Promotion Practice*, *14*(1), 15–23. doi:10.1177/1524839911405850 PMID:21558472

Kotter, J. (1995). Leading change: Why transformation efforts fail. (cover story). *Harvard Business Review*, *73*(2), 59–67.

Kotter, J. (2012). *Leading change. Harvard Business Review.*

Krumholz, H. M. (2014). Big data and new knowledge in medicine: The thinking, training, and tools needed for a learning health system. *Health Affairs*, *33*(7), 1163–1170. doi:10.1377/hlthaff.2014.0053 PMID:25006142

Kuo, T., Sahama, A. W., Kushniruk, E., Borycki, M., & Grunwell, D. K. (2014). Health big data analytics: Current perspectives, challenges and potential solutions. *Int. J. Big Data Intell., 1*(2), 114–126.www.techrepublic.com/article/understanding-the-differences-between-ai-machine-learning-and-deep-learning

Kuza, C. C. (2017). Burnout among critical care nurses and the role of ICU telemedicine (PhD dissertation). University of Pittsburgh. ProQuest Dissertations & Theses Global database. (10831866)

Kuziemsky, C. E., Eynakchi, R., Jibb, L., & Stacey, D. (2019). Digital Process Innovation for Patient Centred Cancer Symptom Management. In ITCH (pp. 250-255). Academic Press.

Langlois, E. V., Campbell, K., Prieur-Richard, A., Karesh, W. B., & Daszak, P. (2012). Towards a better integration of global health and biodiversity in the new Sustainable Development Goals beyond rio+20. *EcoHealth, 9*(4), 381–385. doi:10.100710393-012-0800-8 PMID:23001330

Lannan, K. (2015). *Interpretative phenomenological analysis: Exploring the formative experiences of community college students enrolled in remedial courses* (Doctoral dissertation). Colorado State University. Retrieved from https://dspace.library.colostate.edu/handle/10217/170325

Lawler Iii, E. E. (2014). Sustainable Effectiveness and Organization Development. *OD Practitioner, 46*(4), 65–67.

Lee, K. (2019). Epidemiology is ecosystem science. *Synthese*, 1–29.

Lee, Y. H., Hsieh, Y. C., & Hsu, C. N. (2011). Adding innovation diffusion theory to the technology acceptance model: Supporting employees' intentions to use E-Learning systems. *Journal of Educational Technology & Society, 14*(4), 124–137.

Leggat, S. G. (2007). Effective healthcare teams require effective team members: Defining teamwork competencies. *BMC Health Services Research, 7*(1), 17. doi:10.1186/1472-6963-7-17 PMID:17284324

Lehnbom, E. C., Brien, J. E., & McLachlan, A. J. (2014). Knowledge and attitudes regarding the personally controlled electronic health record: An Australian national survey. *Internal Medicine Journal, 44*(4), 406–409. doi:10.1111/imj.12384 PMID:24754689

Lehnbom, E. C., McLachlan, A., & Brien, J. A. (2012). A qualitative study of Australians' opinions about personally controlled electronic health records. *Studies in Health Technology and Informatics, 178*, 105–110. PMID:22797027

Leonardi, P. M. (2012). Materiality, Sociomateriality, and Socio-Technical Systems: What Do These Terms Mean? How Are They Different? Do We Need Them? *Materiality and Organizing: Social Interaction in a Technological World.*

Leong, C., Pan, S. L., Newell, S., & Cui, L. (2016). The Emergence of Self-Organizing E-Commerce Ecosystems in Remote Villages of China: A Tale of Digital Empowerment for Rural Development. *MIS Quarterly, 40*(2), 475-A8.

Liaw, S. T., & Hannan, T. (2011). Can we trust the PCEHR not to leak? *The Medical Journal of Australia, 195*(4), 222. doi:10.5694/j.1326-5377.2011.tb03287.x PMID:21843131

Linski, C. M. III. (2013). Process consultation and law enforcement: A practitioner's case study report. *Organization Development Journal, 31*(4), 63–73.

Lin, T. C., & Bautista, J. R. (2017). Understanding the Relationships between mHealth Apps' Characteristics, Trialability, and mHealth Literacy. *Journal of Health Communication, 22*(4), 346–354. doi:10.1080/10810730.2017.1296508 PMID:28323546

Liu, W., Wang, Z., Liu, X., Zeng, N., Liu, Y., & Alsaadi, F. E. (2017). A survey of deep neural network architectures and their applications. *Neurocomputing, 234*, 11–26. doi:10.1016/j.neucom.2016.12.038

Lloyd, J., & Ferguson, S. L. (2017). Innovative information technology solutions: Addressing current and emerging nurse shortages and staffing challenges worldwide. *Nursing Economics*, *35*(4), 211–212.

Lopez, A., Detz, A., Ratanawongsa, N., & Sarkar, U. (2012). What patients say about their doctors online: A qualitative content analysis? *Journal of General Internal Medicine*, *27*(6), 685–692. doi:10.100711606-011-1958-4 PMID:22215270

Ludwick, D. A., & Doucette, J. (2009). Adopting electronic medical records in primary care: Lessons learned from health information systems implementation experience in seven countries. *International Journal of Medical Informatics*, *78*(1), 22–31. doi:10.1016/j.ijmedinf.2008.06.005 PMID:18644745

Luna, D., Almerares, A., Mayan, J. C. III, Gonzalez Bernaldo de Quiros, F., & Otero, C. (2014). Health Informatics in Developing Countries: Going beyond Pilot Practices to Sustainable Implementations: A Review of the Current Challenges. *Healthcare Informatics Research*, *20*(1), 3–10. doi:10.4258/hir.2014.20.1.3 PMID:24627813

Lunt, N., & Carrera, P. (2010). Medical-tourism: Assessing the evidence on treatment abroad. *Maturitas*, *66*(1), 27–32. doi:10.1016/j.maturitas.2010.01.017 PMID:20185254

Lunt, N., & Carrera, P. (2011). Systematic review of web sites for prospective medical tourists. *Tourism Review*, *66*(1/2), 57–67. doi:10.1108/16605371111127224

Lunt, N., Hardey, M., & Mannion, R. (2010). Nip, tuck and click- Medical-tourism and the emergence of web-based health information. *The Open Medical Informatics Journal*, *4*(1), 1–11. doi:10.2174/1874431101004010001 PMID:20517465

Lunt, N., Horsfall, D., & Hanefeld, J. (2016). MTm: A snapshot of evidence on treatment abroad. *Maturitas*, *88*, 37–44. doi:10.1016/j.maturitas.2016.03.001 PMID:27105695

Lupton, D. (2014). The Commodification of patient opinion: The digital patient experience economy in the age of big data. *Sociology of Health & Illness*, *36*(6), 856–869. doi:10.1111/1467-9566.12109 PMID:24443847

Lynn, J. (2016). *Value based care hurting most vulnerable hospitals.* http://www.hospitalemrandehr.com/2016/03/25/value-based-care hurting-most-vulnerable-hospitals/

MacColl, I., Cooper, R., Rittenbruch, M., & Viller, S. (2005). Watching Ourselves Watching: Ethical Issues in Ethnographic Action Research. OZCHI 2005 Proceedings, 1–4.

Mace, S. (2015). Mobile patient engagement. *HealthLeaders*, *18*, 62–64.

Mackey, T. K., Kuo, T. T., Gummadi, B., Clauson, K. A., Church, G., Grishin, D., ... Palombini, M. (2019). 'Fit-for-purpose?'–challenges and opportunities for applications of blockchain technology in the future of healthcare. *BMC Medicine*, *17*(1), 68. doi:10.118612916-019-1296-7 PMID:30914045

Madan, M., & Jain, E. (2017). Impact of organizational culture & climate on managerial effectiveness: An empirical study. *Delhi Business Review*, *16*(2), 47–57.

Mahuire, A., Bussmann, S., Kocker, C., Verra, S., Giurgi, L. A., & Ruggeri, K. (2016). Raising concerns about the information provided on medical travel agency websites: A place for policy. *Health Policy and Technology*, *5*(4), 414–422. doi:10.1016/j.hlpt.2016.07.001

Majchrzak, A., & Markus, M. L. (2012). Technology Affordances and Constraints in Management Information Systems (Mis). Encyclopedia of Management Theory, 5.

Majchrzak, A., Faraj, S., Kane, G. C., & Azad, B. (2013). The Contradictory Influence of Social Media Affordances on Online Communal Knowledge Sharing. *Journal of Computer-Mediated Communication*, *19*(1), 38–55.

Majeed, S., & Lu, C. (2017). *Changing Preferences, Moving Places and Third-Party Administrators: A Scoping Review of Medical-tourism Trends (1990-2016).* Almatourism. doi:10.6092/issn.2036-5195/6675

Manganello, J., Gerstner, G., Pergolino, K., Graham, Y., Falisi, A., & Strogatz, D. (2017). The relationship of health literacy with use of digital technology for health information: Implications for public health practice. *Journal of Public Health Management and Practice*, *23*(4), 380–387. doi:10.1097/PHH.0000000000000366 PMID:26672402

Manogaran, G., & Lopez, D. (2018). Health data analytics using scalable logistic regression with stochastic gradient descent. *International Journal of Advanced Intelligence Paradigms*, *10*(1-2), 118–132. doi:10.1504/IJAIP.2018.089494

Marrie, R.A., Patel, R., Figley, C.R., Kornelsen, J., Bolton, J.M., Graff, L., … Fisk, J.D. (2019). Diabetes and anxiety adversely affect cognition in multiple sclerosis. *Multiple Sclerosis and Related Disorder Satellites, 27*(1), 164-170.

Marschang, S. (2014). *Health inqualities and eHealth: 2014 eHealth Forum, Report of the e-Health stakeholder Group.* Retrieved from Athens: http://www.ehealth2014.org/wpcontent/

Marshak, R. J., & Grant, D. (2008). Organizational discourse and new organization development practices. *British Journal of Management, 19*(s1), S7–S19. doi:10.1111/j.1467-8551.2008.00567.x

Martin, R., Ira Ktena, S. & Pawlowski, N. (2018). An Introduction to Biomedical Image Analysis with Tensor Flow and DLT. *Imperial College London*, *29*(1), 82-85.

Maruthappu, M., Sood, H. S., & Keogh, S. B. (2014). The NHS Five Year Forward View: Transforming care. *The British Journal of General Practice*, *64*(629), 635–635. doi:10.3399/bjgp14X682897 PMID:25452525

Mary Norine, W., & Rumsfeld, J. S. (2017). Leading the digital transformation of healthcare. *Journal of the American College of Cardiology*, *70*(21), 2719–2722. doi:10.1016/j.jacc.2017.10.020 PMID:29169479

Masís Vargas, A. (2019). *One hour of device screen time at night could lead to increased sugar consumption.* Society for the Study of Ingestive Behavior (SSIB).

Masís Vargas, A. (2019). *Society for the Study of Ingestive Behavior. Blue light at night increases the consumption of sweets in rats. Science Daily.*

Mason, A., & Wright, K. (2011). Framing medical-tourism: An examination of appeal, risk, convalescence, accreditation, and interactivity in medical-tourism websites. *Journal of Health Communication*, *16*(2), 163–177. doi:10.1080/10810730.2010.535105 PMID:21161812

McAfee, A., Brynjolfsson, E., Davenport, T.H., Patil, D.J., & Barton, D. (2012). Big data: the management revolution. *Harvard Bus Rev*, *90*(1), 60-68.

McCabe, C., & Timmins, F. (2016). Embracing healthcare technology - What is the way forward for nurse education? *Nurse Education in Practice*, *21*, 104–106. doi:10.1016/j.nepr.2016.10.007 PMID:27810650

McConalogue, E., Davis, P., & Connolly, R. (2019). Health Technology Assessment: The Role of Total Cost of Ownership. *Business Systems Research*, *10*(1), 180–187. doi:10.2478/bsrj-2019-0013

McCullough, J. S., Casey, M., Moscovice, I., & Prasad, S. (2010). The effect of health information technology on quality in U.S. hospitals. *Health Affairs*, *29*(4), 647–654. doi:10.1377/hlthaff.2010.0155 PMID:20368594

McKenna, B., Myers, M. D., & Newman, M. (2017). Social Media in Qualitative Research: Challenges and Recommendations. *Information and Organization*, *27*(2), 87–99.

McKinsey & Company. (2013). *The big-data revolution in US healthcare: Accelerating value and innovation.* Available from https://www.mckinsey.com/industries/healthcare-systems-and-services/our-insights/the-big-data-revolution-in-us-health-care

Medhekar, A., Wong, H.Y., & Hall, J.E. (2020). Healthcare Providers Perspective on Value in Medical Travel to India. *Tourism Review*. (forthcoming) DOI 10.1108/TR-06-2019-0276

Medhekar, A. (2014). Government policy initiatives for developing sustainable medical-tourism industry. *Journal on Business Review, 3*(3), 95–105.

Medhekar, A. (2017). The Role of Social Media for Knowledge Dissemination in Medical-tourism - A Case of India. In R. Chugh (Ed.), *Harnessing Social Media as a Knowledge Management Tool* (pp. 25–54). IGI Global. doi:10.4018/978-1-5225-0495-5.ch002

Medhekar, A., & Newby, L. (2012). Information Search for Medical Treatment Abroad. *Journal of Applied Global Research, 5*(13), 53–72.

Medhekar, A., Wong, H. Y., & Hall, J. (2014). Medical-tourism: A Conceptual Framework for an Innovation in Global Healthcare Provision. In A. Goyal (Ed.), *Innovations in Services Marketing and Management: Strategies for Emerging Economies* (pp. 148–169). IGI Global. doi:10.4018/978-1-4666-4671-1.ch009

Medhekar, A., Wong, H. Y., & Hall, J. E. (2019). Factors influencing inbound medical travel to India. *Journal of Health Organization and Management, 33*(2), 155–172. doi:10.1108/JHOM-08-2018-0234 PMID:30950309

Meeker, M., & Wu, L. (2018). *Internet trends 2018*. Academic Press.

Mehta, N., & Pandit, A. (2018). Concurrence of big data analytics and healthcare: A systematic review. *International Journal of Medical Informatics, 114*, 57–65. doi:10.1016/j.ijmedinf.2018.03.013 PMID:29673604

Mendoza, A., Carroll, J., Stern, L., & Linda, S. (2010, Mar.). Software Appropriation Over Time : From Adoption to Stabilization and Beyond. *Australasian Journal of Information Systems*, 5–23.

Menvielle, L., Audrain-Pontevia, A. F., & Menvielle, W. (Eds.). (2017). *The digitization of healthcare: New challenges and opportunities*. Springer. doi:10.1057/978-1-349-95173-4

Merolli, M., Gray, K., & Martin-Sanchez, F. (2013). Health Outcomes and Related Effects of Using Social Media in Chronic Disease Management: A Literature Review and Analysis of Affordances. *Journal of Biomedical Informatics, 46*(6), 957–969.

Merolli, M., Gray, K., Martin-Sanchez, F., & Lopez-Campos, G. (2015). Patient-Reported Outcomes and Therapeutic Affordances of Social Media: Findings from a Global Online Survey of People with Chronic Pain. *Journal of Medical Internet Research, 17*(1), e20.

Meskó, B., Drobni, Z., Bényei, É., Gergely, B., & Győrffy, Z. (2017). Digital health is a cultural transformation of traditional healthcare. *mHealth, 3*, 38–38. doi:10.21037/mhealth.2017.08.07 PMID:29184890

Meskó, B., Radó, N., & Győrffy, Z. (2019). Opinion leader empowered patients about the era of digital health: A qualitative study. *BMJ Open, 9*(3), e025267. doi:10.1136/bmjopen-2018-025267 PMID:30898816

Messum, D., Wilkes, L., Peters, C., & Jackson, D. (2017). Senior Managers' and Recent Graduates' Perceptions of Employability Skills for Health Services Management. *Asia Pacific Journal of Cooperative Education, 18*(2), 115–128.

Miles, M. B., Quarterly, A. S., & Dec, Q. M. (1979). Qualitative Data as an Attractive Nuisance. *The Problem of Analysis, 24*(4), 590–601.

Miles, M. B., Huberman, M. A., & Saldaña, J. (2014). *Qualitative Data Analysis: A Methods Sourcebook*. SAGE Publications, Inc.

Miller, A. R., & Tucker, C. (2013). Active social media management: The case of healthcare. *Information Systems Research, 24*(1), 52–70. doi:10.1287/isre.1120.0466

Minn, R., & Morrow, E. S. (2018). Natural medicines in the clinical management of diabetes. *Natural Medicines*. https://naturalmedicines.therapeuticresearch.com

Mintzberg, H. (2009). *Managing*. Berrett-Koehler Publication, Inc.

Mitchell, B., & Begoray, D. (2010). Electronic Personal Health Records That Promote Self-Management in Chronic Illness. *OJIN: The Online Journal of Issues in Nursing, 15*(3). doi:10.3912/OJIN.Vol15No03PPT01

Moccia, S., De Momi, E., Guarnaschelli, M., Savazzi, M., Laborai, A., Guastini, L., ... Mattos, L. S. (2017). Confident texture-based laryngeal tissue classification for early stage diagnosis support. *Journal of Medical Imaging (Bellingham, Wash.), 4*(3), 34502. doi:10.1117/1.JMI.4.3.034502 PMID:28983494

Moghavvemi, S., Ormond, M., Musa, G., Mohamed-Isa, C. R., & Chandy, J. C. (2017). Connecting with prospective medical-tourists online: A cross-sectional analysis of private hospital websites promoting medical-tourism in India, Malaysia and Thailand. *Tourism Management, 58*(Feb), 154–163. doi:10.1016/j.tourman.2016.10.010

Moghimi, H., de Steiger, R., Schaffer, J., & Wickramasinghe, N. (2013). The benefits of adopting e performance Management Techniques. *Health & Technology, 3*(3), 237-247.

Mohammed, A., & Yunus, A. (2017). Technology Acceptance in Healthcare Service: A Case of Electronic Medical Records (ERM). *International Journal of Academic Research in Business and Social Sciences, 7*(11).

Moorhead, S. A., Hazlett, D. E., Harrison, L., Carroll, J. K., Irwin, A., & Hoving, C. (2013). A New Dimension of Healthcare: Systematic Review of the Uses, Benefits, and Limitations of Social Media for Health Communication. *Journal of Medical Internet Research, 15*(4), e85–e101. doi:10.2196/jmir.1933 PMID:23615206

Moreno-Conde, A., Parra-Calderón, C. L., Sánchez-Seda, S., Escobar-Rodríguez, G. A., López-Otero, M., Cusso, L., ... Albertí-Ibarz, M. (2019). ITEMAS ontology for healthcare technology innovation. *Health Research Policy and Systems, 17*(1), 47. doi:10.118612961-019-0453-y PMID:31046786

Moriarty, J. M. (2014). The modern experience of care: Patient satisfaction as a quality metric after the Affordable Care Act (MA thesis). Boston University. ProQuest Central; ProQuest Dissertations & Theses Global database. (1560379)

Morris, M. (2013). The future of hospitals: Visions of the healthcare landscape in 2035. *Becker's Hospital Review*. Retrieved from https://www.beckershospitalreview.com/hospital-management-administration/the-future-of-hospitals-visions-of-the-healthcare-landscape-in-2035.html

Morse, S. (2018). 82% of clinicians, IT leaders blame burnout on interruptions from tech tools. *Healthcare Finance*. Retrieved from https://www.healthcarefinancenews.com/news/82-clinicians-it-leaders-blame-burnout-interruptions-tech-tools

Murdoch, T. B., & Detsky, A. S. (2013). The inevitable application of big data to healthcare. *Journal of the American Medical Association, 309*(13), 1351–1352. doi:10.1001/jama.2013.393 PMID:23549579

Myers, M. D., & Newman, M. (2007). The Qualitative Interview in IS Research: Examining the Craft. *Information and Organization, 17*(1), 2–26.

Nahavandi, A. (2015). *The art and science of leadership* (7th ed.). Pearson Education, Inc.

Nall, R. (2018). An overview of diabetes types and treatments. *Medical News Today.* https://www.medicalnewstoday.com/articles/323627.php

Nambisan, P., Kreps, G. L., & Polit, S. (2013). Understanding electronic medical record adoption in the United States: Communication and sociocultural perspectives. *Interactive Journal of Medical Research, 2*(1), e5. doi:10.2196/ijmr.2437 PMID:23612390

Nancarrow, S. A. (2015). Six principles to enhance health workforce flexibility. *Human Resources for Health, 13*(1), 9. doi:10.1186/1478-4491-13-9 PMID:26264184

Nanni, L., Brahnam, S., Ghidoni, S., & Lumini, A. (2018). Bioimage Classification with Handcrafted and Learned Features. *IEEE/ACM Transactions on Computational Biology and Bioinformatics.* doi:10.1109/TCBB.2018.2821127 PMID:29994096

Nanni, L., Brahnam, S., Lumini, A., & Barrier, T. (2014). *Ensemble of local phase quantization variants with ternary encoding* (Vol. 506). Studies in Computational Intelligence; doi:10.1007/978-3-642-39289-4_8

Nanni, L., Paci, M., Caetano dos Santos, F. L., Brahnam, S., & Hyttinen, J. (2016). Review on Texture Descriptors for Image Classiðcation. In *Computer Vision and Simulation: Methods, Applications and Technology*. Nova Science Publisher.

Narangajavana, Y., Fiol, C. L. J., Tena, M. A., Artola, R.-M., & Sánchez-García, J. (2017). The influence of social media in creating expectations. An empirical study for a tourist destination. *Annals of Tourism Research, 65*(1), 60–70. doi:10.1016/j.annals.2017.05.002

NaRanong, A., & NaRanong, V. (2011). The effects of medical-tourism: Thailand's experience. *Bulletin of the World Health Organization, 89*(5), 336–344. doi:10.2471/BLT.09.072249 PMID:21556301

Nelson, L. P. (2014). Patient engagement solutions. *Health Management Technology, 35*(11), 18–19. PMID:25622456

NewsRx. (2019a). *Artificial Intelligence; Findings from University College London Hospital update knowledge of Artificial Intelligence (Artificial intelligence and computer-aided diagnosis in colonoscopy: current evidence and future directions). Computer Technology Journal.*

NewsRx. (2019b). *Artificial Intelligence; Investigators at Massachusetts General Hospital Detail Findings in Artificial Intelligence (Artificial Intelligence in Surgery: Promises and Perils). Medical Devices & Surgical Technology Week.*

Newswire. (2016). Digital transformation market in healthcare: Global industry analysis and forecast 2015 - 2025. *PR Newswire.*

Ngai, E. W. T., Tao, S. S. C., & Moon, K. K. L. (2015). Social Media Research: Theories, Constructs, and Conceptual Frameworks. *International Journal of Information Management, 35*(1), 33–44.

Ngai, E., Moon, K. L. K., Lam, S. S., Chin, E. S. K., & Tao, S. S. C. (2015). Social Media Models, Technologies, and Applications: An Academic Review and Case Study. *Industrial Management and Data Systems, 115*(5), 769–802.

Nordqvist, C. (2019). What to know about coronary heart disease. *Medical News Today.* https://www.medicalnewstoday.com/articles/184130.php

Nosaka, R., Ohkawa, Y., & Fukui, K. (2011). Feature extraction based on co-occurrence of adjacent local binary patterns. In Lecture Notes in Computer Science (including subseries Lecture Notes in Artificial Intelligence and Lecture Notes in Bioinformatics). doi:10.1007/978-3-642-25346-1_8

Nosaka, R., & Fukui, K. (2014). HEp-2 cell classification using rotation invariant co-occurrence among local binary patterns. *Pattern Recognition, 47*(7), 2428–2436. doi:10.1016/j.patcog.2013.09.018

O'Driscoll, M. P. P. J. T., & Taylor, P. J. (1992). Congruence between theory and practice in management training needs analysis. *International Journal of Human Resource Management*, *3*(3), 593–603. doi:10.1080/09585199200000167

Office for Civil Rights. (2013). Summary of the HIPAA privacy rule. *U.S. Department of Health & Human Services.* https://www.hhs.gov/hipaa/for-professionals/privacy/laws-regulations/index.html

Office for Official Publications of the European Communities. (2004). *E-Health, Making Healthcare Better for European Citizens: An Action Plan for a European E-health Area.* Author.

Ojala, T., Pietikainen, M., & Maenpaa, T. (2002). Multiresolution gray-scale and rotation invariant texture classification with local binary patterns. *IEEE Transactions on Pattern Analysis and Machine Intelligence*, *24*(7), 971–987. doi:10.1109/TPAMI.2002.1017623

Ojansivu, V., & Heikkilä, J. (2008). Blur insensitive texture classification using local phase quantization. In Lecture Notes in Computer Science (including subseries Lecture Notes in Artificial Intelligence and Lecture Notes in Bioinformatics) (Vol. 5099 LNCS, pp. 236–243). doi:10.1007/978-3-540-69905-7_27

Olden, P. C. (2003). Hospital and community health: Going from stakeholder management to stakeholder collaboration. *Journal of Health and Human Services Administration*, *26*(1/2), 35–57. PMID:15330379

Ommaya, A. K., Cipriano, P. F., Hoyt, D. B., Horvath, K. A., Tang, P., Paz, H. L., . . . Sinsky, C. A. (2018). *Care-centered clinical documentation in the digital environment: Solutions to alleviate burnout.* NAM Perspectives. Discussion Paper, National Academy of Medicine. doi:10.31478/201801c

ONC. (2014). *Connecting health and care for the nation: A shared national wide interoperability roadmap.* Office of the National Coordinator for Health Information Technology (ONC). Retrieved from https://www.healthit.gov/sites/default/files/hie-interoperability/nationwide-interoperability-roadmap-final-version-1.0.pdf

Orlikowski, W. J., & Iacono, C. S. (2001). Research Commentary: Desperately Seeking the 'IT' in IT Research - A Call to Theorizing the IT Artifact. *Information Systems Research*, *12*(2), 121–134.

Orlikowski, W. J., & Scott, S. V. (2015). The Algorithm and the Crowd: Considering the Materiality of Service Innovation. *MIS Quarterly*, *39*(1), 201–216.

Orlikowski, W. J., Iacono, S., & Iacono, C. S. (2006). Desperately Seeking the 'IT'in IT Research: A Call to Theorizing the IT Artifact. *Information Systems: The State of the Field*, *34*(2), 19.

Otte-Trojel, T., de Bont, A., Rundall, T. G., & van de Klundert, J. (2014). How outcomes are achieved through patient portals: A realist review. *Journal of the American Medical Informatics Association*, *21*(4), 751–757. doi:10.1136/amiajnl-2013-002501 PMID:24503882

Oussous, A., Benjelloun, F. Z., Lahcen, A. A., & Belfkih, S. (2018). Big Data technologies: A survey. *Journal of King Saud University-Computer and Information Sciences*, *30*(4), 431–448. doi:10.1016/j.jksuci.2017.06.001

Paasche-Orlow, M., Parker, R., Gazmararian, J., Nielsen-Bohlman, L., & Rudd, R. (2005). The prevalence of limited health literacy. *Journal of General Internal Medicine*, *20*(2), 175–184. doi:10.1111/j.1525-1497.2005.40245.x PMID:15836552

Panahi, S., Watson, J., & Partridge, H. (2012). Social Media and Tacit Knowledge Sharing : Developing a Conceptual Model. Academic Press.

Panch, T., Szolovits, P., & Atun, R. (2018, December). Artificial intelligence, machine learning and health systems. *Journal of Global Health*, *8*(2), 020303. doi:10.7189/jogh.08.020303 PMID:30405904

Park, S., Parwani, A., Aller, R., Banach, L., Becich, M., Borkenfeld, S., ... Pantanowitz, L. (2013). The history of pathology informatics: A global perspective. *Journal of Pathology Informatics*, *4*(1), 7–7. doi:10.4103/2153-3539.112689

Parra-López, E., Bulchand-Gidumal, J., Gutiérrez-Taño, D., & Díaz-Armas, R. (2011). Intentions to use social media in organizing and taking vacation trips. *Computers in Human Behavior*, *27*(2), 640–654. doi:10.1016/j.chb.2010.05.022

Passos, N. R., Rodrigues, A. F., Macedo, H. T., Prado, B. O., da Silva, G. J., & Matos, L. N. (2019, May). Open Data Extraction, Transformation, and Loading as a Tool for Supporting 2018 Elections' Voters. In *Proceedings of the XV Brazilian Symposium on Information Systems* (p. 23). ACM. 10.1145/3330204.3330232

Patel, R., Chang, T., Greysen, S. R., & Chopra, V. (2015). Social Media Use in Chronic Disease: A Systematic Review and Novel Taxonomy. *American Journal of Medicine*, *128*(12), 1335–1350.

Patrick, K., Hekler, E.B., Estrin, D., Mohr, D.C., Riper, H., Crane, D., Godino, J., & Riley, W.T., (2016). *The pace of technologic change: implications for digital health behavior intervention research*. Academic Press.

Pearce, C., & Bainbridge, M. (2014). A personally controlled electronic health record for Australia. *Journal of the American Medical Informatics Association*, *21*(4), 707–713. doi:10.1136/amiajnl-2013-002068 PMID:24650635

Pearlstein, S. (2005, June 8). Free Market Philosophy doesn't always work for healthcare. *Washington Post*.

Pendse, S., Benson, J. J., Maurya, P., & Miller, M. J. (2019). *U.S. Patent Application No. 15/725,630*. US Patent Office.

Pereira, R., & Pereira, E. G. (2015). Future internet: Trends and challenges. *International Journal of Space-Based and Situated Computing*, *5*(3), 159–167. doi:10.1504/IJSSC.2015.070952

Pinkney, L. M. (2013). *Healthcare reform: Innovative and other proven strategies for successfully managing and implementing organizational change*. University of Maryland University College. ProQuest Central; ProQuest Dissertations & Theses Global database. (3608771)

Piotrzkowska-Wróblewska, H., Dobruch-Sobczak, K., & Byra Michałand Nowicki, A. (2017). Open access database of raw ultrasonic signals acquired from malignant and benign breast lesions. *Medical Physics*, *44*(11), 6105–6109. doi:10.1002/mp.12538 PMID:28859252

Placidway. (2019). *The Power of digital health in medical-tourism*. Available from http://www.placidsolutions.com/infographics-power-digital-health-medical-tourism/

Plant, L., Noriega, B., Sonti, A., Constant, N., & Mankodiya, K. (2016). Smart E-textile gloves for quantified measurements in movement disorders. *Proceedings of the IEEE MIT Undergraduate Research Technology Conference (URTC)*, 1–4. 10.1109/URTC.2016.8284077

PMP. (2018). The Project Manager of the Future. *The Project Management Institute*. Retrieved from https://www.pmi.org/-/media/pmi/documents/public/pdf/learning/thought-leadership/pulse/digital-pm-skills.pdf?sc_lang_temp=en

Pocock, N. S., & Phua, K. H. (2011). Medical-tourism and policy implications for health systems: A conceptual framework from a comparative study of Thailand, Singapore and Malaysia. *Globalization and Health*, *7*(1), 12. doi:10.1186/1744-8603-7-12 PMID:21539751

Polyakova, A. G., Loginov, M. P., Serebrennikova, A. I., & Thalassinos, E. (2019). *Design of a socio-economic processes monitoring system based on network analysis and big data*. Academic Press.

Pontefract, S. K., & Wilson, K. (2019). Using electronic patient records: Defining learning outcomes for undergraduate education. *BMC Medical Education*, *19*(1), 30. doi:10.118612909-019-1466-5 PMID:30670000

Porter, M., & Lee, T. (2013). *The strategy that will fix healthcare*. Harvard Business Review Reprint R1310B.

Porter, M. (2010). What is value in healthcare? *The New England Journal of Medicine*, *2010*(26), 2477–2481. doi:10.1056/NEJMp1011024 PMID:21142528

Porter, M., & Teisberg, E. (2009). *Redefining Healthcare*. Harvard Business Review Press.

Pousti, H., Urquhart, C., & Linger, H. (2014). Exploring the Role of Social Media in Chronic Care Management. IFIP Advances in Information and Communication Technology, 446, 163–185. doi:10.1007/978-3-662-45708-5_11

Queensland Health. (2017). *Digital Health Strategic Vision for Queensland 2026*. Author.

Queensland Health. (2017). *Digital Health Strategic Vision for Queensland 2026*. State of Queensland: Queensland Health. Available from https://www.health.qld.gov.au/__data/assets/pdf_file/0016/645010/digital-health-strat-vision.pdf

Raj, A., & D'Souza, R. (2019). *A Review on Hadoop Eco System for Big Data*. Academic Press.

Rasmus, A., Valpola, H., Honkala, M., Berglund, M., & Raiko, T. (2015). Semi-supervised learning with Ladder networks. Advances in Neural Information Processing Systems.

Rastogi, R., Chaturvedi, D. K., Satya, S., Arora, N., Yadav, V., Chauhan, S., & Sharma, P. (2018). SF- 36 Scores Analysis for EMG and GSR Therapy on Audio, Visual and Audio Visual Modes for Chronic TTH. In Proceedings of the IC-CIDA-2018. Springer.

Rastogi, R., Chaturvedi, D. K., Arora, N., Trivedi, P., & Mishra, V. (2017). Swarm Intelligent Optimized Method of Development of Noble Life in the perspective of Indian Scientific Philosophy and Psychology. *Proceedings of NSC-2017(National system conference).*

Rauh, S., Wadsworth, E., & Weinstein, H. (2013). The Unintended consequences of Bundled Payments By weeks. *Annals of Internal Medicine*, *158*(1), 62–64. doi:10.7326/0003-4819-158-1-201301010-00012 PMID:23277901

Reifsteck, M. W., & Reese, M. L. (2016). The digital health explosion. A comprehensive strategy is required to remain relevant and responsive. *Healthcare Executive*, *31*(3), 66–67. PMID:27319110

Rich, E., & Miah, A. (2014). Understanding digital health as public pedagogy: A critical framework. *Societies (Basel, Switzerland)*, *4*(2), 296–315. doi:10.3390oc4020296

Robbins, S. P., & Judge, T. A. (2017). *Organizational behavior*. Pearson Education, Inc.

Rodrigues, R. J., & Risk, A. (2003). eHealth in Latin America and the Caribbean: Development and policy issues. *Journal of Medical Internet Research*, *5*(1), e4–e4. doi:10.2196/jmir.5.1.e4 PMID:12746209

Rogers, E. M. (2003). *Diffusion of innovations*. New York, NY: Simon and Schuster.

Romanow, D., Cho, S., & Straub, D. W. (2012). Riding the Wave: Past Trends and Future Directions for Health IT Research. *MIS Quarterly*, *36*(3). doi:10.2307/41703474

Roth, M., & Keller, B. (2019). Modernization through digital transformation. *TD: Talent Development*, *73*(1), 32.

Rozenblum, R., & Bates, D. W. (2013). Patient-Centred Healthcare, Social Media and the Internet: The Perfect Storm? *BMJ Quality & Safety*, *22*(3), 183–6.

Russo, E., Sittig, D. F., Murphy, D. R., & Singh, H. (2018). Challenges in patient safety improvement research in the era of electronic health records. *Health Care*, *4*(4), 285–290. PMID:27473472

Sachin, S., Goyal, S. K., Avinash, S., & Kamal, K. (2019). Nuts and Bolts of ETL in Data Warehouse. In *Emerging Trends in Expert Applications and Security* (pp. 1–9). Singapore: Springer. doi:10.1007/978-981-13-2285-3_1

Saini, H., Rastogi, R., Chaturvedi, D. K., Satya, S. N., Gupta, M., & Verma, H. (2019). An Optimized Biofeedback EMG and GSR Biofeedback Therapy for Chronic TTH on SF-36 Scores of Different MMBD Modes on Various Medical Symptoms. In Hybrid Machine Intelligence for Medical Image Analysis, Studies Comp. Intelligence. Springer Nature Singapore, Pte Ltd. doi:10.1007/978-981-13-8930-6_8

Saini, H., Rastogi, R., Chaturvedi, D. K., Satya, S., Arora, N., Verma, H., & Mehlyan, K. (2018). Comparative Efficacy Analysis of Electromyography and Galvanic Skin Resistance Biofeedback on Audio Mode for Chronic TTH on Various Indicators. In *Proceedings of ICCIIoT- 2018*. Elsevier.

Saldana, J. (2009). An Introduction to Codes and Coding. The Coding Manual for Qualitative Researchers, 1–31.

Saldana, J. (2009). *The Coding Manual for Qualitative Researchers*. Academic Press.

Saliba, V., Legido-Quigley, H., Hallik, R., Aaviksoo, A., Car, J., & McKee, M. (2012). Telemedicine across borders: A systematic review of factors that hinder or support implementation. *International Journal of Medical Informatics*, *81*(12), 793–809. doi:10.1016/j.ijmedinf.2012.08.003 PMID:22975018

Samhan, B., Crampton, T., & Ruane, R. (2018). The Trajectory of IT in Healthcare at HICSS: A Literature Review, Analysis, and Future Directions. *Communications of the Association for Information Systems*, *43*, 1. doi:10.17705/1CAIS.04341

Sandhu. (2020). Digital Systems Innovation for Health Data Analytics. In *Handbook of Research on Optimizing Healthcare Management Techniques*. IGI Global.

Sandhu, K., & Corbitt, B. (2008). A framework for electronic services system. *International Journal of Electronic Customer Relationship Management*, *2*(1), 50. doi:10.1504/IJECRM.2008.019568

Sandoz. (2019). *How digital tools are improving access to healthcare*. Available from https://www.sandoz.com/stories/access-healthcare/how-digital-tools-are-improving-access-healthcare

Sareah, F. (2015). *Interesting Statistics for the Top 10 Social Media Sites*. Academic Press.

Sarkar, U., Karter, A., Liu, J., Adler, E., Nguyen, R., Lopez, A., & Schilling, D. J. (2011). Social disparities in internet patient portal use in diabetes: Evidence that the digital divide extends beyond access. *J. Am Med Infrom Assoc*, *2011*(18), 318–321. doi:10.1136/jamia.2010.006015

Sarker, S. K., Bhas, G., Paul, R., Pal, H., Yusuf, M. A., & Eva, E. O. (2019). E-Pharmacy Utilization on the Spectrum of Digital Pharmaceutical Practices, Patterns and Challenges in Bangladesh. *Journal of Shaheed Suhrawardy Medical College*, *11*(1), 43–47. doi:10.3329/jssmc.v11i1.43178

Sarrami, F. P., Travaglia, J., Debono, D., & Braithwaite, J. (2014). Implementing strategies in consumer and community engagement in healthcare: Results of a large-scale, scoping meta-review. *BMC Health Services Research*, *14*(1), 402. doi:10.1186/1472-6963-14-402 PMID:25230846

Saxena, M., Kumar, B., & Matharu, S. (2018). Impact of Yagya on Particulate Matters. *Interdisciplinary Journal of Yagya Research*, *1*(1), 1-8.

Saxena, M., Sengupta, B. & Pandya, P. (2008). Controlling the Microflora in Outdoor Environment: Effect of Yagya. *Indian Journal of Air Pollution Control*, *8*(2), 30 – 36.

Saxena, M., Sharma, M., Sain, M.K., Bohra, G., & Sinha, R. (2018). Yagya reduced level of indoor Electro-Magnetic Radiations (EMR). *Interdisciplinary Journal of Yagya Research*, *1*(2), 231-239.

Scheer, V. (2016). Process Improvement for Implementing and Sustaining Change in Healthcare (Master's thesis). The College of St. Scholastica. ProQuest Dissertations & Theses Global database. (10125146)

Schein, E. H. (2004). Organizational culture and leadership (3rd ed.). The Jossey-Bass Business & Management Series.

Schultze, U., & Avital, M. (2011). Designing Interviews to Generate Rich Data for Information Systems Research. *Information and Organization*, *21*(1), 1–16.

Schultze, U. (2011). *The Avatar as Sociomaterial Entanglement: A Performative Perspective on Identity, Agency and World-Making in Virtual Worlds*. ICIS.

Schwarzmüller, T., Brosi, P., Duman, D., & Welpe, I. M. (2018). How does the digital transformation affect organizations? Key themes of change in work design and leadership. *Management Review*, *29*(2), 114–138. doi:10.5771/0935-9915-2018-2-114

Serra, G., Grana, C., Manfredi, M., & Cucchiara, R. (2015). Gold: Gaussians of local descriptors for image representation. *Computer Vision and Image Understanding*, *134*, 22–32. doi:10.1016/j.cviu.2015.01.005

Shafran, R. F. (2017). Leading organizational change: A phenomenological study of the nonlinear strategies used by female leaders in global companies (EdD dissertation). Pepperdine University. ProQuest Dissertations & Theses Global database. (10635765 Ed.D.)

Sharma, A., Rastogi, R., Chaturvedi, D. K., Satya, S., Arora, N., Trivedi, P., ... Singh, A. (2019). *Intelligent Analysis for Personality Detection on Various Indicators by Clinical Reliable Psychological TTH and Stress Surveys. In Proceedings of CIPR 2019 at Indian Institute of Engineering Science and Technology*. Springer-AISC Series.

Sharma, H. (2014). Importance and performance of managerial training in Indian companies–an empirical study. *Journal of Management Development*, *33*(2), 75–89. doi:10.1108/JMD-11-2013-0144

Sharma, P., Rastogi, R., Chaturvedi, D. K., Satya, S., Arora, N., Yadav, V., & Chauhan, S. (2018). *Analytical Comparison of Efficacy for Electromyography and Galvanic Skin Resistance Biofeedback on Audio- Visual Mode for Chronic TTH on Various Attributes. In Proceedings of the ICCIDA-2018. Springer.*

Shaw, T., Hines, M., & Kielly-Carroll, C. (2017). *Impact of Digital Health on the Safety and Quality of Healthcare*. Sydney: ACSQHC Available from https://www.safetyandquality.gov.au/

Shaw, J., Agarwal, P., Desveaux, L., Palma, D. C., Stamenova, V., Jamieson, T., ... Bhattacharya, O. (2018). Beyond "Implementation": Digital health innovation and service design. *Digital Media*, *48*(1), 1–5. doi:10.103841746-018-0059-8 PMID:31304327

Sheldon, L. K. (2005). Communication in oncology care: The effectiveness of skills training workshops for healthcare providers. *Clinical Journal of Oncology Nursing*, *9*(3), 305–312. doi:10.1188/05.CJON.305-312 PMID:15973840

Sheri-Lynne, L., & Singh, P. (2007). Leadership development: Learning from best practices. *Leadership and Organization Development Journal*, *28*(5), 444–464. doi:10.1108/01437730710761742

Shuck, B., Twyford, D., Reio, T. G. Jr, & Shuck, A. (2014). Human resource development practices and employee engagement: Examining the connection with employee turnover intentions. *Human Resource Development Quarterly*, *25*(2), 239–270. doi:10.1002/hrdq.21190

Shuwandy, M. L., Zaidan, B. B., Zaidan, A. A., & Albahri, A. S. (2019). Sensor-based mHealth authentication for real-time remote healthcare monitoring system: A multilayer systematic review. *Journal of Medical Systems*, *43*(2), 33. doi:10.100710916-018-1149-5 PMID:30612191

Sikka, R., Morath, J. M., & Leape, L. (2015). The Quadruple Aim: Care, health, cost and meaning in work. *BMJ Quality & Safety*, *24*(10), 608–610. doi:10.1136/bmjqs-2015-004160 PMID:26038586

Simoni, J. M., Kutner, B. A., & Horvath, K. J. (2015). Opportunities and challenges of digital technology for HIV treatment and prevention. *Current HIV/AIDS Reports, 12*(4), 437–440. doi:10.100711904-015-0289-1 PMID:26412082

Simonyan, K., & Zisserman, A. (2015). *Very Deep Convolutional Networks for Large-Scale Image Recognition.* CoRR, abs/1409.1

Singh, G. K. G., & Singh, S. K. G. (2008). Malaysian graduates' employability skills. *UNITAR e-Journal, 4*(1), 15-45.

Singh, N., & Singh, B. N. (2014). Recent Trends in Training and Developments in Indian Health-Care Sectors in the Changed Economic Scenario. International Journal of Scientific and Research Publications, 20.

Singh, P., Rastogi, R., Chaturvedi, D. K., Arora, N., Trivedi, P., & Vyas, P. (2018). Study on Efficacy of Electromyography and Electroencephalography Biofeedback with Mindful Meditation on Mental health of Youths. *Proceedings of the 12th INDIACom,* 84-89.

Singh, V., Rastogi, R., Chaturvedi, D. K., Satya, S., Arora, N., Sirohi, H., . . . Verma, P. (2018). Which One is Best: Electromyography Biofeedback Efficacy Analysis on Audio, Visual and Audio- Visual Modes for Chronic TTH on Different Characteristics. In *Proceedings of ICCIIoT-2018.* Elsevier.

Singh, A., Rastogi, R., Chaturvedi, D. K., Satya, S., Arora, N., Sharma, A., & Singh, A. (2019). Intelligent Personality Analysis on Indicators in IoT-MMBD Enabled Environment. In *Multimedia Big Data Computing for IoT Applications: Concepts, Paradigms, and Solutions.* Springer. doi:10.1007/978-981-13-8759-3_7

Singhal, P., Rastogi, R., Chaturvedi, D. K., Satya, S., Arora, N., Gupta, M., . . . Gulati, M. (2019). Statistical Analysis of Exponential and Polynomial Models of EMG & GSR Biofeedback for Correlation between Subjects Medications Movement & Medication Scores. *IJITEE, 8*(6S), 625-635. https://www.ijitee.org/download/volume-8-issue-6S/

Sittig, D. F. (2002). Personal health records on the internet: A snapshot of the pioneers at the end of the 20th Century. *International Journal of Medical Informatics, 65*(1), 1–6. doi:10.1016/S1386-5056(01)00215-5 PMID:11904243

Sittig, D. F., Belmont, E., & Singh, H. (2018). Improving the safety of health information technology requires shared responsibility: It is time we all step up. *Health Care, 6*(1), 7–12. PMID:28716376

Smith, J. A. (2011). Evaluating the contribution of interpretative phenomenological analysis. *Health Psychology Review, 5*(1), 9–27. doi:10.1080/17437199.2010.510659

Smith, S., & Saleem, H. (2013). *What has HCI done to institutionalize improvement? A report from 17 countries. USAID Healthcare Improvement Project.* HCI.

Smollan, R. K., & Sayers, J. G. (2009). Organizational culture, change, and emotions: A qualitative study. *Journal of Change Management, 9*(4), 435–457. doi:10.1080/14697010903360632

Song, T., Li, H., Meng, F., Wu, Q., & Cai, J. (2017). LETRIST: Locally Encoded Transform Feature Histogram for Rotation-Invariant Texture Classification. *IEEE Transactions on Circuits and Systems for Video Technology.* doi:10.1109/TCSVT.2017.2671899

Sowmya, B. J., Shetty, C., Cholappagol, N. V., & Seema, S. (2019). IOT and Data Analytics Solution for Smart Agriculture. In *The Rise of Fog Computing in the Digital Era* (pp. 210–237). IGI Global. doi:10.4018/978-1-5225-6070-8.ch010

Spagnoletti, P., Resca, A., & Sæbø, Ø. (2015). Design for Social Media Engagement: Insights from Elderly Care Assistance. *The Journal of Strategic Information Systems, 24*(2), 128–145.

Speier, A. R. (2011). Brokers, consumers and the Internet: How North American consumers navigate their infertility journeys. *Reproductive Biomedicine Online, 23*(5), 592–599. doi:10.1016/j.rbmo.2011.07.005 PMID:21955489

Spriggs, M., Arnold, M. V., Pearce, C. M., & Fry, C. (2012). Ethical questions must be considered for electronic health records. *Journal of Medical Ethics*, *38*(9), 535–539. doi:10.1136/medethics-2011-100413 PMID:22573881

Springer, P. J., Clark, C. M., Faan, A., Strohfus, P., & Belcheir, M. (2012). Using transformational change to improve organizational culture and climate in a school of nursing. *The Journal of Nursing Education*, *51*(2), 81–88. doi:10.3928/01484834-20111230-02 PMID:22201273

Srinivasan, C. R., Rajesh, B., Saikalyan, P., Premsagar, K., & Yadav, E. S. (2019). A review on the different types of Internet of Things (IoT). *Journal of Advanced Research in Dynamical and Control Systems*, *11*(1), 154–158.

Stensaker, I., & Meyer, C. (2011). *Change experience and employee reactions: Developing capabilities for change* (Vol. 41). Academic Press.

Stevenson, J. E., & Nilsson, G. (2012). Nurses' perceptions of an electronic patient record from a patient safety perspective: A qualitative study. *Journal of Advanced Nursing*, *68*(3), 667–676. doi:10.1111/j.1365-2648.2011.05786.x PMID:21781148

Strauss, A. L., Corbin, J. M., & Strauss, A. L. (2008). Basics of Qualitative Research. Academic Press.

Strauss, A., & Corbin, J. (2008). Basics of Qualitative Research: Techniques and Procedures for Developing Grounded Theory. In *Basics of Qualitative Research Grounded Theory Procedures and Techniques* (Vol. 3). Academic Press.

Subramaniyaswamy, V., Manogaran, G., Logesh, R., Vijayakumar, V., Chilamkurti, N., Malathi, D., & Senthilselvan, N. (2019). An ontology-driven personalized food recommendation in IoT-based healthcare system. *The Journal of Supercomputing*, *75*(6), 3184–3216. doi:10.100711227-018-2331-8

Szegedy, C., Liu, W., Jia, Y., Sermanet, P., Reed, S., Anguelov, D., … Rabinovich, A. (2015). Going deeper with convolutions. In *Proceedings of the IEEE conference on computer vision and pattern recognition* (pp. 1–9). IEEE.

Tait, I. E. (2013). Comparison of project management software tool use in healthcare and other industries (PhD dissertation). Capella University. ProQuest Central; ProQuest Dissertations & Theses Global database. (3607024)

Tenhunen, H. (2015). Smart e-health gateway: bringing intelligence to Internet-of-Things-based ubiquitous healthcare systems. In *Proceedings of the Annual IEEE Consumer Communications and Networking Conference*. IEEE.

Thackeray, R., Neiger, B. L., Hanson, C. L., & Mckenzie, J. F. (2008). Enhancing Promotional Strategies within Social Marketing Programs: Use of Web 2.0 Social Media. *Health Promotion Practice*, *9*(4), 338–343. doi:10.1177/1524839908325335 PMID:18936268

The Brookings Initiative on artificial intelligence and emerging technologies seeks to establish a proper societal framework for the impending "digitalization of everything." (n.d.). https://www.brookings.edu/research/the-opportunities-and-challenges-of-data-analytics-in-health-care/

Thimbleby, H. (2013). Technology and the future of healthcare. *Journal of Public Health Research*, *2*(3), 28. doi:10.4081/jphr.2013.e28 PMID:25170499

Thind, J. S., & Simon, R. (2019, June). Implementation of Big Data in Cloud Computing with optimized Apache Hadoop. In *2019 3rd International conference on Electronics, Communication and Aerospace Technology (ICECA)* (pp. 997-1001). IEEE. 10.1109/ICECA.2019.8821854

Thomas, D. (2014). Leading under pressure, coping practices of executives: A mixed methods study (EdD dissertation). Pepperdine University. ProQuest Central; ProQuest Dissertations & Theses Global database. (3668392)

Timian, A., Rupcic, S., Kachnowski, S., & Luisi, P. (2013). Do patients “like” good care? Measuring hospital quality via Facebook. *American Journal of Medical Quality*, *28*(5), 374–382. doi:10.1177/1062860612474839 PMID:23378059

Tomlinson, J. (2019). My Health Record implementation in private specialist practice. *The Medical Journal of Australia*, *210*(6), S32–S34. doi:10.5694/mja2.50030 PMID:30927474

Torous, J., Chan, S., Luo, J., Boland, R., & Hilty, D. (2018). Clinical Informatics in Psychiatric Training: Preparing Today’s Trainees for the Already Present Future. *Academic Psychiatry*, *42*(5), 694–697. doi:10.100740596-017-0811-4 PMID:29047074

Torrens, E., & Walker, S. M. (2017). Demographic characteristics of Australian health consumers who were early registrants for opt-in personally controlled electronic health records. *The HIM Journal*, *46*(3), 127–133. doi:10.1177/1833358317699341 PMID:28537210

Treem, J. W., & Leonardi, P. M. (2012). Social Media Use in Organizations: Exploring the Affordances of Visibility, Editability, Persistence, and Association. *Annals of the International Communication Association*, (36), 143–189.

Trochimiuk, R. (2015). Professional Development of Older Employees in Small and Medium Enterprises. *Journal of Management and Business Administration. Central Europe*, *23*(1), 80–95.

Tsai, H. C., Cohly, H., & Chaturvedi, D. K. (2013). Towards the Consciousness of the Mind, Towards a Science of Consciousness. *Dayalbagh Conference Proceeding*, *1*(1), 20-29.

Tsang, E. W. K. (2013). Case Study Methodology: Causal Explanation, Contextualization, and Theorizing. *Journal of International Management*, *19*(2), 195–202.

Turner, L. (2010). Medical-tourism and the global market place in health services: US patients, international hospitals and the search for affordable healthcare. *International Journal of Health Services*, *40*(3), 443–467. doi:10.2190/HS.40.3.d PMID:20799670

Turner, L. (2011). Canadian medical-tourism companies that have exited the marketplace: Content analysis of websites used to market transnational medical travel. *Globalization and Health*, *7*(40), 1–16. doi:10.1186/1744-8603-7-40 PMID:21995598

United Nations. (1948). *Universal Declaration of Human Rights*. Author.

United Nations. (n.d.). *Communication Materials*. Retrieved from https://www.un.org/sustainabledevelopment/news/communications-material/.

Urquhart, C., & Vaast, E. (2012). *Building Social Media Theory from Case Studies: A New Frontier for IS Research*. ICIS.

Vaast, E., Safadi, H., Lapointe, L., & Negoita, B. (2017). Social Media Affordances for Connective Action: An Examination of Microblogging Use During the Gulf of Mexico Oil Spill. *MIS Quarterly*, *41*(4), 1179–1205.

ValueCenter. (n.d.). Change vs. Transformation. *Better Value Center.* Retrieved from https://www.valuescentre.com/

Van de Belt, T. H., Berben, A. S., Samsom, M., Engelen, L. P., & Schoonhoven, L. (2012). Use of Social Media by Western European Hospitals: Longitudinal Study. *Journal of Medical Internet Research*, *14*(3), e61–e71. doi:10.2196/jmir.1992 PMID:22549016

van Dooren, K., Lennox, N., & Stewart, M. (2013). Improving access to electronic health records for people with intellectual disability: A qualitative study. *Australian Journal of Primary Health*, *19*(4), 336–342. doi:10.1071/PY13042 PMID:23962451

Van Fleet, D. D., & Peterson, T. O. (2016). Improving healthcare practice behaviors. *International Journal of Health Care Quality Assurance*, *29*(2), 141–161. doi:10.1108/IJHCQA-07-2015-0089 PMID:26959895

Van Gemert-Pijnen, J. E., Nijland, N., van Limburg, M., Ossebaard, H. C., Kelders, S. M., Eysenbach, G., & Seydel, E. R. (2011). A Holistic Framework to Improve the Uptake and Impact of eHealth Technologies. *Journal of Medical Internet Research*, *13*(4). doi:10.2196/jmir.1672

van Harten, J., Knies, E., & Leisink, P. (2016). Employer's investments in hospital workers' employability and employment opportunities. *Personnel Review*, *45*(1), 84–102. doi:10.1108/PR-05-2014-0115

Venkatesh, V., & Davis, F. D. (2000). A theoretical extension of the technology acceptance model: Four longitudinal field studies. *Management Science*, *46*(2), 186–204. doi:10.1287/mnsc.46.2.186.11926

VerticalNews. (2019). Artificial Intelligence; Researchers at Royal Adelaide Hospital Target Artificial Intelligence (Artificial Intelligence for Sex Determination of Skeletal Remains: Application of a Deep Learning Artificial Neural Network To Human Skulls). *Journal of Robotics & Machine Learning,* 2367.

Vest, J. R., & Gamm, L. D. (2010). Health information exchange: Persistent challenges and new strategies. *Journal of the American Medical Informatics Association*, *17*(3), 288–294. doi:10.1136/jamia.2010.003673 PMID:20442146

Vladimir, R.-B., Jorge, G.-M., Martín, L.-N., Yaroslava, R.-B., Javier, C.-R., Diego, Q.-P., ... Verónica Cevallos, L.-W. (2018). A Hybrid System to Support the Psychological Intervention for Children With Autism: A Proposal Based on Knowledge Modeling and Intelligent Technologies. *International Journal of E-Services and Mobile Applications*, *10*(4), 74–100. doi:10.4018/IJESMA.2018100105

von Wagner, C., Steptoe, A., Wolf, M. S., & Wardle, J. (2009). Health literacy and health actions: A review and a framework from health psychology. *Health Education & Behavior*, *36*(5), 860–877. doi:10.1177/1090198108322819 PMID:18728119

Vukovic, V., Favaretti, C., Ricciardi, W., & de Waure, C. (2018). Health Technology Assessment evidence on e-health/m-health technologies: Evaluating the transparency and thoroughness. *International Journal of Technology Assessment in Health Care*, *34*(1), 87–96. doi:10.1017/S0266462317004512 PMID:29455685

Vyas, P., Rastogi, R., Chaturvedi, D. K., Satya, S., Arora, N., & Singh, P. (2018). Statistical Analysis for Effect of Positive Thinking on Stress Management and Creative Problem Solving for Adolescents. *Proceedings of the 12th INDIACom*, 245-251.

Wade, V. A., Taylor, A. D., Kidd, M. R., & Carati, C. (2016). Transitioning a home telehealth project into a sustainable, large-scale service: A qualitative study. *BMC Health Services Research*, *16*(1), 1–10. doi:10.118612913-016-1436-0 PMID:27185041

Walker, D., Mora, A., Demosthenidy, M., Menachemi, N., & Diana, M. (2009). Meaningful Use of EHRs among Hospitals Ineligible for Incentives Lags Behind that of other hospitals, 2009-13. *Health Affairs, 35*(3), 495-501.

Walsham, G. (1995, May). Interpretive Case Studies in IS Research: Nature and Method. *European Journal of Information Systems*, 74–81.

Walsham, G. (2006). Doing Interpretive Research. *European Journal of Information Systems*, *15*(3), 320–330.

Walsh, I., Gettler-Summa, M., & Kalika, M. (2016). Expectable Use: An Important Facet of IT Usage. *The Journal of Strategic Information Systems*, *25*(3), 177–210. doi:10.1016/j.jsis.2016.01.003

Walsh, L., Hemsley, B., Allan, M., Dahm, M., Balandin, S., Georgiou, A., ... Hill, S. (2019). Assessing the quality and usability of 'MyHRC' within a health literacy framework: What's changed since 2016? *The HIM Journal*, 1–13. doi:10.1177/1833358319864734 PMID:31370712

Walsh, L., Hill, S., Allan, M., Balandin, S., Georgiou, A., Higgins, I., ... Hemsley, B. (2018). A content analysis of the consumer-facing online information about 'MyHRC': Implications for increasing knowledge and awareness to facilitate uptake and use. *The HIM Journal*, *4*(6), 106–116. doi:10.1177/1833358317712200 PMID:28589741

Wang, X., Parameswaran, S., Bagul, D. M., & Kishore, R. (2017). Does Online Social Support Work in Stigmatized Chronic Diseases? A Study of the Impacts of Different Facets of Informational and Emotional Support on Self-Care Behavior in an HIV Online Forum. ICIS'2017.

Wang, L., & Alexander, C. A. (2013). Automated identification technology and information security in digital hospitals. *International Journal of Information and Network Security*, *2*(5), 348–359. doi:10.11591/ijins.v2i5.3914

We are social. (2019). *Digital 2019, Q2 Global Digital Statshot*. Retrieved from https://wearesocial.com/blog/2019/04/the-state-of-digital-in-april-2019-all-the-numbers-you-need-to-know

Weiner, L. J. (2016). Improving physician engagement. *HealthLeaders, 19,* 8-10.

Weinstein, R. S., Lopez, A. M., Krupinski, E. A., Beinar, S. J., Holcomb, M., McNeely, R. A., ... Barker, G. (2008). Integrating telemedicine and telehealth: Putting it all together. *Studies in Health Technology and Informatics*, *131*, 23–38. PMID:18305320

Westbrook, J. I., Woods, A., Rob, M. I., Dunsmuir, W. T., & Day, R. O. (2010). Association of interruptions with an increased risk and severity of medication administration errors. *Archives of Internal Medicine*, *170*(8), 683–690. doi:10.1001/archinternmed.2010.65 PMID:20421552

Weston, S. (2017). The real challenge for digital transformation is not your technology. *CIO*.

WHO. (2016). *Integrated Care Models: An Overview*. Health Services Delivery Programme.

WHO. (2019). *Healthcare Service Delivery.* Available at https://www.who.int/healthsystems/topics/delivery/en/

Wickramasinghe, N., Troshani, I., Hill SR., Hague W., & Goldberg, S. (2011). A transaction cost assessment of a pervasive technology solution for gestational diabetes. *International Journal of Healthcare Information Systems and Informatics, 6*(4), 60-76.

Wickramasinghe, S., Kliman, L., Vogel, D., & Goldberg, S. (2014). *Exploring the Possibility for a Pervasive Technology Solution to Facilitate Effective Diabetes Selfcare for Patients with GDM*. Paper presented at 2014 ECIS, Tel Aviv, Israel.

Wickramasinghe, N., John, B., George, J., & Vogel, D. (2019). Achieving Value-Based Care in Chronic Disease Management. *Intervention Study JMIR Diabetes*, *4*(2), e10368. doi:10.2196/10368 PMID:31066699

Wicks, P., Stamford, J., Grootenhuis, M. A., Haverman, L., & Ahmed, S. (2014). Innovations in e-health. *Quality of Life Research: An International Journal of Quality of Life Aspects of Treatment, Care and Rehabilitation*, *23*(1), 195–203. doi:10.100711136-013-0458-x PMID:23852096

Williams, S., & Cooper (2006). Culture-based Literacy and Aboriginal Health. *Canadian Journal of Public Health*, *97*(S21).

Wood, S., Schwartz, E., Tuepker, A., Pres, N. A., Nazi, K. M., Turvery, C., & Nichol, W. P. (2013). Patient Experiences with Full Electronic Access to Health Records and Clinical Notes Through the My HealtheVet Personal Health Record Pilot: Qualitative Study. *Journal of Medical Internet Research*, *15*(3), e65. doi:10.2196/jmir.2356 PMID:23535584

Wootton, R., Kvedar, J., & Dimmick, S. L. (2006). *Home Telehealth: Connecting care within community*. London: Royal Society of Medicine Press.

World Health Organisation (WHO). (2019). *Defining Health Literacy*. Available from https://www.who.int/healthpromotion/conferences/7gchp/track2/en/

World Health Organisation. (2011). mHealth: New horizons for health through mobile technologies. Author.

World Health Organisation. (2016). *Global diffusion of eHealth: Making universal health coverage achievable. Report of the third global survey on eHealth*. Retrieved from Geneva, Switzerland: https://apps.who.int/iris/bitstream/10665/252529/1/9789241511780- eng.pdf?ua=1

World Health Organisation. (2016). *Global diffusion of eHealth: Making universal health coverage achievable*. Report of the third global survey on eHealth. Retrieved from Geneva: https://apps.who.int/iris/bitstream/10665/252529/1/9789241511780-

World Health Organisation. (2019). *Global Strategy on Digital Health 2020-2024*. Author.

World Health Organisation. (2019). https://www.who.int/behealthy/digital-health

World Health Organisation. (2019). Retrieved Apr 21, 2019 from https://www.who.int/behealthy/digital-health

World Health Organization. (2011). *m-Health New horizons for health through mobile technologies*. World Health Organziation.

World Health Organization. (2011). mHealth: New horizons for health through mobile technologies; Global Observatory for eHealth series. Author.

Wu, W., & Haick, H. (2018). Healthcare Monitoring: Materials and Wearable Devices for Autonomous Monitoring of Physiological Markers. *Advanced Materials*, *30*(41), 1870309. doi:10.1002/adma.201870309 PMID:29498115

Xiang, Z., & Gretzel, U. (2010). Role of social media in online travel information search. *Tourism Management*, *31*(2), 179–188. doi:10.1016/j.tourman.2009.02.016

Yadav, V., Rastogi, R., Chaturvedi, D. K., Satya, S., Arora, N., & Bansal, I. (2018). Intelligent Analysis for Detection of Complex Human Personality by Clinical Reliable Psychological Surveys on Various Indicators. *The national Conference on 3rd MDNCPDR-2018 at DEI.*

Yadav, V., Rastogi, R., Chaturvedi, D. K., Satya, S., Arora, N., Gupta, M., . . . Sharma, P. (2019). Chronic TTH Analysis by EMG & GSR Biofeedback on Various Modes and Various Medical Symptoms Using IoT. In Advances in ubiquitous sensing applications for healthcare. Book-Big Data Analytics for Intelligent Healthcare Management.

Yadav, V., Rastogi, R., Chaturvedi, D.K., Satya, S., Arora, N., Yadav, V., Sharma, P., & Chauhan, S. (2018). Statistical Analysis of EMG & GSR Biofeedback Efficacy on Different Modes for Chronic TTH on Various Indicators. *Int. J. Advanced Intelligence Paradigms, 13*(1), 251-275. Doi:10.1504/IJAIP.2019.10021825

Yamin, C., Emani, S., Williams, D., Lipsitz, S., Karson, A., Wald, J., & Bates, D. (2011). The digital divide in adoption and use of a personal health record. *Intern Med, 171*(6), 568-574

Yang, H., Cheung, C., & Fang, C. C. (2015). An empirical study of hospitality employability skills: Perceptions of entry-level hotel staff in china. *Journal of Hospitality & Tourism Education*, *27*(4), 161–170. doi:10.1080/10963758.2015.1089510

Yazdanpanah, A., Parsaei, A., & Jeihooni, A. K. (2018). The role of digital marketing in medical-tourism industry in point of view of medical-tourism policy makers of Shiraz in 2017. *Universal Journal of Pharmaceutical Research*, *3*(1), 1–6. doi:10.22270/ujpr.v3i2.128

Yin, R. K. (2013). *Case Study Research: Design and Methods* (Vol. 5). Academic Press.

Yin, R. K. (2017). *Case study research and applications: Design and Methods*. Thousand Oaks, CA: SAGE Publications.

Yogesan, K., Bos, L., Brett, P., & Gibbons, M. C. (2009). *Handbook of Digital Homecare*. Springer-Verlag Berlin Heidelberg.

Yoo, Y. (2010). Computing in Everyday Life: A Call for Research on Experiential Computing. *MIS Quarterly*, *34*(2), 213.

Yoo, S., Kim, S., & Lee, K. H. (2013). A study of user requests regarding the fully electronic health record system at Seoul National University Bundang Hospital. *Studies in Health Technology and Informatics*, *192*, 1015. PMID:23920789

Yoo, Y., Henfridsson, O., & Lyytinen, K. (2010). Research commentary—the new organizing logic of digital innovation: An agenda for information systems research. *Information Systems Research*, *21*(4), 724–735. doi:10.1287/isre.1100.0322

Ženko, Z., Mulej, M., & Potocan, V. (2017). Knowledge-cum-values Management belongs to the Way out from Global Crisis. *Business Systems Research*, *8*(1), 113–123. doi:10.1515/bsrj-2017-0009

Zhong, H., Zhu, W., Xu, Y., & Cui, J. (2018). Multi-authority attribute-based encryption access control scheme with policy hidden for cloud storage. *Soft Computing*, *22*(1), 243–251. doi:10.100700500-016-2330-8

Zulman, D., Nazi, K. M., Turvey, C. L., Wagner, T. H., Woods, S., & An, L. C. (2011). Patient, interest in sharing personal health record information: A web-based survey. *Annals of Internal Medicine*, *155*(12), 805–810. doi:10.7326/0003-4819-155-12-201112200-00002 PMID:22184687

Zurita, L., & Nøhr, C. (2004). Patient opinion–EHR assessment from the user's perspective. *Studies in Health Technology and Informatics*, *107*(2), 1333–1336. PMID:15361031

Zuvekas, S., & Cohen, J. (2016). Fee-for-service, while much maligned, remains the dominant payment method for physician visits. *Health Affairs, 35*(3), 411-414.

About the Contributors

Kamaljeet Sandhu is an an active, experienced researcher and is passionate about research in Digital Innovation and Strategy, Business Analytics, Digital Health, AI, IoT, Cryptocurrency, Blockchain, Cloud Computing, IT Startup, FinTech, Cybersecurity, Accounting, Corporate Governance and CSR, Supply Chain, ERP, SMEs, and Entrepreneurship. The editor held multiple leadership positions including Senior Research Fellow at the University of South Australia and Senior Academic position in Canada at the University of Northern British Columbia and in Australia that include University of Wollongong, Charles Darwin University, Deakin University, and in Fiji at the University of South Pacific. As a PhD Principal Supervisor, the editor has supervised and mentored several PhD research students to successful completion, and students have successfully gained academic and research appointments at international universities and other organizations. The PhD student research is funded by international government and industry scholarships. The editor has multidisciplinary experience working across different Faculties such as Business, Accounting, Finance, Management, Economics, IT and IS, Software, and Computer Science.

* * *

D. K. Chaturvedi is working in Dept. of Elect. Engg, Faculty of Engg, D.E.I., Dayalbagh, Agra since 1989. Presently he is Professor. He did his B.E. from Govt. Engineering College Ujjain, M.P. then he did his M.Tech. and Ph.D. from D.E.I. Dayalbagh. He is gold medalist and received Young Scientists Fellowship from DST, Government of India in 2001-2002 for postdoctoral research at the Univ. of Calgary, Canada. Also, he had research collaboration with different organizations at national and international level. He is the Fellow - The Institution of Engineers (India), Fellow - Aeronautical Society of India, Fellow - IETE, Sr. Member IEEE, USA and a Member of many National and International professional bodies such as IET, U.K., ISTE, Delhi, ISCE, Roorkee, IIIE, Mumbai and SSI etc. The IEE, U.K. recognized his work in the area of Power System Stabilizer and awarded honorary membership to him in 2006. He did many R&D projects of MHRD, UGC, AICTE etc. and consultancy projects of DRDO. He contributed in the national mission of ICT of Govt. of India as Virtual Power Lab Developer. He has guided 10 Ph.Ds., 65 M.Tech. Dissertations and published more than 300 International and National Papers. He has chaired and Co-Chaired many International and National Conferences. He is referee of many International Journals including IEE Proceedings and IEEE Transactions. He is Head of Dept. of Footwear Technology, Convener, Faculty Training and Placement Cell, and Advisor, IEI Students' Chapter (Elect. Engg.), D.E.I. Dayalbagh, Agra.

Sisira Edirippulige is a Senior Lecturer and the Program Director of Digital Health postgraduate programs delivered at the Centre for Online Health. His main professional interests include e-health/ telemedicine, and education and training. In his role as senior academic at the centre, he has been involved in a number significant research projects and the development of a number of education and training programs relating to Telehealth/e-Health/m-Health.

Steve Goldberg is the founder and CEO of Inet Intl Inc, Canada.

Mayank Gupta is acting as System and IT Analyst in Tata Consultancy services, Noida and expert of Data sciences and Business Analytics. He has skill to visualize the situations from different perspectives and explore the real facts through critical Analysis. He has deep interest in Human health domains.

Esha Jain Esha Jain has qualified Doctorate as well as UGC-NET in Management and has more than 13 years of work experience including both the Industry and Academics. A Certified Technical Analyst (in Stock Market) from Government of NCT of Delhi and Government of India, and Amazon Trained E-commerce Specialist, she has also qualified a module of Financial Markets with Distinction organized by (NSE) National Stock Exchange of India. She has also achieved a Statement of Accomplishment with Distinction in the certification course on 'Personal and Family Financial Planning' from the University of Florida. An awardee of 'Eminent Educationist Award', 'Asia Pacific Gold Star Award', 'Young Woman Educator and Scholar Award', 'Excellence Award 2017', she was also selected for "Rajiv Gandhi Education Excellence Award" and 'Bharat Vidya Shiromani Award'. She is the Resource Person for Various Faculty Development Programmes in the field of Academics, Research and SPSS. She is also awarded 27 Honors and Awards, including 15 Best Research Paper Awards and a Dean Committee Choice Award in various International Conferences of repute. She has been invited by IIM Indore for review of 'Institutional Development Plans (IDPs)' under the World Bank-supported Madhya Pradesh Higher Education Quality Improvement Project (MPHEQIP) to be submitted to Department of Higher Education, Government of Madhya Pradesh, and also took webinar sessions for Financial Management and Taxation Management (PG level) of Sikkim Manipal University Distance Learning Education. She has taken modules of Chartered Institute of Management Accountants (CIMA), London, UK and certified by the Institute of Chartered Accountants of India (ICAI) for conducting 'Investor Awareness Programmes' in institutions and organizations. She has published five (5) patents with the Government of India. More than 70 of her research papers are published in various International Journals and Conference Proceedings of repute as well as authored two (2) books, one is on 'Foreign Exchange Management' & other one is on 'Principles of Management with text and cases' under reputed Brands and also contributed chapters in another book on 'Corporate Social Responsibility'. She has also presented around 80 research papers and cases at various national and international conferences as well as has chaired various National and International Seminars and Conferences as Session Chair, Keynote Speaker and Panelist in Panel Discussions. She has also associated 12 various International Journals as Editorial Board Member, Academic Advisor, Research Paper Reviewer & Editor-in-Chief. She is also an External Examiner for evaluating Ph.D. Thesis for Jain University, Bengaluru and Pune University.

Alessandra Lumini is an Associate Researcher at the Department of Computer Science and Engineering of the University of Bologna. She received a degree in Computer Science from the University of Bologna, Italy, on March 26th, 1996. In 2001 she received her Ph.D. degree for her work on "Image

Databases". Now she is an Associate Researcher at the University of Bologna. She is a member of the Biometric Systems Lab and of the Smart City Lab. She is interested in Biometric Systems, Pattern Recognition, Machine Learning, Image Databases, Multidimensional Data Structures, Digital Image Watermarking, Bioinformatics.

Gianluca Maguolo received his Master Degree in Mathematics from the University of Padua in 2017. He is currently a Ph.D. student in Information Engineering at the University of Padua. His research mainly focuses on ensembles of convolutional neural networks for image classification.

Anita Medhekar is a senior lecturer in economics and holds a PhD from Deakin University, Australia. She has taught at undergraduate and post graduate levels in India, Indonesia and Australia. Currently, she is teaching at Central Queensland University, Rockhampton, Australia. Her research interest is in applied Micro and Macroeconomics, International Trade, Development Economics, Public Finance, South-Asia, Health Economics, Tourism Economics, Bilateral Trade and Development for Peace, Public Policy, and Public-Private Partnerships. She has presented papers at numerous international conferences and has numerous publications to her credit as refereed conference proceedings, book chapters, and journal articles.

Julie Nguyen is a lecturer in Podiatry at CQUniversity. She received her Bachelor of Podiatry degree from La Trobe University and the Master of Public Health degree from the University of Melbourne. She has extensive clinical experience in the area of high risk foot and diabetic foot. She has worked in the acute care setting for numerous years as well as outreach, public and private sector. Julie has also worked in various roles such as Lead Project Officer in Public Affairs and Communication, Health Promotion and Healthcare projects including Department of Health and Human Services funded projects. Julie is currently involved in research in the area of 3 dimensional printed orthotic therapy, simulation education, health policy, ageing in home, telemedicine, and health technology. Julie is a member of the CQUniversity Human Research Ethics Committee.

Rohit Rastogi received his B.E. degree in Computer Science and Engineering from C.C.S.Univ. Meerut in 2003, the M.E. degree in Computer Science from NITTTR-Chandigarh (National Institute of Technical Teachers Training and Research-affiliated to MHRD, Govt. of India), Punjab Univ. Chandigarh in 2010. Currently he is pursuing his Ph.D. In computer science from Dayalbagh Educational Institute, Agra under renowned professor of Electrical Engineering Dr. D.K. Chaturvedi in area of spiritual consciousness. Dr. Santosh Satya of IIT-Delhi and dr. Navneet Arora of IIT-Roorkee have happily consented him to co supervise. He is also working presently with Dr. Piyush Trivedi of DSVV Hardwar, India in center of Scientific spirituality. He is a Associate Professor of CSE Dept. in ABES Engineering. College, Ghaziabad (U.P.-India), affiliated to Dr. A.P. J. Abdul Kalam Technical Univ. Lucknow (earlier Uttar Pradesh Tech. University). Also, He is preparing some interesting algorithms on Swarm Intelligence approaches like PSO, ACO and BCO, etc. Rohit Rastogi is involved actively with Vichaar Krnati Abhiyaan and strongly believe that transformation starts within self.

Buddhika Senanayake is a visiting researcher from Sri Lanka. He is a public health researcher affiliated with the Ministry of Health in Sri Lanka and currently do research relating to telehealth at the Centre for Health Services Research, The University of Queensland, Australia.

Parul Singhal received her B.TECHdegree from AKTU Univ. Presently She is M.Tech. Second year student of CSE in ABESEC, Ghaziabad. She is a Teaching Assistant in the CSE department of ABES Engineering. Ghaziabad, India. She is presently working on data mining (DM) and machine learning (ML). She is also working on TTH and stress. She has keen interest in Google surfing. Her hobbies are playing badminton and reading books. She is young, talented and dynamic.

Nirupama Tyagi is a Master of Philosophy candidate at the University of Queensland. Her main area of interest is the digital health workforce development.

Nilmini Wickramasinghe, after completing five degrees at the University of Melbourne, Australia, accepted a full scholarship to undertake PhD studies at Case Western Reserve University's Weatherhead School of Management in Cleveland, Ohio USA in health informatics management and later completed an executive program in value-based healthcare at Harvard Business School. For over 20 years she has been actively, researching and teaching within various aspects of digital health in both US and Australia Professor Wickramasinghe collaborates with leading scholars at various premier healthcare organizations and universities throughout Australasia, US and Europe and is well published with more than 400 referred scholarly articles, more than 10 books, numerous book chapters, an encyclopaedia and a well established funded research track record. She holds a patent around analytics solution for managing healthcare data and is the editor-in-chief of two scholarly journals.

Xiaoyun Zhou is a PhD candidate at the University of Queensland. Her area of research interest is the use of online methods for delivering education and training.

Dina Ziadlou is a university instructor, mentor, and expert specializing in digital healthcare transformation. She has over 16 years of speciated expertise in the healthcare industry. She holds the position of Chair of Digital Transformation Leadership (DTL) in the International Society for Telemedicine and e-Health (ISfTeH) and she is part of the WHO Digital Health Technical Advisory Group (DHTAG) and Roster of Experts. She earned her doctorate in Healthcare Management and Leadership from Colorado Technical University, USA, Ph.D. in Medical IT from TMU, MS in IT Management from TMU, and BS in Biomedical Engineering from SRU. She has been awarded for several successful projects in Telemedicine, HIT, and digital health projects and has widely been consulted internationally. She has several national and international publications in telemedicine, digital health, and digital transformation leadership. She is an ambassador of PCORI (Patient-Centered Outcomes Research Institute), a member of HIMSS (Healthcare Information and Management Systems Society) and RISE Health Association and mentor-coach of California Association Healthcare Leaders (CAHL).

Index

A

Adoption 2, 8-9, 14-15, 17-18, 24-25, 28-29, 39-40, 49, 55-56, 58, 60-61, 68, 79-80, 105, 112, 131-133, 137, 139-143, 172, 177, 180, 185
Affordances/Constraints 55
Analytical 73, 113, 116, 119-121, 123, 125, 212-213
Appropriation 36-37, 39-41, 45-50, 56
Artificial Intelligence in Health (AIH) 1
AUC 158, 161-163, 167
Australia 2, 6, 58, 104, 106, 131-132, 134-139, 141, 143, 174, 177, 180

B

Big Data 4, 26, 72-73, 75, 78, 104-105, 181, 186-190, 192-193, 197, 200, 202, 208
Breast Cancer 151-152, 157

C

Change Leadership 72, 74, 77, 88-89
chronic conditions 56-59, 63, 66-68, 97, 101, 103-104, 107
Chronic Diseases 38, 56, 59, 66
Chronic illness 36-41, 45-46, 48-50, 56, 63, 68
co-morbidities 59
Convolutional Neural Networks 151-152, 167
Culture Development 77-78, 81-83

D

Deep Learning 152, 161, 164, 167
diabetes 9, 21, 38, 58-59, 64-66, 68, 197, 202-216
Digital Health 2-10, 13-19, 21-22, 24-29, 35, 57-60, 66, 68, 73-74, 79-81, 83-86, 89, 97-105, 107, 131-133, 135-137, 139, 141, 143, 150, 170-175, 177-182, 199
Digital Health Innovation 2-4, 6-10, 13-14, 24-26, 29, 35, 132-133, 137, 139
Digital Health Literacy 29, 35, 135, 143
digital health solutions 57-60, 68, 104, 179, 181
digital health usefulness 6
Digital Systems Innovation 1-2, 5, 9
digital technologies 1-2, 14-15, 17, 28-29, 35, 37, 73-74, 77, 79-88, 99, 101, 131-132, 136, 143, 174, 179, 197
Digital Technology Management 84, 86
Digital Transformation 66, 72-74, 76-80, 82-83, 85, 89, 98
Digitization 114, 187, 189

E

e-Health 2, 14-19, 21-22, 27-29, 35, 58, 61, 98-99, 102, 104-107, 112, 131-137, 139-143, 150, 180-181, 185
E-Health Literacy 35, 141-142, 150
Electronic Health Record 2, 102, 112, 135, 137-138, 177, 185
Employability Skills 113-115, 119-121, 124
Employees' Engagement 78
empowerment 9, 13-14, 49, 76, 78, 80-82, 88-89, 131-132, 135-137, 142-143
Ensembles of Classifiers 167

G

Globalization 60, 74, 82, 88, 90

H

Health data analytics 1-2, 5-7, 10, 13
Health Informatics 15, 80, 99-100, 107, 112, 132, 173, 175, 178, 181, 185
Health Information Sources 35

Health Innovation 2-4, 6-10, 13-14, 24-26, 29, 35, 132-133, 137, 139, 150
Health Literacy 29, 35, 67, 83, 132, 134-136, 143, 150
Health System 3-4, 86-87, 99, 102, 104, 107, 112, 133-134, 176, 180, 185
health workforce 97, 99, 101, 171, 173, 175, 180-181
Healthcare 2-4, 9, 13-19, 21-22, 24-29, 35, 37-39, 56-64, 66-68, 72-89, 97-100, 102-107, 112-116, 119-125, 131-143, 150, 170-176, 178-182, 185-193, 197, 201-202, 213, 216
Healthcare Industry 2, 60, 62, 72, 98, 107, 113-115, 119-120, 122, 124-125, 187, 189-190, 193, 213
Human Resource Empowerment 76, 78, 80

I

Illness Management 36-37, 39-41, 43, 45-50, 56
innovation 1-10, 13-14, 24-26, 28-29, 35, 38, 60, 82, 86, 98, 113, 117, 120, 131-133, 137, 139, 141-142, 150, 152, 171-172, 179
IT Artefact 37, 39-40, 56

K

k-Fold-Cross Validation 167

L

Leave-One-Out Testing Protocol 167

M

Machine Learning 152, 167, 190, 201, 213-214, 216
Materiality 56
medical education 98, 104-105, 112, 180, 185
medical tourist 13-14, 35
Medical travel 13-19, 21-22, 24-25, 27-28, 35
Medical-Tourism 16, 19, 22, 25-29, 35
mobile health 15, 60-64, 78, 81, 99-101, 112, 132-134, 150, 173, 181, 185
modes of delivery 15, 180
My Health Record 131-132, 137-139, 150, 177-178

O

Online Communities 16, 24, 41, 56, 60
Online Social Networks 56

P

patient experience 13-14, 19, 21, 27, 29, 35, 60, 66, 68, 75, 107, 132, 135
Process Analytics 186, 192-193

Q

Quadruple Aims 72-76, 88-89

R

ROC Curve 167

S

Self-Management 36-39, 56, 61, 64, 66-68, 79, 81, 102-103, 107, 113, 120-121, 125, 129, 133, 135-138, 141-143
Social Media 7-8, 13-15, 17-19, 21-22, 24-25, 29, 35-41, 43, 45, 49-50, 56, 60, 200
Social media appropriation 40
Social media tool 43
Sustainability 59, 87, 133

T

Teamwork 113, 116, 118-122, 124
Technology features 37, 50
Technology Use 55-56, 134
Telehealth 75, 82, 84, 86, 98-100, 103, 105, 112, 172, 174, 180, 185
Telemedicine 78, 80-81, 84, 88, 98-100, 102, 105-106, 112, 172-173, 175, 181, 185
training 64, 77, 79, 97-98, 101-102, 105-107, 113-120, 123-125, 134-135, 156-159, 161-164, 168, 170, 173, 179-182
Training Need Analysis 114-115

W

Work Engagement 113, 120, 122, 124
workforce readiness 170, 173, 179

www.ingramcontent.com/pod-product-compliance
Lightning Source LLC
LaVergne TN
LVHW060306011026
849161LV00011B/2780